Pathology Practicals

Pathology Practicals

Santosh Kumar Mondal MBBS, MD
Associate Professor
Department of Pathology
Bankura Sammilani Medical College
Bankura, WB

ex-Associate Professor
Department of Pathology
Medical College, College Street
Kolkata, WB

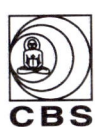

CBS Publishers & Distributors Pvt Ltd

New Delhi • Bengaluru • Chennai • Kochi • Kolkata • Mumbai

Bhopal • Bhubaneswar • Hyderabad • Jharkhand • Nagpur • Patna • Pune • Uttarakhand • Dhaka (Bangladesh) • Kathmandu (Nepal)

Disclaimer

Science and technology are constantly changing fields. New research and experience broaden the scope of information and knowledge. The author has tried his best in giving information available to him while preparing the material for this book. Although all efforts have been made to ensure optimum accuracy of the material, yet it is quite possible some errors might have been left uncorrected. The publisher, the printer and the author will not be held responsible for any inadvertent errors or inaccuracies.

Pathology Practicals

ISBN: 978-93-87964-34-1

Copyright © Author and Publisher

First Edition: 2019
Reprint: 2020

All rights reserved. No part of this book may be reproduced or transmitted in any form or by any means, electronic or mechanical, including photocopying, recording, or any information storage and retrieval system without permission, in writing, from the author and the publisher.

Published by Satish Kumar Jain and Produced by Varun Jain for
CBS Publishers & Distributors Pvt Ltd
4819/XI Prahlad Street, 24 Ansari Road, Daryaganj, New Delhi 110 002, India.
Ph: 011-23289259, 23266861, 23266867 Fax: 011-23243014   Website: www.cbspd.com
e-mail: delhi@cbspd.com; cbspubs@airtelmail.in.
Corporate Office: 204 FIE, Industrial Area, Patparganj, Delhi 110 092
Ph: 011-4934 4934   Fax: 011-4934 4935   e-mail: publishing@cbspd.com; publicity@cbspd.com

Branches

- **Bengaluru:** Seema House 2975, 17th Cross, K.R. Road, Banasankari 2nd Stage, Bengaluru 560 070, Karnataka
  Ph: +91-80-26771678/79   Fax: +91-80-26771680   e-mail: bangalore@cbspd.com
- **Chennai:** 7, Subbaraya Street, Shenoy Nagar, Chennai 600 030, Tamil Nadu
  Ph: +91-44-26680620, 26681266   Fax: +91-44-42032115   e-mail: chennai@cbspd.com
- **Kochi:** 42/1325, 1326, Power House Road, Opposite KSEB Power House, Ernakulam 682 018, Kochi, Kerala
  Ph: +91-484-4059061-65   Fax: +91-484-4059065   e-mail: kochi@cbspd.com
- **Kolkata:** 6/B, Ground Floor, Rameswar Shaw Road, Kolkata 700 014, West Bengal
  Ph: +91-33-22891126, 22891127, 22891128   e-mail: kolkata@cbspd.com
- **Mumbai:** 83-C, Dr E Moses Road, Worli, Mumbai 400018, Maharashtra
  Ph: +91-22-24902340/41   Fax: +91-22-24902342   e-mail: mumbai@cbspd.com

Representatives

• Bhopal	0-8319310552	• Bhubaneswar	0-9911037372	• Hyderabad	0-9885175004
• Jharkhand	0-9811541605	• Nagpur	0-9421945513	• Patna	0-9334159340
• Pune	0-9623451994	• Uttarakhand	0-9716462459	• Dhaka (Bangladesh)	01912-003485
• Kathmandu (Nepal)	977-9818742655				

Printed At : Goyal Offset Works (P) Limited

to
_____

*four important persons in my life:
my parents, Mr Nitai Chandra Mondal and
Smt Jyotsna Mondal
and
my wife Shampa Mondal and
son Soumyadeep Mondal*

Preface

Francis Bacon once said "Some books to be tasted, others swallowed and some few to be chewed and digested". But books like friends should be a few and well chosen.

Clarifying concepts and inculcating the fundamental tenets in pathology practicals are daunting tasks for any medical teacher. Pathology is a rapidly expanding field of medicine with new techniques. In modern era, tremendous growth is in progress in diagnostic pathology.

In this book, five sections (Haematology, Clinical Pathology, Histopathology and Cytopathology, Museum Techniques and Mounted Surgical Specimens and Problem Cards and Discussion) with a total of 16 chapters have been included. All these chapters are related to pathology practicals. Not only the practical aspect of a test or technique has been described but also the theoretical concept with regard to that particular test has been explained. At the end of every chapter, viva voce questions related to that particular topic have been included that will help the medical students face the examiner during pathology practical examinations.

Real mounted surgical specimens and their gross/macroscopic features will enhance the students' understanding. The problem cards will help to build logical thinking among the medical students. For easy understanding, many colour as well as black and white pictures/microphotographs, flow charts, diagrams, and tables have been included.

I thank my parents, my wife Shampa and son Soumyadeep for their constant support to complete this work. I thank Dr Debashis Chakrabarty, Associate Professor, Department of Pathology, SSKM Hospital, Kolkata, West Bengal, for helping me during preparation of this book. I also thank my postgraduate students Dr Bidhan Chandra Nayak and Dr Saptarshi Bhattacharya of Bankura Sammilani Medical College for their great help.

Despite our best efforts, some mistakes might creep in. I request all the readers to kindly bring to my notice if there is any mistake or typing error. Your positive criticism, appreciations and suggestions are valuable to us and are most welcome.

Santosh Kumar Mondal
E-mail: dr_santoshkumar@hotmail.com

Contents

Preface   *vii*

Part I: Haematology

1. Blood Collection and Anticoagulants	3
2. Blood and Bone Marrow Smear Preparation and Staining Methods	14
3. Marrow Puncture Needle and Examination of Bone Marrow	35
4. Total Count of WBC, RBC and Platelets	46
5. Erythrocyte Sedimentation Rate (ESR) and Packed Cell Volume (PCV)	56
6. Haemoglobin Estimation	65
7. Bleeding Time (BT), Clotting Time (CT) Prothrombin Time (PT) and APTT Time	76
8. Blood Grouping and Rh Typing	85

Part II: Clinical Pathology

9. Urine Examination	103
10. Lumbar Puncture Needle, Cerebrospinal Fluid and Other Body Fluids	129

Part III: Histopathology and Cytopathology

11. Histological Techniques	145
12. H and E (Haematoxylin and Eosin) and Other Special Stains	158
13. HP Slides (Light Microscopy)	168
14. Cytology: Exfoliative and FNAC	181

Part IV: Museum Techniques and Mounted Surgical Specimens

15. Museum Specimens	205

Part V: Problem Cards and Discussion

16. Problem Cards	239

Appendices   263

- Appendix I: Common Instruments in Pathology 263
- Appendix II: Reference Values (Range) 273

Index   *277*

Part I

Haematology

1. Blood Collection and Anticoagulants
2. Blood and Bone Marrow Smear Preparation and Staining Methods
3. Marrow Puncture Needle and Examination of Bone Marrow
4. Total Count of WBC, RBC, and Platelets
5. Erythrocyte Sedimentation Rate (ESR) and Packed Cell Volume (PCV)
6. Haemoglobin Estimation
7. Bleeding Time, Clotting Time, Prothrombin Time and APTT Time
8. Blood Grouping and Rh Typing

1
Blood Collection and Anticoagulants

Blood is the most frequent body fluid used for analytical purpose. Blood is a mesenchymal tissue consisting of a liquid portion called plasma and particulate or formed elements (RBCs, WBCs, platelets) which are suspended in plasma.

Plasma

Blood plasma is a straw-coloured fluid component of blood which normally holds the blood cells in suspension. So, plasma can be called extracellular matrix of blood cells. It makes near about 55% of the total blood value. It is composed mostly of water (up to 95% by volume) and dissolved proteins (6–8%). These proteins are albumin (4.5 gm%), globulins (2.5 gm%) and fibrinogens (0.3 gm%). Apart from proteins, glucose, clotting factors, electrolytes (Na^+, Mg^{2+}, Ca^{2+}, Cl^-, HCO_3^-, etc.). Hormones, carbon dioxide and oxygen are present in the plasma.

Serum

When blood is collected in the test tube or vial without addition of anticoagulants, then blood is clotted. The clot is formed by using blood cells, clotting factor like fibrinogen. The fluid is separated from clot. So, this fluid contains proteins and other elements but lacks fibrinogen (used in the formation of clot).

So, serum is plasma minus fibrinogen.

BLOOD COLLECTION AND PROCESSING

Three general procedures for obtaining blood are:
1. Venipuncture for venous blood
2. Arterial puncture for arterial blood
3. Skin puncture for capillary (peripheral) blood

Venous blood is preferred for most haematological examinations.

Venipuncture or Venous Puncture

Venous blood is best withdrawn from an antecubital vein by means of a dry glass syringe or disposable plastic syringe. The steps are:
  i. Position the patient properly, depending on whether the patient is sitting or prone (ambulatory or non-ambulatory). This is to make sure for easy access to the antecubital fossa.
 ii. The patient is asked to make a fist, so that veins become more prominent and more palpable.
iii. Select a suitable vein for venipuncture. For veins of the antecubital fossa, the median cubital and cephalic veins may be used alternatively. In case, the patient has an intravenous line, draw venous blood from other arm.
 iv. Cleanse the venipuncture site with 70% alcohol (isopropanol) or 1% iodine-

saturated swab stick. Allow the area to dry.

v. Apply a tourniquet few inches above the puncture site. But remember, do not keep the tourniquet for more than one minute.
vi. Hold the vein firmly, both above and below the puncture site. For this, use either thumb and middle finger or thumb and index finger.
vii. Perform the venipuncture. Enter the syringe needle (19 or 20 gauge) at approximately 15° angle to the arm. If using the evacuated system or vacuotainer as soon as the needle is inserted in the vein, ease the collection tube forward in the holder as far as possible, firmly securing the needle holder in place.
viii. Release the tourniquet when blood begins flow.
ix. After blood collection, place a clean cotton ball or gauze lightly over the site. Withdraw the needle, then apply pressure to site.
x. Now apply an adhesive bandage strip over the cotton ball or gauze to stop bleeding or formation of haematoma.

Note
i. The needles should not be too fine or too long, those of 19 or 20 SWG British standard, American standard 19 SWG = 18 (1.016 mm), 20 SWG = 19 (0.914 mm) are suitable.
ii. If the veins are very small then 23 SWG (= 22 or 0.610) to be used to collect at least 2 ml venous blood.
iii. If veins are selected from dorsum of the hand, it tends to bleed easily. So, care must be taken.
iv. Beware of haemolysis of blood during collection. It can be avoided or minimized by using clean apparatus, withdrawing the blood slowly, not using too fine needle, delivering the blood slowly into the receiver and avoiding frothing during the withdrawal of the blood and subsequent mixing with the anticoagulant.

2. Arterial Puncture

Arterial blood is used rarely. It is used to measure oxygen and carbon dioxide tension, as well as pH (arterial blood gases or ABGs). These blood gas measurements are critical in the assessment of oxygenation problems encountered in patients with pneumonia, pneumonitis and pulmonary embolism. Also

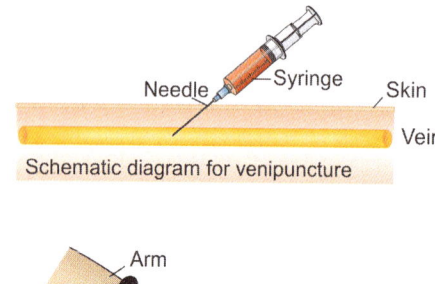

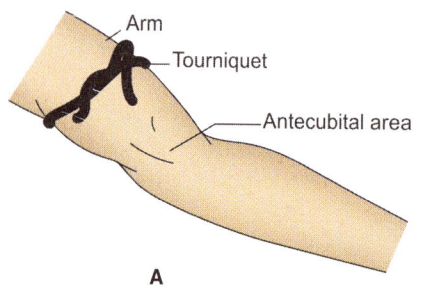

A

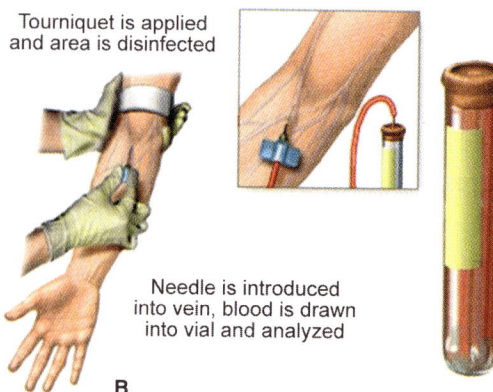

B

Fig. 1.1A and B: Blood collection procedure

critically ill cardiovascular patients and patients who are undergoing cardiac or pulmonary surgery are monitored for hypoxaemia.

Arterial puncture is technically more difficult than venous puncture. Increased pressure of the flowing blood, makes it more difficult to stop bleeding with the undesired development of a haematoma. The arteries selected for arterial punctures are radial, brachial and femoral arteries in order of choice. Unsuitable sites are oedematous, irritated, near a wound, or in an area of an arteriovenous (AV) shunt or fistula. Although venous blood yields adequate pH values if properly collected but venous blood yields incorrect values for arterial oxygen saturation and alveolar pCO_2.

Skin Puncture (Capillary Blood)

Skin puncture is the method of choice in paediatric patients especially infants. The large amount of blood collected from repeated venipuncture may cause anemia (iatrogenic), especially in premature infants. Skin puncture is also preferred in geriatric patients because of thinness of skin and loss of skin elasticity which cause venipuncture difficult.

In the neonates and infants, the heel is often used for skin puncture. A deep heel prick is made at the distal edge of the calcaneal protuberance following 5–10 minutes prior exposure to prewarmed water. In the older paediatric population, and in geriatric patients, ear lobes or finger are preferred.

This capillary blood collected by skin puncture is good for making blood smear or for a single routine haematological test. A blood smear prepared from capillary blood without anticoagulant gives better information about blood cell morphology and differential count. But the total count is not very accurate. This is because of dilution by the tissue fluid and sometimes also due to lack of free flow of capillary blood. But if free flow capillary blood is received, then it is as satisfactory as venous blood.

Capillary blood obtained from heel puncture is not good for pCO_2 and pO_2 determination in the first day of life, probably owing to vasoconstriction and poor perfusion of the extremities. In infants with respiratory distress syndrome, heel blood deviates significantly from arterial blood in all parameters except standard bicarbonate and base excess.

The discrepancies between peripheral (capillary) and venous blood are more pronounced if ear lobe than finger is chosen for skin puncture. However, if the ear is rubbed well with a piece of cotton or lint until ear is warm and pink, then a good spontaneous flow of blood can be obtained using sterile lancets as prickers. In this case, RBC count, leukocyte count and haemoglobin content almost close to venous blood.

Heel Puncture Method (Fig. 1.2)

A deep puncture in the heel is made after heel is really warm (5–10 minutes prior

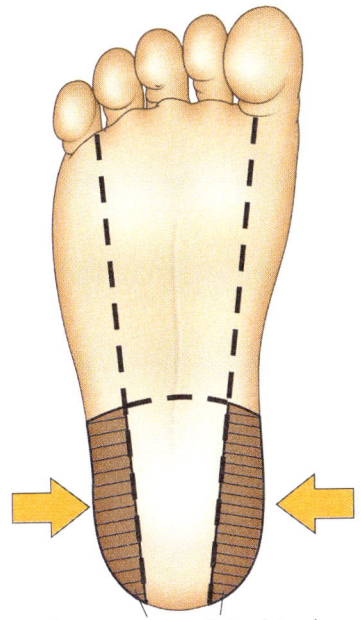

Proper area (medial or lateral parts of plantar surface)

Fig. 1.2: Heel puncture method

exposure to prewarmed water) by using a steel lancet. Ideal sites are the medial or lateral parts of the plantar surface of the heel. Remember, the central plantar area and posterior curvature are not chosen in infants because of risk of injury to the underlying tarsal bones.

Ear Lobe Puncture Method

Rub the ear until it becomes warm and pink. Then with a sterile lancet prick the ear lobe (as it has no bone or cartilage) to a depth of 2–3 mm by a single stab. Wipe and discard first few drops of blood. Collect the blood sample when it flows spontaneously (usually in about 30 seconds). Always use different lancet for different patients.

Finger Prick (Stick) Procedure

The best locations for finger sticks are the 3rd (middle) and 4th (ring) finger of the non-dominated hand. Do not select tip of the finger or the centre of the finger. The second (index) finger tends to have thicker and calloused skin, so not preferred. The fifth finger (little finger) tends to have less soft tissue overlying the bone.

1. After selection of site of the finger, put on gloves and cleanse the puncture site with 70% alcohol (isopropanol).
2. Massage the finger toward the selected site prior to puncture.
3. Then with a sterile safety lancet make a skin puncture just off the finger pad.
4. Wipe away the first drop of blood which contains excess tissue fluid/plasma. Take subsequent blood drop into collection tube/device by gentle pressure on the finger; or put the blood drop onto a glass slide.

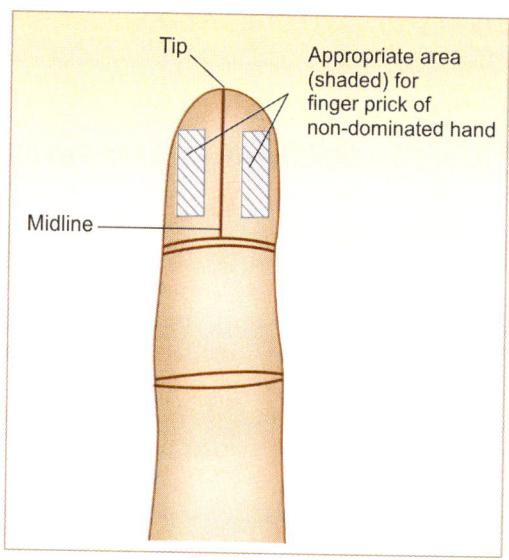

Fig. 1.3: Finger prick (stick) procedure

5. Cap, rotate and invert the collection device/tube.
6. Label it.

Differences Between Venous and Peripheral (Capillary) Blood

- The platelet count is usually higher in venous than in peripheral blood (average 9% higher, but may go up to 32%). This is probably due to adhesion of platelets to the skin puncture site resulting in lower platelet count in peripheral blood.
- Venous blood and peripheral blood are not same, even though capillary blood is free-flowing which comes from arterioles after skin puncture.
- The RBC count, haemoglobin content and packed cell volume (PCV) is slightly higher in peripheral blood than venous blood. The total leukocyte count (TLC) and neutrophil counts are also higher about 8%, and monocyte count by 12% in peripheral blood. In children, it may be up to 100% higher, both for heel and ear lobe punctured capillary blood.
- But the monocytes and neutrophils tend to accumulate in the ear lobe if the blood is not free-flowing.

ANTICOAGULANTS

The anticoagulants prevent blood from clotting and as a result, plasma is formed. Most anticoagulants bind with calcium ions (Ca^{2+}) and remove it by calcium chelating. Calcium is a factor in the coagulation cascade. As the calcium is chelated it cannot work. So, clot is not formed. Heparin, on the other hand, directly interferes in the coagulation process by destroying thrombin as well as thromboplastin.

Platelets + clotting factors + calcium → thrombin which convents fibrinogen → fibrin clot.

1. EDTA (Ethylenediamine Tetra-acetic Acid)

It is also called sequestrene and probably the best anticoagulant for routine haematological investigations.

Mechanism of action: It is a powerful calcium chelating or binding agent and acts by binding the calcium in blood. So, active calcium ions are not available for coagulation process.

Concentration of EDTA: A concentration of 1.2 mg of anhydrous salt per ml of blood is required. For dipotassium salt, a concentration of 1.5 ± 0.25 mg/ml of blood is recommended as per International Council for Standardization in Haematology (ICSH). The dipotassium salt is very soluble and is preferred over disodium salt which is less soluble.

Advantages of EDTA
i. Very good anticoagulant for routine haematological investigations. EDTA has the advantage over oxalate anticoagulant because it prevents clumping of platelets *in vitro*. So, platelet count can also be performed on venous blood.
ii. The dilithium salt of EDTA has the advantage that same blood sample can be used for chemical investigations apart from haematological investigations. But dilithium salt is less soluble compared to dipotassium salt and is less preferred.

Disadvantages of EDTA: Excess of EDTA (>2 mg/ml), irrespective of its salts, cause shrinkage and degenerative changes in RBCs and WBCs. Also, excess salt causes significant decrease in PCV and increase in MCHC (mean corpuscular haemoglobin concentration). Excess EDTA causes platelets to swell and then disintegrate, resulting in spuriously high platelet count as the swollen platelet fragments are large enough to be counted as normal platelets.

2. Trisodium Citrate

A 3.8% aqueous solution of trisodium citrate ($Na_3 C_6H_5O_7, 2H_2O$) is the anticoagulant of choice **for coagulation studies**. It is also most widely used anticoagulant **for ESR** (erythrocyte sedimentation rate) also. But for coagulation studies (prothrombin time) 9:1 blood to anticoagulant is used, whereas in ESR determination 4:1 venous blood to anticoagulant is used.

Mechanism of action: Coagulation is prevented by precipitation of blood calcium in the form of a double salt (calcium sodium salt) which is very weakly dissociated.

3. Heparin

Heparin powder or liquid is used in a concentration of 10–20 IU (0.1–0.2 mg) per ml of blood.

Mechanism of action: It acts by inhibiting thromboplastin formation. Also it has antithrombin activity, i.e. inhibiting the action of thrombin on fibrinogen in the presence of plasma of co-factor antithrombin III.

Uses
i. Osmotic fragility test
ii. Chemical investigation like plasma iron estimation
iii. Demonstration of LE cell in SLE patients
iv. Lymphocyte culture for karyotyping/genetic study
v. Lymphoma/leukaemia panel for flow cytometry or immunophenotyping

vi. Nitro blue tetrazolium (NBT) test to assess phagocytic activity of phagocytes.

Advantage: It is an effective anticoagulant and does not alter the size of RBCs. It minimizes chances of haemolysis. Some consider heparin in the form of lithium salt is the ideal universal anticoagulant for blood.

Disadvantages
i. It is expensive
ii. It is inferior to EDTA as anticoagulant
iii. Heparinized blood should not be used for making blood films as it gives a faint blue colouration to the background when blood smears are stained with Romanowsky stains. Also, it causes leukocytes to clump, so TLC and DLC will be erroneous.

4. Oxalate

Potassium, sodium and ammonium oxalates act as calcium chelating agent like EDTA and trisodium citrate. They interact with blood calcium and form calcium oxalate after chelation.

i. Potassium and sodium oxalate: Used mainly for chemical analysis. Concentration of anticoagulant 2 mg/ml of blood.
ii. Double oxalate (Wintrobe's mixture): It is a mixture of two types of oxalates (ammonium oxalate and potassium oxalate in a ratio of 3:2). It is used in a concentration of 2 mg/ml of blood. Preparation of double oxalate mixture is as follows:

Ammonium oxalate: 1.2 gm

Potassium oxalate: 0.8 gm

Distilled water: 100 ml

This solution contains 20 mg of oxalates (both ammonium and potassium oxalate)/ml solution. So, 0.2 ml of this solution containing 4 mg of oxalates is sufficient for 2 ml of blood (up to 5 ml blood) as anticoagulants.

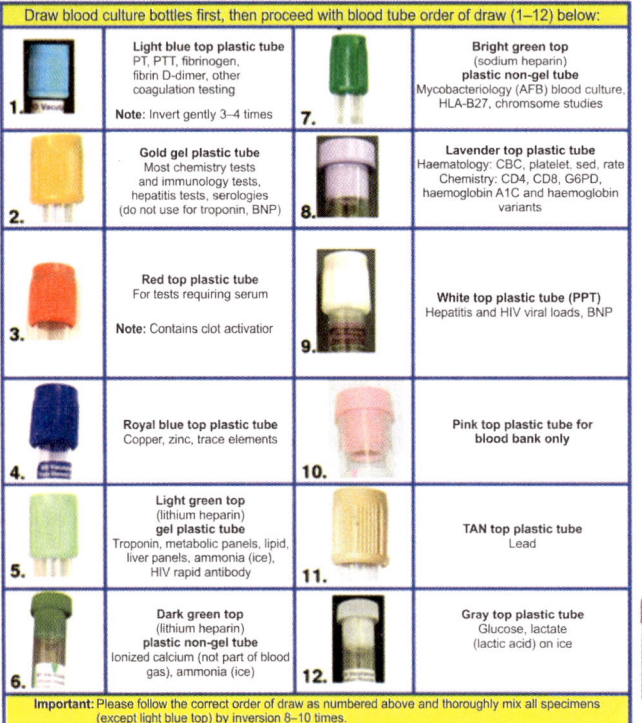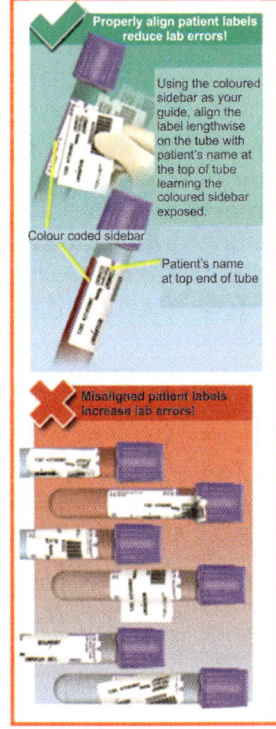

Fig. 1.4: Colour code of top of blood tube/vial and their significance

Uses

i. Determination of haematocrit value or PCV.
ii. Determination of haemoglobin and total leukocyte count (TLC)
iii. Determination of specific gravity of whole blood or plasma.
iv. Single powder in the form of sodium or potassium oxalate can be used for blood urea and creatine estimation.

5. Sodium Fluoride

It is used in the concentration of 30 mg powder/5 ml of blood or 6 mg powder/ml of blood. **Mechanism of action:** (i) It chelates calcium and forms calcium fluoride, (ii) it prevents glycolysis by blocking acid phosphorylase enzymes in RBCs but increases amylase activity.

Uses: It is anticoagulant of choice for blood sugar estimation.

Table 1.1: Some blood anticoagulants and their use

Name of anticoagulants (requirement per ml of blood)	Mechanism of action	Diagnostic use
1. No anticoagulant for serum in plain vial/tube	No anticoagulant; blood is clotted	Serum: Liver function test (protein, bilirubin, SGOT/AST, SGPT/ALT, alkaline phosphatase, γGT, etc.), lipid profile (cholesterol, triglyceride, HDL, LDL, VLDL), area, creatine, etc.
2. EDTA (1–1.5 mg/ml)	Binds Ca^{2+} and chelates it	Haemoglobin estimation, PCV, TLC, DLC, platelet count, parasite detection (microfilaria, malaria)
3. Trisodium citrate (3.8% aqueous solution; blood to anticoagulant ratio of 9:1 or 4:1 for coagulation studies and ESR respectively)	Binds Ca^{2+} and precipitates it as double salt (calcium sodium salt)	Coagulation studies, prothrombin time, ESR
4. Heparin (0.1–0.2 mg/ml)	Inhibits thrombin in the presence of antithrombin III. Also, it inhibits thromboplastin formation	• Osmotic fragility test • Plasma iron estimation • Demonstration of LE cells • Lymphocyte culture for karyotyping/genetic studies • Lymphoma/leukaemia panel for flow cytometry/immunophenotyping
5. Sodium or potassium oxalate (2 mg/ml)	Binds Ca^{2+} and chelates it	Blood urea and creatine
6. Double oxalate (ammonium and potassium oxalate, 2 mg/ml)	Binds Ca^{2+} and chelates it	Hb, TLC, DLC, MCV, ESR
7. Sodium fluoride (6 mg powder/ml of blood)	• Blocks RBC enzymes for glycolytic inhibition of glucose • Also, chelates calcium	Blood glucose (sugar) estimation

For glucose estimation, fluoride may be added to heparin also.

> **Note**
> Fluoride inhibits glycolysis of blood cells (RBCs) which may otherwise destroy glucose at the rate of about 5%/hour.

BLOOD COLLECTION TUBES/VIALS AND COLOUR CODE

1. **Red or gold top clot tube:** Contains no anticoagulant. Blood will clot and serum will be formed.
2. **Purple top tube:** Contains EDTA anticoagulant.
3. **Blue top tube:** Contains 3.8% buffered sodium citrate anticoagulant for coagulation studies.
4. **Black top tube:** Contains 3.8% sodium citrate for ESR only
5. **Light green top tube:** Contains lithium heparin anticoagulant.
6. **Dark green top tube:** Contains sodium heparin anticoagulant used for amino acid and cytogenetic studies.
7. **Gray top tube:** Contains glycolytic inhibitor or sodium fluoride for glucose estimation.
8. **Yellow tube:** Contains acid citrate dextrose (used in blood banking).

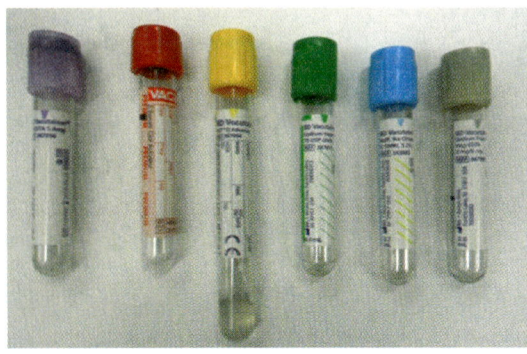

Fig. 1.5

SOURCES OF BLOOD COLLECTION ERROR

1. Wrong patient identification or labelling error
2. Haemoconcentration: Prolonged tourniquet time (>1 minute) restricts blood flow causing false high results, e.g. cell counts.
3. Haemodilution: If blood is collected from an arm with an IV (intravenous), the blood can be diluted and/or contaminated causing false low cell counts.
4. Haemolysis: Caused by traumatic blood drawing technique, vigorous shaking of the blood tube or forcing the blood through syringe needle into the tube. Rupture of blood cells causes release of cell constituents like potassium, tissue factors and responsible for low RBC counts.
5. Use of wrong anticoagulant/tube: As for example, heparin causes platelet clumping. Hence, unsuitable for platelet counts.
6. Partially clotted blood draws improper mixing of anticoagulant containing tubes or blood obtained using poor blood drawing technique (e.g. too slow) may clot. Cells are trapped in the fibrin clot causing falsely low cell counts.
7. Insufficient fill: All tubes should have minimum draw amounts to maintain the proper anticoagulant concentration to blood volume. As for example, blue top tubes for coagulation test must be full.
8. Proper instruction for the said test not followed, e.g. certain tests have time limits for testing.

EFFECT OF STORAGE OF BLOOD

- When blood is kept in room temperature (18–25°C) for prolonged time, certain changes take place regardless of the anticoagulant use.

- This is obvious in EDTA blood (tripotassium salt > dipotassium salt).
- RBCs begin to swell; as a result, MCV increases, osmotic fragility and prothrombin time increase slowly and ESR decreases.
- The TLC and platelet count gradually fall. It is best to perform TLC and platelet count within 2 hours.
- The fall in leukocyte count is more if there is excessive amount of EDTA (>4.5 mg/ml).
- Reticulocyte count is unchanged for 24 hours at 4°C but at room temperature, it begins to fall within 6 hours.
- Nucleated RBCs (normoblasts) disappear from stored blood within 1–2 days at room temperature.
- Haemoglobin content is relatively stable for days unless it is infected.

For different investigations, blood is collected in tubes with or without anticoagulants. If there is anticoagulant, after mixing the blood cells of whole blood can be analyzed. Centrifugation of whole blood separates the cells from fluid plasma. In the bottom there will be RBCs. Above, there will be plasma containing fibrinogen. In between these two layers, there will be a **buffy coat** containing WBCs and platelets.

If there is no anticoagulant, fibrinogen will be used up to form fibrin strands which entrap blood cells. Centrifugation of this blood will separate the clot from the fluid serum. Serum lacks fibrinogen.

Serum and plasma can be obtained on standing also and they can be taken out by micropipette without disturbing fibrin clot or blood cells respectively. But, centrifugation will give better quality serum or plasma.

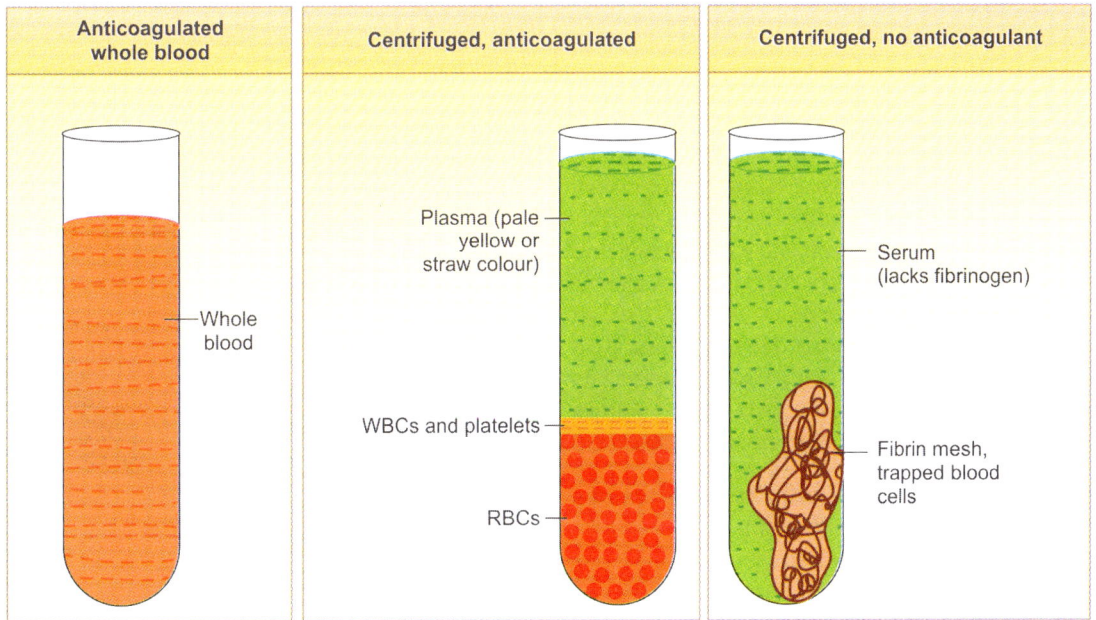

Fig. 1.6: Left tube contains anticoagulated whole blood, middle tube showing plasma and last tube showing serum

VIVA VOCE

Q1. What are differences between serum and plasma?

Ans:

Serum	Plasma
1. Serum is formed as supernatant when blood undergoes clotting	1. Plasma is obtained by centrifugation of anticoagulant mixed blood. Anticoagulant mixed blood after standing may also give plasma but of poor quality compared to plasma after centrifugation.
2. Serum does not contain fibrinogen, prothrombin and other clotting factors like V, VII, VIII, IX, X, XI and XII which have been used in clotting.	2. It contains all the clotting factors including fibrinogen. But calcium ion is absent.
3. It is used to estimate different biochemical parameters and serum enzymes like uric acid, electrolytes, urea, creatinine, SGOT, SGPT, alkaline phosphatase, etc.	3. It is used mainly for coagulation studies like PT, APTT, TT, etc. Also used for detection of plasma glucose, plasma calcium, plasma ammonia, etc.
4. Serum is clear fluid.	4. Plasma is yellowish or straw coloured.

Q2. What is the ideal gauge needle (bore size) for collection of venous blood?

Ans: If the needle is too large for the vein for which it is intended, it will tear the vein and cause bleeding (haematoma). If the needle, is too small, it will damage the blood cells especially RBCs. So, laboratory tests which require whole blood cells or haemoglobin or plasma will give inaccurate results.

The gauge refers to the inner measurement or opening of the needle. Usually needle gauge of 21G to 23G is preferred for venous blood collection. Small bore needles of 25G or less cannot be recommended and reserved only for problematic venous accesses and newborns. Usually 25G or lesser size may cause haemolysis and inaccurate results of electrolytes especially potassium. Nonetheless, 21G needles are most commonly used for routine tests.

Q3. Why is middle or ring finger preferred for capillary blood collection?

Ans: The best locations for finger sticks are the 3rd (middle) and 4th (ring) finger of the non-dominated hand. Do not select tip of the finger or the centre of the finger. The second (index) finger tends to have thicker and calloused skin, so not preferred. The fifth finger (little finger) tends to have less soft tissue overlying the bone. Ulnar side of the tip of ring finger is comparatively less innervated. So, needle prick is less painful to the patients.

Q4. Why too much pressure is not given during blood collection from finger prick?

Ans: Needle prick should be deep enough so that free flow blood comes out. Gentle pressure may be applied to start the blood. But too much pressure to finger tip should not be given as tissue fluid will come out which will dilute the blood. So, haematological values will be lowered.

Q5. Why double oxalate is preferred over single oxalate as an anticoagulant?

Ans: Ammonium salt (ammonium oxalate) causes swelling of RBCs while potassium salt (potassium oxalate) causes shrinkage of RBCs. Hence, mixture of these two salts or double oxalate will cause neither RBC swelling nor RBC shrinkage. Normal shape and size of RBCs are maintained. Potassium oxalate: Ammonium oxalate = 2:3.

But oxalates are not preferred as anticoagulant for Hb/TLC/platelet count as they induce morphologic alterations in WBCs and RBCs. So, smear morphology cannot be studied.

Q6. Why excess EDTA is bad as anticoagulant?

Ans: Excess of EDTA (>2 mg/ml), irrespective of its salts, cause shrinkage and degenerative changes in RBCs and WBCs. Also, excess salt cause significant decrease in PCV and increase in MCHC (mean corpuscular haemoglobin concentration). Excess EDTA causes platelets to swell and then disintegrate, resulting in spuriously high platelet count as the swollen platelet fragments are large enough to be counted as normal platelets.

Q7. What is a vacutainer?

Ans: Vacutainer: This is a blood collection tube which is sterile glass tube with a coloured rubber stopper creating a vaccum seal inside of the tube facilitating the drawing of a predetermined volume of blood/liquid. Vacutainer tubes may contain anticoagulant/additives to stabilize and preserve the blood/liquid specimen prior to analytical testing. Tubes containing gel can be easily handled and transported after centrifugation without the blood cells and serum mixing.

Vacutainer tubes were invented by Joseph Kleiner and Becton Dickinson in 1949.

Q8. What are different vacutainers used in haematology?

Anticoagulant/additives	Colour	Blood volume	Uses
1. Plain	Red	6 ml	Most biochemistry including drug levels, serological tests, which uses serum, cross-matching.
2. EDTA-K2	Purple	3 ml	Most haematological tests, HbA1C, molecular genetics tests using blood DNA.
3. Lithium heparin	Green	4 ml	Cytogenetic tests using blood DNA, osmotic fragility test, STAT biochemistry like electrolytes, renal screen, ammonia, etc. After blood is drawn inside by vacuum, it should be inverted gently at least 6 times to prevent clotting.
4. Sodium citrate	Blue	2.7 ml	Coagulation studies. This tube should be inverted at least 3–4 times.
5. Sodium fluoride/potassium oxalate	Grey	6 ml	Glucose test. It should be inverted gently at least 6 times.
6. SST II, clot activator and serum gel separator, plain	Yellow	5 ml	All tests requiring serum except those few that need red cells as well

2

Blood and Bone Marrow Smear Preparation and Staining Methods

Examination of blood and bone marrow smear/film are important haematologic evaluation and to diagnose a haematologic disease. Blood or bone marrow smears should be prepared immediately as delay can cause spurious results.

Here, three methods of making blood smears/films are described

1. Wedge method
2. Spinner or spin method
3. Cover glass method

WEDGE METHOD

This is perhaps the most common method to prepare a blood film. Place a small drop of blood (2–3 mm in diameter) about 1–2 cm from the end of a clean, dust-free slide which is on flat surface. Then without any delay, a spreader (second slide) is hold between thumb and forefinger of the right hand against the surface of the first slide at an angle of 30–45° and move it back to make contact with the blood drop to spread it. Then push the spreader slide at a moderate speed forward until all the blood has been spreaded over the first slide forming a moderately thin film. Ideally, the spreader slide should be clean, dry and slightly narrower than the first slide so that blood does not cross the edge of the first slide and edges of blood film can be examined under the microscope.

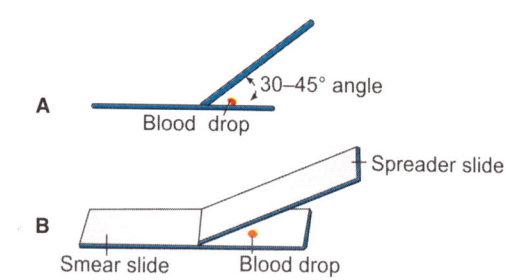
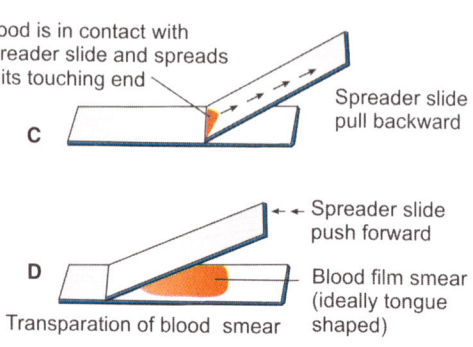

Fig. 2.1A to D: Preparation of blood smears. (A) small blood drop from 1 to 2 cm from one end of glass slide; (B) Place the spreader slide at an angle of 30° to 45° over the smear slide; (C) Pull back the spreader slide so that it touches the blood drop and spreads throughout the edge of the spreader slide; (D) Push forward to make blood/smear

Blood and Bone Marrow Smear Preparation and Staining Methods

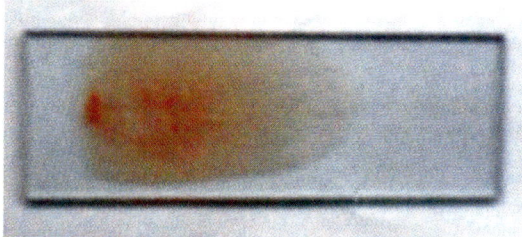

Fig. 2.2: Ideal thin blood smear

Note

a. The blood drop should be such that it can produce the blood film 3–4 cm in length.

b. The ideal thickness of blood film should be such that there will be some overlap of RBC (red blood cells) throughout much of the blood film's length. But the RBCs are separated at the tail end of the film.

c. The film should not cover the entire surface of glass slide.

d. Ideally, there will be a thick portion and a thin portion in a good film and there will be gradual transition from one to the other.

e. The blood film should have an even, smooth appearance and should be free ridges, waves or holes.

f. The edge of spreader slide must be very smooth. Roughed edges will produce ragged tails containing many leukocytes (WBCs).

g. The thickness of blood film can be adjusted by changing the speed of spreading or by changing the angle of the spreader slide or by using a larger or smaller blood drop.

h. At a given angle, increasing the speed of spreader slide will cause increase in the thickness of the film.

i. At a given speed, increasing the angle of spreader slide will also cause increase in the thickness of the film.

j. The faster the blood film is air dried, the better the spreading of the individual cells on glass slide. Slow drying of film (as in humid weather) may cause contraction artifacts of the cells.

k. There may be disproportionate monocytes at the tip of the feather (tail) edge or neutrophils just in from the feather edge and both at the lateral edges of the film.

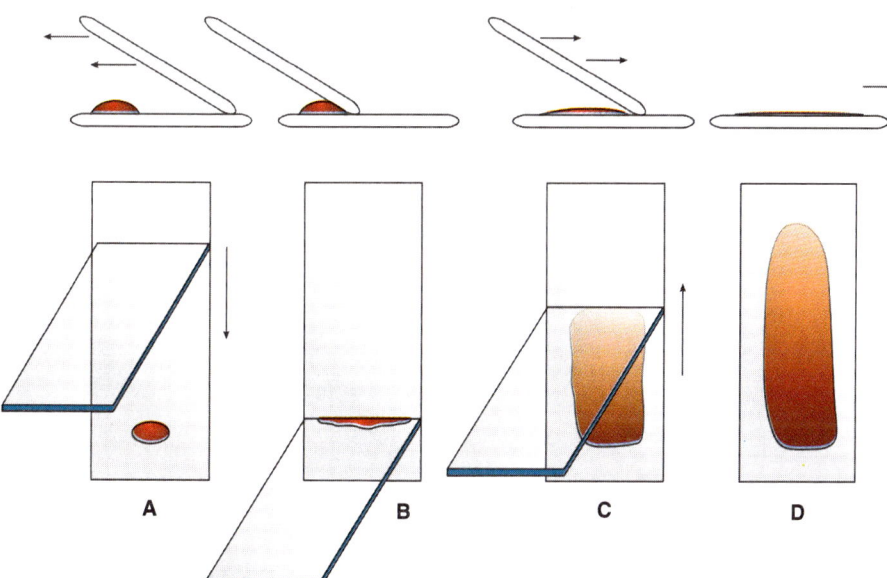

Fig. 2.3A to D: Upper row showing side view of different steps of making a thin blood film. Lower row showing front view of different steps of making a thin blood film

Thin film

- Good preparation—feathered end of the film should be centrally located on the slide with free margins on both sides, when properly prepared, it will be only one cell layer thick at this end.

- Badly prepared smears can cause presence of streaks—as a result of chipped spreader.

- Holes in the film indicate faulty preparation and dirty or greasy slides, respectively.

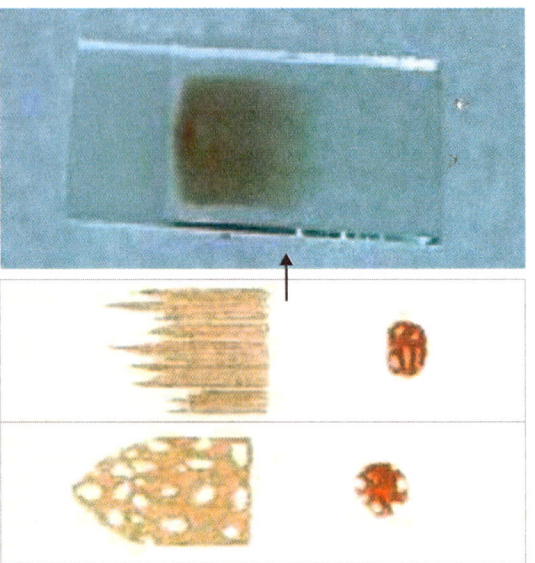

Fig. 2.4: Good and badly prepared thin blood film

SPINNER OR SPIN METHOD

Spinner or spin method is an automated method in which 1–2 drops of blood drops are placed in the centre of a glass slide. Then it is spun at a high speed in a spherical centrifuge (e.g. cytospin) for a short period. The blood drops are spreaded on the glass slide in a monolayer. With this method leukocytes and platelets are distributed uniformly without any distortion.

Note

1. The RBCs may be distorted. To overcome this problem, mix one volume of 9 gm/L NaCl (sodium chloride) to 2 volumes of blood for diluting the blood and then put the diluted blood on the glass slide.

2. White blood cells (WBCs) can be easily examined on any spot in the film made by spinner method.

3. Unlike wedge method, it does not produce disproportionate monocytes and/or neutrophils at the tail or lateral edges.

COVER GLASS METHOD

For this, 22 mm square (number one or one and a half cover glasses) are recommended. Touch a cover glass to the top of a small blood drop without touching the skin. Now place it, blood side down crosswise onto another cover glass, so that the corners appear as an eight point star. The small blood drop will spread out quickly and evenly in a thin layer between the two surfaces. Prepare blood film by pulling the cover glasses quickly and firmly apart on a plane parallel to their surfaces. After that, cover glasses are placed on clean paper (film side up) and are air dried.

Blood film from venous blood may be prepared likewise by placing a blood drop on a coverslip and follow the above mentioned steps.

THICK SMEAR AND ITS PREPARATION

While the blood film mentioned above, is suitable for studies of cellular morphology, sometimes thick smears are prepared to detect microfilariae and malarial parasites.

Thick smears are very useful when parasites (malaria and microfilaria) are scanty but identification of the parasites is less than thin films. Mixed infection (both *Plasmodium vivax* and *falciparum*) may also be missed. Thick smear is also useful when there is severe leukopenia. It helps to perform differential count or at least the proportion of polymorphonuclear to mononuclear cells.

Preparation of Thick Film

A drop of blood is placed in the centre of a glass slide and is spreaded out with a corner of another slide to cover an area about four times its original area. The film may be air-dried or dried at 37°C for 30 minutes in an incubator. If the film is satisfactory, then printed matter (small print of newspaper) is just visible.

Alternatively, four small blood drops may be taken in the mid-portion of a glass slide. They are joined together to form a blood film (square shaped) in the mid-portion of the slide.

Sinton proposed to make thin and thick smears onto a glass slide. For this, a large blood drop is taken near one end to make thick smear and one small blood drop is taken in the centre of the slide. Thick smear is prepared from the large blood drop (square shaped) while thin smear is prepared from the small blood drop (tongue shaped) in the same manner as previously described.

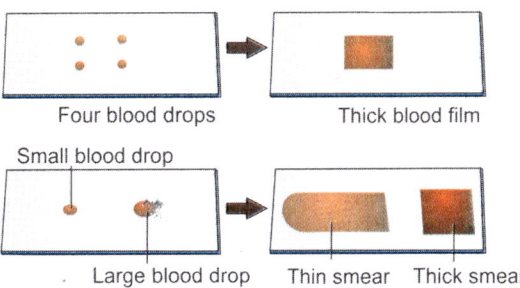

Fig. 2.5: Preparation of thick and thin blood films in the upper panel. Preparation of both thin and thick blood films on the same slide.

Fixation of Blood Films

Blood films need to be fixed before staining to prevent haemolysis when they come in contact with water during water-based (aqueous) stains or water is poured during staining. For this, blood films are coated with

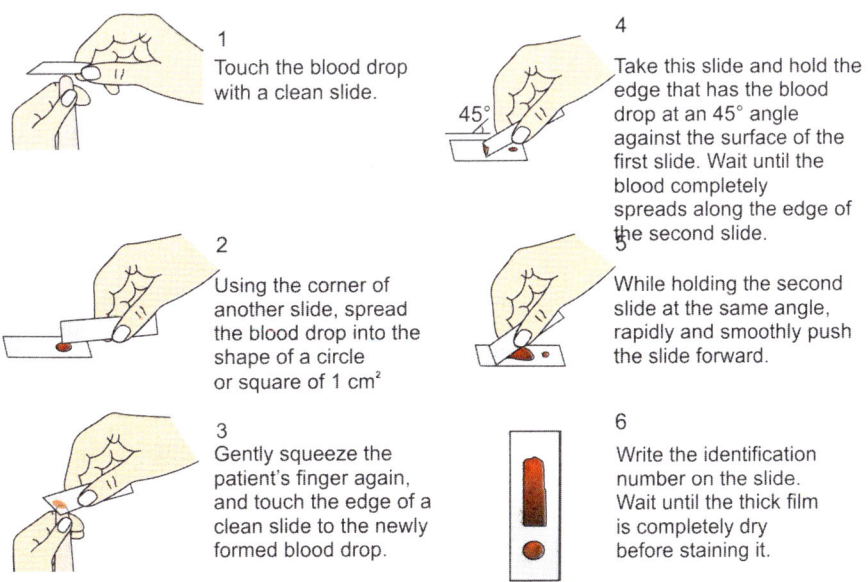

Fig. 2.6: Preparation of a thin and a thick blood film on the same slide

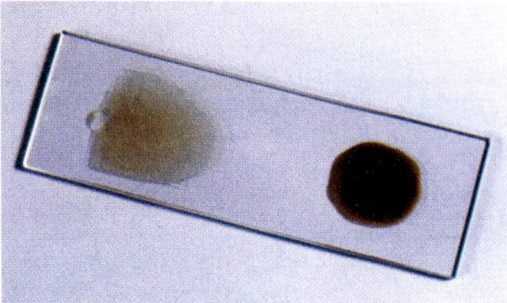

Fig. 2.7: Thin and thick blood films on the same slide. Thin blood film is typically tongue-shaped while thick blood film is circular or square shaped

acetone-free methyl alcohol for 1–2 minutes. This alcohol (methyl alcohol) denatures the proteins present in the blood and hardens the blood cells. As Leishman's stain and Wright's stain contain acetone-free methyl alcohol in the staining solution, the blood films do not require prefixation with alcohol. But Giemsa staining needs prefixation with alcohol as the ready to use staining solution contains only 5% alcohol (suboptimal for fixation).

BONE MARROW ASPIRATE FOR EXAMINATION

1. **Bone marrow films:** Put one drop of aspirate onto slides about 1 cm from one end. Then quickly suck off most of blood present in the aspirate with the help of a fine Pasteur pipette applied to the edge of each drop. Alternatively, keep the glass slides on a slope (to tilt them) for draining away of the blood.

    While the blood is removed, the irregularly shaped marrow fragments adhere to the slide. After that make bone marrow films which will be 3–5 cm in length by using a smooth edged glass spreader of less than 2 cm width. The marrow fragments are dragged behind the spreader and place the marrow cells trailing behind the spreader (trail of cells). The differential count should be made in these cellular trails, starting from the marrow fragment and working back towards the head of the film.

    Fix the bone marrow films and stain them with Romanowsky dyes as for peripheral blood films. But for high quality, a longer fixation time is needed (>20 minutes in methanol).

    Some advocate to add the aspirated marrow material to an anticoagulant like EDTA in a tube and to prepare a marrow films on returning to the laboratory. But there may be a possibility of using excess anticoagulant (only 0.2 to 0.3 ml of marrow aspirate compared to 2–5 ml of blood). The stained marrow film may show pink-staining amorphous material and some of the erythroblasts and reticulocytes may clump together due to excess anticoagulants.

2. **Bone marrow imprints:** Bone marrow fragments/particles of imprints may also be used for preparation of imprints. One or more visible particles are picked up with a capillary pipette, a toothpick or the broken end of a wooden applicator. The bone marrow particle (s) are transferred immediately to a slide and made to adhere to it by a gentle smearing motion. The slide is air dried rapidly by waving it and then is stained.

3. **Crush preparations:** A small drop aspirate containing a slide near one end. Another slide is placed over the first slide. Slight pressure is given to crush the bone marrow and the slides are separated by pulling them apart in a direction parallel to their surfaces.

    All bone marrow films should be dried quickly by moving them in the air (air dried) or by exposing them to a fan.

    As the bone marrow aspirate is being spreaded, the fat appears as irregular holes and make it sure that the marrow, material not only the blood has been aspirated.

POOR BLOOD SMEARS AND ITS COMMON CAUSES

1. The glass slides should be very clean as dirty slides do not give an even smear.

2. Put an appropriate size of blood drop onto glass slide and make the smear immediately. Delay will cause uneven distribution of WBCs.
3. The spreader slide should be moved steadily and confidently. Jerky movement or loss of contact between spreader slide and smear slide will give poor smears.
4. Angle between the spreader slide and smear slide should be 30° to 45°. Increasing the angle may result in a thick smear, whereas decreasing the result in a thin smear.

FIXING AND STAINING OF BLOOD SMEAR

The smears should be stained immediately after the preparation. Methanol (acetone-free) present in the common Romanowsky stains fix the smear slides in the staining procedure. If staining is delayed then smears must be fixed with methanol for 2–3 minutes. Fixation of smears will prevent distortion of blood cells and smears can be stored for future staining.

In the blood cells, some structural components are acidic while others are basic. Acidic substances stain with basic stain like methylene blue, azure B, etc. and are called basophilic. Examples of basophilic substances are nuclei and nucleic acids. Some basic structures like haemoglobin are stained with acid stains like eosin and are called acidophilic or eosinophilic. Other structures stained by combination of the two are called neutrophilic.

Stains which are composed of both acid and basic dyes are known as "Romanowsky" stains. These stains have the ability to make subtle distinctions during staining of cell and can stain the granules differentially. Neutrophilic granules are weakly stained by azure complexes, whereas eosinophilic granules get stained by acidic component of the dye and basophilic granules which contain acid heparin are stained by basic component of the dye.

The thiazine's basic component consists of methylene blue (tetramethyl thionine) and in varying proportions, its analogues produced by oxidative demethylation: Azure B (trimethyl thionine); azure A (asymmetric dimethylthionine), azure C (monomethyl thionine) and symmetric dimethlyl thionine.

As already said most Romanowsky stains are dissolved in methyl alcohol and combine fixation with staining. Various modifications of the original Romanowsky combination of methylene blue (basic stain) and eosin (acid stain) are now used. Usually combination of azure B and eosin Y is used as Romanowsky stain. Common Romanowsky stains are:
1. Leishman's stain
2. Wright's stain
3. Giemsa stain
4. May-Grünwald-Giemsa (MGG) stain
5. Field's stain
6. Jenner's stain
7. MacNeal stain

Leishman's stain is mostly used in the routine staining of blood film though wright's stain and Giemsa stain are also very popular. Giemsa stain is ideal for staining and detecting malarial parasites and other protozoa. Field's stain is used for staining thick film to detect malarial parasites and it offers rapid staining and screening of blood smears. MGG stains are used not only for blood/bone marrow films but also for cytology/FNAC smears.

Leishman's Stain

Reagents
1. Leishman powder (eosin-methylene blue powder): 0.15 gm
2. Methyl alcohol (acetone-free): 100 ml

The Leishman powder is placed in a conical flask to which methyl alcohol is added. Then the mixture is warmed to 50°C for 10–15 minutes. It is then filtered. The dye is ripened by keeping the filtrate in sunlight for 3–4 days or in an incubator at 37°C for 7 days.

Method: Dry the film in the air and flood the slide with the stain. After 2 minutes, add double the volume of water and stain the film for 7–10 minutes. Then wash the smear in a stream of buffered water until it has acquired a pinkish tinge (up to 2 minutes). After the back of the slide has been wiped clean, set it up right to dry.

Wright's Stain

Reagents
1. Wright's stain powder: 0.2 gm
2. Methyl alcohol (acetone-free): 100 ml

The solution is kept at 37°C for a few days before use.

Method: Almost same as in Leishman's staining. When the stain is ripe, a scum of film is formed over the surface of the stain.

Giemsa Stain

Reagents
- Giemsa powder: 0.6 gm
- Glycerol: 50 ml
- Acetone-free methyl alcohol: 50 ml

Giemsa powder (0.6 gm) is placed in a conical flask. Then 50 ml of glycerol is added. This mixture is warmed at 50°C for 15 minutes with occasional shaking and then 50 ml methanol is added to the mixture. It is now filtered and filtrate is ready for use. But before use the stain should be diluted 1:10.

Method: Unlike Leishman or Wright stain, here the blood films should be fixed with methyl alcohol (acetone-free) separately for 3–5 minutes and then dried. Diluted Giemsa stain (1:10) is poured on the fixed smear and kept for 20–30 minutes. Wash the smear with neutral/distilled water and dry.

May-Grünwald-Giemsa Stain

Reagents
1. May-Grünwald powder: 0.3 gm
2. Acetone-free methyl alcohol: 100 ml

Dissolve the 0.3 gm powder (dye) in 100 ml methyl alcohol and warm it at 50°C for 10 minutes. During warming shake it from time to time, filter after 24 hours.

Method: Fixed the smear in methyl alcohol for 3–5 minutes. Then stain the film with diluted (1:10) May-Grünwald stain for 5 minutes. Then stain the film with diluted (1:10) Giemsa stain for 15–20 minutes. Wash with buffered water and dry in the air.

Field's Stain

Reagents

1. **Stain A (polychromed methylene blue)**
   a. Methylene blue: 0.26 gm
   b. Azure B (optional): 0.1 gm
   c. Disodium hydrogen phosphate: 2.5 gm
   d. Potassium dihydrogen phosphate: 1.25 gm
   e. Water: 100 ml

   Dissolve the phosphates in warm freshly boiled water. Then mix the azure B with phosphate solution and dissolve it well. Lastly the dyes (methylene blue) are added and mix well. Filter it.

2. **Stain B (eosin)**
   a. Eosin Y (yellow eosin, water soluble): 0.26 gm
   b. Disodium hydrogen phosphate: 2.5 gm
   c. Potassium dihydrogen phosphate: 1.25 gm
   d. Water: 100 ml

   Dissolve the phosphates in warm freshly boiled water. Then mix the dye (eosin Y) with phosphate solution and dissolve it well, filter it.

Staining Method

1. Fix the film for 10–15 seconds in methanol.
2. Pour off the methanol and put 12 drops of diluted stain B (1:4 dilution in water)
3. Immediately add 12 drops of stain A.
4. Agitate the slides to mix the stains.
5. After 1 minute, rinse the slide in water.
6. Differentiate the slide in phosphate buffer for 5–10 seconds at pH 6.6.
7. Wash the slide in water.
8. Place it on end to drain and then dry.

Table 2.1: Common causes of faulty staining and their corrections

Faulty staining pattern	Causes	Corrections
1. Excessive blue stain	Thick films, prolonged staining time, inadequate washing or too high alkaline pH of stain or diluent.	Staining for less time or using less stain and more diluent. The pH of the buffer should be lowered.
2. Excessive pink stain	Insufficient staining, prolonged washing time, mounting the coverslips before they are dry, too high acidity (very low pH) of the diluents buffer or stain.	Staining time or washing time as advocated pH of buffer and stain should be adjusted.
3. Precipitates on the film	Drying during period of staining, inadequate washing of slide after staining, inadequate filtration of the stain, dust particles on smear or slide and use of unclean slides.	Act as per the cause

Note
i. A pH to the alkaline side of neutrality accentuates the azure component of Romanowsky stain at the expenses of the eosin and vice versa.
ii. A pH of 6.8 is usually recommended for general or routine use.
iii. To look, malarial parasites a pH of 7.2 is recommended in order to detect Schuffer's dots of *Plasmodium vivax, ovale* and *malariae*. (Remember Maurer's dots in *P. falciparum* and Ziemann's dots in *P. malariae*).

Chemical Theory of Romanowsky Staining

The mechanism by which certain components or structure of a cell stain with particular dye, depends on complex differences between the different dyes. As for example, azure B in dimer form is bound to anionic molecules, e.g. phosphate groups of DNA, whereas eosin Y is bound as a monomer to cationic sites of proteins.

As early as the dyes are bound to particular structure of the cell, either electron interaction occurs with dye-dye aggregation or the eosin Y molecule is inserted between the azure B molecules and the complex is held together by charge effect.

So, the acidic groupings of the nucleic acids and proteins of the cell nuclei and primitive cytoplasm determine their uptake of the basic dyes (like azure B). On the other hand, the presence of basic groupings on the haemoglobin molecules determines its affinity for acidic dyes and its staining with eosin (acid dye).

Examination of Romanowsky Stained Blood Smear

At first, examine the stained blood smear under low power for screening. Note the background colour and distribution of WBCs. In an ideal stained smear, three zones can be indentified visually. The starting area or the "head" of the smear (where blood drop was originally placed), following which is the "body" and the thin end of the smear known as "tail".

At the tail end, RBCs lie singly and the neutrophils and monocytes predominate. In the body, RBCs overlap each other to a certain extent and lymphocytes predominate. The ideal area is in-between these "body" and "tail" of the smear where blood

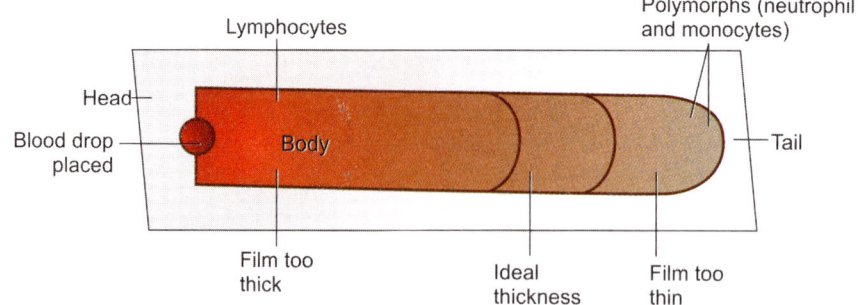

Fig. 2.8: Three zones in stained smears. The head, body and tail

cells are uniformly distributed. Here, the RBCs do not overlap and touch each other slightly.

For differential count of WBCs, two methods can be adopted:
1. The original drop of blood spreaded out between spreader and slide (C-C1). The film is made in such a way that representative strips of film like A-A1 and B-B1 are formed from point of application A and B respectively. In order to make an accurate differential count, all leukocytes in one or more strips (like A-A1, B-B1, etc.) should be inspected and classified.

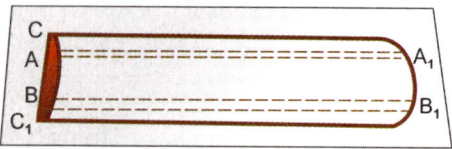

Differential count

Fig. 2.9: Linear or straight line method of differential count of WBC

2. Choose the ideal thickness of the stained smear. Then inspect and classify all the leukocytes in a serpentine counting pattern (shown diagrammatically).

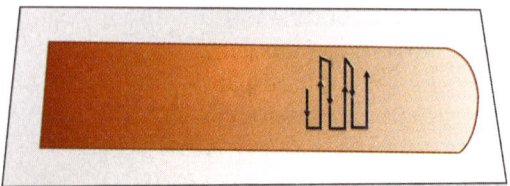

Fig. 2.10: Serpentine counting pattern (area is in between body and tail end of smear)

EXAMINATION OF STAINED BLOOD FILMS

Erythrocytes

The erythrocytes when not crowded together, appear as circular, homogenous discs of nearly uniform size, ranging from 6–8.5 mm in diameter. As for haemoglobinization, normally a small area of central pallor is seen (central 1/3rd) in RBCs.

Colour

1. **Normochromia:** Normal RBC appears pinkish brown due to presence of haemoglobin. Peripheral part looks deep brown while the central part (1/3rd) is pale because of biconcave shape of RBC.
2. **Hypochromia:** When RBC contains less haemoglobin, the central pale area becomes larger and paler. The MCHCs are also decreased. Example: **Iron deficiency anaemia.**
3. **Hyperchromia:** The RBCs become thicker and larger and they stain deeply and less central pallor because of increased haemoglobin content (MCH), but the haemoglobin concentration (MCHC) is normal. Example: **Megaloblastic anaemia.**
4. **Polychromasia:** Theoretically means many colours but practically RBCs appear bluish grey. This is due to presence of residual RNA in RBC (normally absent in mature RBC). So, young red cell shows polychromasia and larger than mature red cell and may lack central pallor. These

young red cells are called reticulocytes. It is most marked in **haemolysis and blood loss**.
4. **Anisochromia:** It means unequal haemoglobin content due to different populations of RBCs. Hence, different staining patterns of individual RBC. Example: **Iron deficiency anaemia treated with blood transfusion**.

Size

1. Normocytes: **Normal RBC** (6–8 µm in diameter, average 7–7.5 µm)
2. Microcytes: Decrease in size of RBC which may result from fragmentation of normally sized red cells (normocytes) or larger red cells (macrocytes). It occurs in many types of abnormal erythropoiesis, **e.g. iron deficiency anaemia and thalassaemia**.
3. Macrocytes: They are lage RBCs having a diameter more than 8 micro mm, a MCV (mean corpuscular volume) more than 95 fl and higher than normal Hb concentration (MCHC). Example: **Megaloblastic anaemia, chronic liver diseases.**
4. Anisocytosis: This is a general term which describes any variation in size of RBC. Example: **Anaemias, thalassaemias**.

Shape

i. **Poikilocytosis:** This is a general term which describe any variation in the shape of RBC.
ii. **Spherocytes:** They are nearly spherical RBC in contrast to normal biconcave disc. Their diameter is smaller than normal and thickness greater than normal. Tiny bits of membrane (in excess of Hb) are removed from adult RBC resulting the cell with a decreased surface/volume ratio. Example: Hereditary spherocytosis and in some cases of autoimmune haemolytic anaemia.
iii. **Target cells (leptocytes):** These refers to leptocytes (unusually thin red cells), and when stained show a peripheral ring of Hb with a dark, central, Hb containing area. Example: Haemoglobinopathies like thalassaemia, chronic liver disease, following splenectomy, HbC disease.
iv. **Schistocytes (cell fragment):** It indicates the presence of haemolysis as seen in severe burn, megaloblastic anaemia or in microangiopathic haemolytic anaemia.
v. **Acanthocytes**: These are irregularly spiculated RBCs in which ends of spicules are bulbous and rounded. Examples: Abetalipoproteinaemia, certain liver diseases.
vi. **Burr cells**: These are small cells or cell fragments bearing one or few spines or spicules (unlike acanthocytes where spicules are seen all over RBC surface). Examples: Microangiopathic haemolytic anaemia, severe burns.

Structure or Content

i. **Basophilic stippling (punctate basophilia):** It is characterized by presence within erythrocytes of irregular basophilic granules which vary from fine to coarse. Fine stippling is seen when there is increased red cell production and therefore increased polychromatophilia. Coarse basophilic stippling may be seen in lead poisoning, megaloblastic anaemia or pyrimidine-5-nucleotidase deficiency. This is attributed to an abnormal instability of the RNA in the young red cell.
ii. **Pappenheimer bodies:** These are abnormal granules of iron found inside RBCs and stained by Wright stain and/or Giemsa stain. These bodies are a type of inclusion body formed by phagosomes that have engulfed excessive amounts of iron. They appear as dense, blue-purple granules within RBCs and are usually only one or two, located in the cell periphery. Examples: Sideroblastic anaemia, haemolytic anaemia, and sickle cell disease.

iii. **Cabot rings:** These are ring shaped, figure of eight or loop-shaped structures. These rings are probably microtubules remaining from a mitotic spindle (due to defective erythropoiesis). Examples: Pernicious anaemia, lead poisoning
iv. **Howell-Jolly bodies:** These are smooth, round remnants of nuclear chromatin. Single Howell-Jolly bodies may be seen in haemolytic anaemia, megaloblastic anaemia and after splenectomy. Multiple Howell-Jolly bodies in a single RBC usually indicate megaloblastic anaemia or defective erythropoiesis.
v. **Rouleax formation:** Rouleax formation is the alignment of RBCs on one another so that they resemble stack of coins. Examples: Multiple myeloma, other para-proteinaemia (monoclonal gammopathy) and macroglobulinaemia.

White Blood Cells (WBCs)

Differential leukocyte count (DLC): The DLC is done on the basis of size, cytoplasm with or without granules and type of neucleus of WBCs. The WBC may be divided into:
- **Granulocytes** (WBC with cytoplasmic granules): Neutrophils, eosinophils and basophils.
- **Agranulocytes** (WBC without granules): Lymphocytes and monocytes.

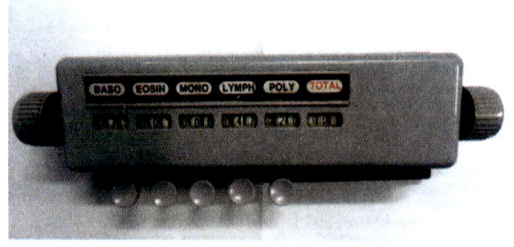

Fig. 2.11: DLC counter (manual) for differential leukocyte count (DLC)

Total leukocyte count (TLC): Normal total leukocyte count in adult person is 4000–11000/mm^3. Leukocytosis refers to TLC more than 11000/mm^3. Leukopenia less than 4000/mm^3.

Neutrophils (Polymorphs)

This leukocyte averages 12 μm in diameter, they are smaller than monocytes and eosinophils and slightly larger than basophils. **Segmented neutrophil** has at least two of its lobes separated by a filament. **Band neutrophil** has either a U-shaped nucleus of uniform thickness or a strand of nuclear material thicker than a filament connecting the lobes (appearance of "telephonic receiver").

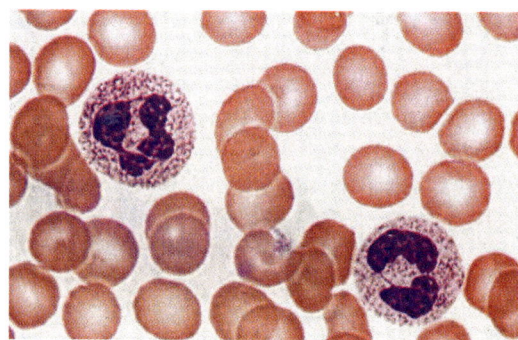

Fig. 2.12: Neutrophils

- The cytoplasm is filled up with tiny granules (0.2–0.3 μm) which stain tan to pink or orange with Romanowsky stains.
- Normal segmented neutrophils: 56% of leukocytes (DLC)
- Normal band neutrophils: 03% of leukocytes (up to 8% may be seen)
- Two lobes neutrophils: 10–30% of neutrophils
- Three lobes neutrophils: 40–50% of neutrophils
- Four lobes neutrophils: 10–20% of neutrophils
- Five lobes neutrophils: ≤5% of neutrophils
- In women, 2–3% of circulating neutrophils show an appendage at a terminal nuclear segment. This 'drumstick' is connected to the nucleus by a short stalk

and is about 1.5 µm in diameter. It indicates the inactive X chromosome and corresponds to **Barr body**.

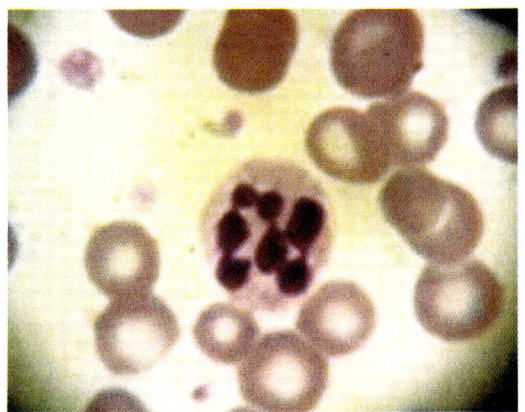

Fig. 2.13: Hypersegmented neutrophils (7 lobes) in megaloblastic anaemia

Hypersegmented neutrophils: If the peripheral smear shows ≥5% of neutrophils having 5 lobes or ≥1% of neutrophils having 6 lobes, then the neutrophils are called hypersegmented.

Causes
1. Megaloblastic anaemia
2. Uraemia
3. Hydroxyurea treatment
4. Cytotoxic treatment especially with methotrexate treatment

Stages of neutrophilic maturation

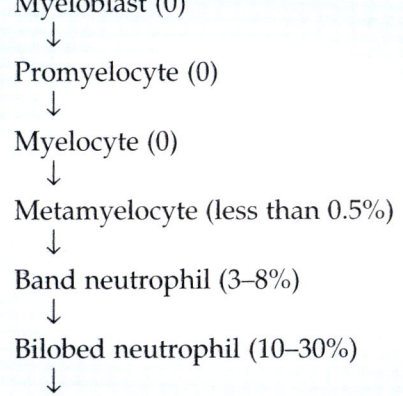

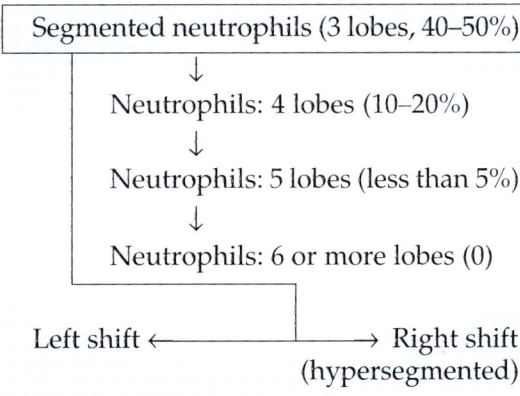

Segmentation of the nucleus of the neutrophil is a normal separation process. With the three-lobed neutrophil as a marker, shift to the left (less nature) or to the right (hypermature) can be understood. A left shift with band neutrophils, metamyelocytes and occasional myelocytes is common in sepsis and usually neutrophils contain toxic granules in cytoplasm. If myeloblast and promyelocytes are seen in peripheral blood, the causes may be leukaemia or leukoerythroblastic anaemia. Sometimes in pregnancy, a significant number of band forms is seen.

Arneth count: Neutrophils are divided in five groups according to number of lobe(s), it possesses:
1. Group I : One lobe
2. Group II: Two Lobes
3. Group III: Three lobes
4. Group IV: Four lobes
5. Group V: Five lobes.

One hundred neutrophils are counted in peripheral smear and number of each group of neutrophil is expressed as a percentage.

If there is increase in the group I and II neutrophils (as seen in sepsis) then there is a shift to left. Whereas, if there is more hypersegmented neutrophils (as seen in megaloblastic anaemia), then there is shift to right.

Arneth index: Percentage of neutrophils in groups I, II and ½ of group III is about 60 (normal range 51–65).

Schilling count: In this count, all the granular leukocytes are divided into four groups and the number of each group is expressed as a percentage of the WBCs. The four groups are:
1. Myelocytes
2. Metamyelocytes
3. Band neutrophils
4. Segmented neutrophils

A dividing line is drawn (usually segmented neutrophils' number). A shift to left happens when the number in percent increases, to the left of the dividing line.

Morphologic alterations in neutrophils

Toxic granules: These are dark blue to purple cytoplasmic granules seen in neutrophils (also in metamyelocytes and band forms). Toxic granules are seen in severe bacterial infections and in other causes of inflammation or toxic conditions. These are myeloperoxidase positive and may be numerous or few in number. Toxic granules are azurophil granules that have retained their basophilic staining reaction by lack of maturation or have developed increased basophilia in mature neutrophils. Toxic granules like azurophilic granules seen in neutrophils with prolonged staining time or decreased pH of staining reaction.

Döhle bodies: Döhle inclusion bodies are small, round or oval pale blue-gray structure, usually found at the peripheral cytoplasm of neutrophil. They consist of decomposed ribosomes and endoplasmic reticulum. Originally they were described in scarlet fever, but they are seen in any other infections, in aplastic anaemia, following administration of toxic agents and in burns.

Cytoplasmic vacuoles: It usually indicates severe sepsis, when toxic granules are also present. Cytoplasmic vacuoles will develop as an artifacts with prolonged standing of the blood before smears are made.

May-Hegglin anomaly: Autosomal dominant disease in which pale blue inclusions resembling Döhle bodies are seen. But the inclusions are larger and more prominent than Döhle bodies, Also, they are found in all leukocytes except lymphocytes.

Pelger-Huet anomaly: It is a benign inherited condition in which neutrophil nuclei fail to segment properly. Most of the neutrophils nuclei have two discrete equal-sized lobes connecting by a thin chromatin bridge. The chromatin is coarsely granular and cytoplasmic granular content is normal.

A similar type acquired morphological anomaly, known as pseudo-Pelger cells may be seen in acute myeloid leukaemia (AML). Here, the neutrophils are hypogranular and have irregular nuclear pattern.

Neutrophilia

Definition: When absolute neutrophil count 7500/mm^3 or 72% of DLC.

Relative neutrophilia: It can be divided into primary (clonal) and secondary.

Primary neutrophilia: Myeloproliferative neoplasms (chronic myeloid leukaemia, acute myeloid leukaemia), neutrophilic leukaemia, hereditary neutrophilia.

Secondary neutrophilia: Localized acute infections (pneumonia, tonsillitis, meningitis, acute otitis media), systemic infection (e.g. septicemia), acute rheumatic fever, vasculitis, acute myocardial infarction, burns, leukoerythroblastic reaction.

Leukoerythroblastic reaction: The presence of normoblasts, tear drop cells and immature cells of neutrophilic series, (promyelocytes, myelocytes, metamyelocytes, band forms) along with neutrophilia in the blood is known as leukoerythroblastic reaction. It often indicates space-occupying disturbances of the bone marrow such as myelofibrosis with myeloid metaplasia, metastatic carcinoma, leukaemias, multiple myelomas, Gaucher's disease, TB and other granulomatous diseases.

Neutropenia

Definition: When neutrophil count is < 43% of leukocytes or an absolute neutrophil and band from <1500/mm^3.

Causes of neutropenia

1. Decreased bone marrow production of neutrophils: Myelodysplastic syndromes, chemotherapy, acute leukaemia, aplastic anaemia.
2. Increased bone marrow production but decreased survival of neutrophils: Hypersplenism, SLE, rheumatoid arthritis, autoimmune and isoimmune neutropenia.
3. Viral infections: Measles, influenza, infectious mononucleosis, HIV infection, hepatitis.
4. Bacterial infection: Miliary TB, overwhelming sepsis, typhoid and paratyphoid, brucellosis, tularemia.
5. Drugs: Antibiotics (chloramphenicol, cephalosporin, vancomycin), sulfa drugs, antimalarials (chloroquine, quinine), antifungal agents (amphotericin B, flucytosine).

Agranulocytosis

Definition: It theoretically means total absence of granulocytes in the peripheral blood.

But severe granulocytopenia (neutrophils and bands <500/mm^3) also referred as agranulocytosis casually.

Causes: Peripheral destruction of polymorphs or neutrophils (often drugs related).
i. Severe bone marrow failure.

A neutrophil and band count <500/mm^3 is high risk factor for sepsis, whereas a count <200/mm^3 leads to overwhelming bacterial infections.

Lymphocytes

At birth, in normal individuals, the absolute numbers of lymphocytes and T cells are highest and may represent 90% of all leukocytes. Thereafter, B cells begin to rise and T cell decreases. In adolescence and adulthood B cells (15%) and T cells (85%) stabilized and lymphocytes constitute 20–40% of all leukocytes. Normally, majority of circulating lymphocytes are small and ≤10% are large.

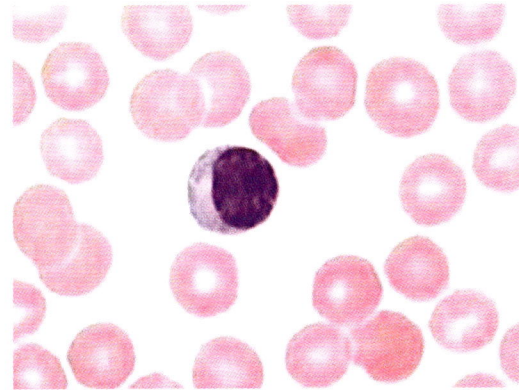

Fig. 2.14: Lymphocyte

The small lymphocytes have a thin rim cytoplasm occasionally containing scanty azurophilic granules. Nuclei are uniform in size (9 μm in diameter) which provides a useful guide for estimating red cell size (average 7–8 μm in diameter). The large lymphocytes (9–15 μm in diameter) have abundant pale blue cytoplasm containing azurophil granules. Because of this, these are known as large granular lymphocytes (LGL) and basically they are activated B lymphocytes or NK (natural killer) cells. The nuclei of lymphocytes have homogeneous chromatin with some clumping at the periphery.

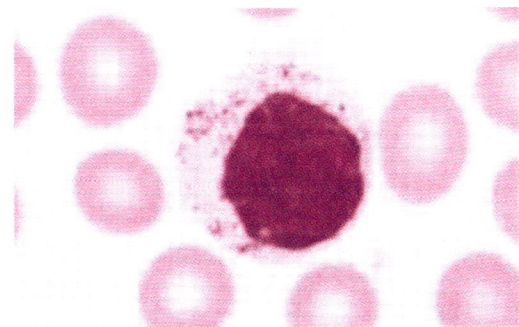

Fig. 2.15: Large granular lymphocyte

Türk cells: In bacterial and viral infections, transforming lymphocytes are present. These Türk cells are immunoblastosis (10 μm in diameter) with a round nucleus and abundant deeply basophilic cytoplasm. Ultimately these cells will transform into plasmacytoid lymphocytes or plasma cells. Occasionally they may be seen in PBS.

Activated lymphocytes: These cells are seen in PBS in virals infections. These cells have slightly larger nuclei and more open chromatin (less dense) and abundant cytoplasm which may be irregular. Example: Infectious mononucleosis or glandular fever.

Lymphocytosis

Definition: It is defined as on absolute lymphocyte count >4000/mm^3 (or >43%) in adults, >7200/mm^3 in adolescents and >9000/mm^3 in young children and infants.

Spurious lymphocytosis: When there is neutropenia with relative lymphocytosis, but normal absolute lymphocyte count (e.g. typhoid fever, thyrotoxicosis, agranulocytosis).

Causes of lymphocytosis

i. *Viral causes:* Influenza, infectious hepatic viral infection, in various exanthemata like measles, mumps, chickenpox, rubella and infectious mononucleosis.
ii. *Bacterial causes:* Enteric or typhoid fever, tuberculosis, pertusis (whooping cough), secondary syphilis, brucellosis.
iii. *Protozoal causes:* Toxoplasmosis.
iv. *Malignancy:* Chronic lymphocytic leukaemia (CLL), acute lymphoblastic leukaemia (ALL), prolymphocytic leukaemia, hairy cell leukaemia, large granular lymphocytic leukaemia, leukemic phase of follicular, mantle cell and splenic marginal zone lymphoma.
v. *Miscellaneous:* Thyrotoxicosis, myasthenia gravis, hypopituitarism, hypersensitivity reaction, stress and drugs (efalizumab).

Lymphocytopenia

Definition: When lymphocyte count is <1500/mm^3 (<18%) in adults, and <3000/mm^3 in children.

Causes: Corticosteroid therapy, Cushing syndrome, sarcoidosis, chemotherapy and radiotherapy, neoplastic conditions especially Hodgkin lymphoma, epinephrine injection, few infections (e.g. acute and chronic retroviral infections of HIV, TB).

Monocytes

Monocytes are the largest of the circulating leukocytes; 15–18 µm in diameter and constitute 2–10% of leukocytes in PBS.

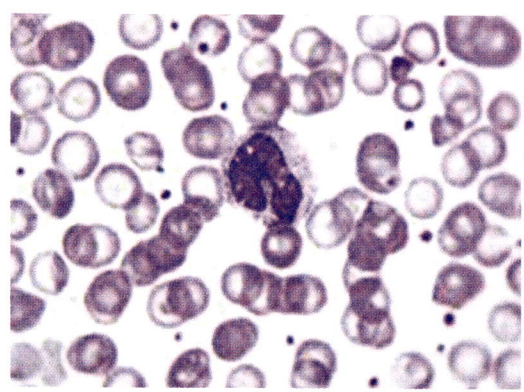

Fig. 2.16: Monocyte

Monocytes are characterized by a large, eccentrically placed nucleus which is stained less intensely than that of other leukocytes. Nuclear shape is variable but there is often a deep indentation giving a horseshoe or even bilobed appearance. The chromatin is finer and more evenly distributed compared to neutrophils. The abundant cytoplasm stains pale grayish-blue with Romanowsky stains. The cytoplasm contains numerous small pink-purple stained lysosomal granules and cytoplasmic vacuoles which may confer "frosted-glass" appearance. Monocytes are highly motile and phagocytic cells are the precursors of macrophages or histiocytes (found in different tissues). Examples: Kupffer cells in liver, Langerhans cells of skin, osteoclast in bone and microglia in CNS.

Monocytosis

Definition: Absolute monocyte count is >500/mm^3 or >12% of DLC.

Causes

i. Bacterial infections: TB, syphilis, brucellosis, bacterial endocarditis.
ii. Protozoan infections: Malaria, kala-azar, trypanosomiasis
iii. Rickettsial infections: Typhus, Rocky Mountain spotted fever.
iv. Malignancy: Acute monocytic or myelomonocytic leukaemia, chronic myelomonocytic leukaemia, myeloproliferative neoplasms, Hodgkin and non-Hodgkin lymphoma, multiple myeloma.
v. Carcinomas: Ovary, breast, stomach
vi. Miscellaneous: Ulcerative colitis, Crohn's disease, sprue, sarcoidosis.

Eosinophils

Eosinophils are a little larger than neutrophils; 12–17 µm in diameter (average 13 µm). They usually have two lobes in the nuclei bit may have three or four lobes also. The cytoplasm is packed with distinctive spherical gold/orange (eosinophilic) granules. They average 3% of the leukocytes in adults.

The most characteristic ultrastructural features of eosinophils are presence of large, ovoid, specific granules each containing an elongated crystalloid in the cytoplasm. These specific granules are membrane bound and of uniform size and the matrix contains a variety of hydrolytic enzymes including histaminase. These crystalloids have a cubic lattice structure and consist of an extremely alkaline or basic protein, known as **major basic protein.**

In comparison to neutrophils, eosinophils are easily differentiated by the colour and size of the cytoplasmic granules. Eosinophilic granules are bright red with eosin and a more brick-red with Romanowsky stains. The cytoplasm is colourless. The nucleus stains less deeply compared to neutrophils and most eosinophils have two lobes or segments, rarely more than three.

Eosinophils are phagocytic cells but compared to neutrophils, they have greater oxidative capacity via the hexose monophosphate shunt. Eosinophils have particular phagocytic activity for antigen–antibody complexes.

Eosinophilia

Definition: Absolute eosinophil count >600/mm^3 or >8% of DLC.

Causes

i. Allergic diseases: Bronchial asthma, seasonal rhinitis (hay fever).
ii. Skin disorders: Atopic dermatitis, eczema, pemphigus eosinophilia.
iii. Parasitic infestations: Trichinosis, tapeworm, cysticercosis, visceral larva migrans (due to roundworm) creeping eruption (due to hookworm), Löeffler's syndrome, pulmonary eosinophilia (due to roundworm), tropical pulmonary eosinophilia (due to hyperimmune reaction caused by microfilariae).
iv. Infections: Scarlet fever, Echinococcus infection, early phase of *Pneumococcus pneumoniae*, fungal infections.
v. Neoplastic disorders: Chronic eosinophilic leukaemia, myelomonocytic leukaemia with inversion, mastocytosis, T cell lymphoma, Hodgkin lymphoma.

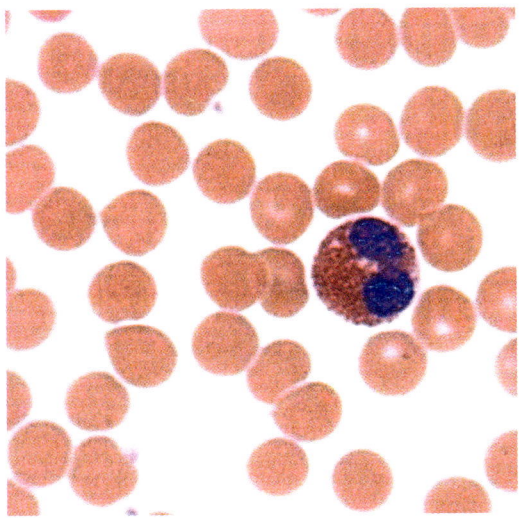

Fig. 2.17: Eosinophil

vi. Drugs: Pilocarpine, digitalis, physostigmine, sulfonamide, etc.

Basophils

Basophils are the rarest (<1%) of the circulating leukocytes. The basophils are intermediate in a size between neutrophils and eosinophils. Like the eosinophils, basophil has a bilobed nucleus but this is usually obscured by numerous large, densely basophilic (deep blue) specific granules which are larger, but fewer in number than those of eosinophils. In few basophils, most of these granules may be missed as these granules are highly soluble in water and tend to be dissolved away during common blood smear preparation. When basophils are stained with the basic dye, like to toluidine blue, the granules bind the basic dye and the dye changes colour to red. This phenomenon is called **metachromasia** and the granules are called metachromatic granules. The cytoplasmic granules of basophils and mast cells contain proteoglycans consisting of sulphated glycosaminoglycans linked to protein core, this accounts for their metachromatic staining characteristic.

Major function of basophils and mast cells is probably immunological response to certain parasites and allergens. Release of histamine and other vasoactive mediators are responsible for the so-called immediate hypersensitivity (anaphylactoid) reaction, which is characteristic of allergic rhinitis (hay fever), urticaria, some forms of asthma and anaphylactic shock.

Basophilia

Definition: Basophil count is >200/mm^3 or >2% of DLC.

Causes
i. Neoplastic conditions: Myeloproliferative syndromes (chronic myeloid leukaemia, myeloid metaplasia, polycythemia vera), acute basophilic leukaemia, Hodgkin lymphoma.
ii. Infections: Chickenpox, small pox
iii. Hypersensitivity states: Drugs, food, foreign protein injection
iv. Others: Hypothyroidism, nephrotic syndrome, chronic haemolytic anaemia following splenectomy, chronic sinusitis and transient basophilia following irradiation.

Leukemoid Reactions

Definition: A leukocyte count of >50,000/mm^3 in non-leukemic condition.

The PBS (peripheral blood smear) shows an increase in and shift to the left of myeloid cells (band neutrophils, metamyelocytes, myelocytes, some promyelocytes and mye-

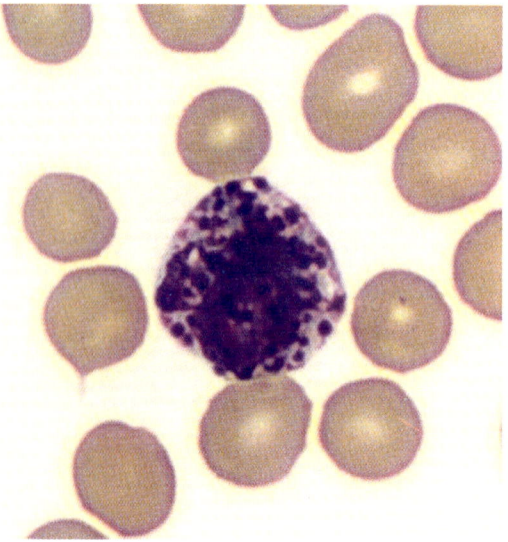

Fig. 2.18: Basophil

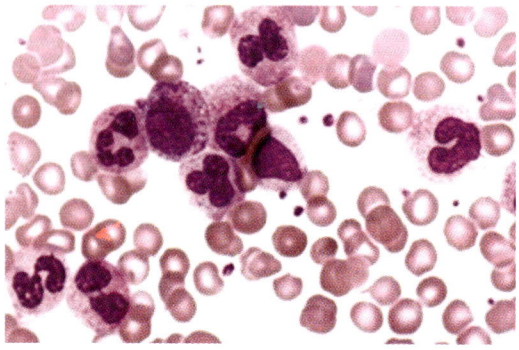

Fig. 2.19: Leukemoid reactions (neutrophilic)

loblasts); and similar quantitative and quantitative changes in lymphocytes, or eosinophils or monocytes. Depending on the predominant cell, leukemoid reactions may be neutrophilic (most common), lymphocytic, eosinophilic or monocytic.

Neutrophilic leukemoid reactions: Excessive neutrophilia along with left shift of myeloid cells. It may occur in many situations like haemolysis, hemorrhage, Hodgkin lymphoma, myelofibrosis, malignancy with bone marrow involvement, severe burns, eclampsia, certain intoxications, and infections (especially tuberculosis).

Examination of PBS is more helpful than bone marrow examination. Increased primary granules (azurophilic granules) in the myeloid cells known as toxic granules, Döhle bodies and cytoplasmic vacuolization may be seen.

Lymphocytic leukemoid reactions: Very high count of normal-appearing or mature lmphocytes may occur in measles, chickenpox, CMV, pertusis and in infectious mononucleosis. When atypical lymphocytes are many or immature lymphocytes (which may be seen in infectious mononucleosis) then the distinction from lymphocytic leukaemia may be difficult. In tuberculosis, normal-appearing or atypical lymphocytes may be found.

Examination of bone marrow is often helpful, because lymphocytes are minimally increased if at all in marrow, in contrast to PBS. If lymphocytes are increased in both PBS and marrow, then it is lymphocytic leukaemia (when fulfill other criteria).

Eosinophilic leukemoid reactions: Blood cells as immature as eosinophilic myelocytes rarely appear in PBS in reactive eosinophilia, in which the TLC may exceed $50 \times 10^3/mm^3$. Eosinophilic leukemoid reactions usually occur in children usually caused by parasitic infections. In adults, the idiopathic hypereosinophilic syndrome may be a cause.

Leukemoid reaction is differentiated from leukemia by
i. Absence of hepatosplenomegaly, lymphadenopathy and hemorrhage.
ii. Presence of blasts/immature cells <5% (in acute leukaemia, blasts ≥20%)
iii. Presence of toxic granules and Döhle bodies in neutrophils (in leukaemia Döhle bodies are absent).
iv. Presence of increased LAP (leukocyte alkaline phosphatase) score but in leukaemia LAP score is decreased.

Platelets (Thrombocytes)

Platelets (thrombocytes) are small, non-nucleated cells formed in the bone marrow from the cytoplasm of very large cells called megakaryocytes. In blood films from EDTA to blood and stained with Romanowsky stains, platelets are round to oval 2–4 μm in diameter. They are irregular in outline with fine red granules which may be scattered or centralized in the cell. A small number of larger platelets, up to 5 μm in diameter may be seen in normal persons.

Their number in circulating blood range from 150,000 to 400,000/mm³. If the platelet count is normal, then on the average, one platelet is found per 10–30 RBCs. At 1000X or in oil immersion, this is equivalent to 7–20 platelets per oil immersion field.

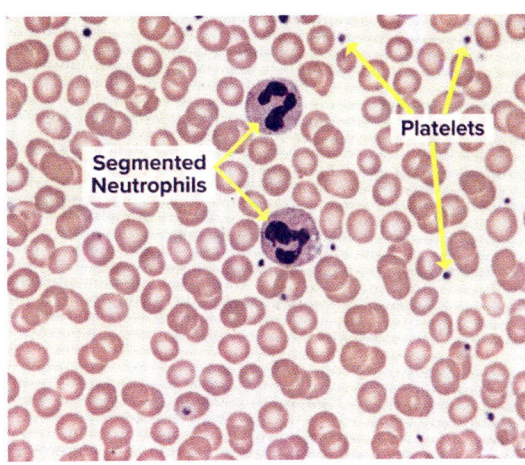

Fig. 2.20: Platelets

Platelet Functions

i. They from plugs to occlude sites of vascular damage by adhering to collagenous tissue at the margin of the wound. Later the platelet plug is replaced by fibrin.
ii. They promote clot formation by providing a surface for the assembly of coagulation protein complexes which are responsible for thrombin formation.
iii. They secrete factors which are involved in vascular repair.

Thrombocytopenia

Thrombocytopenia refers to decrease in the number of platelets in peripheral blood below normal (1.5 lacs/mm^3). But practically a count below 1 lac/mm^3 is considered thrombocytopenia.

Causes

1. *Increased destruction of platelets*
   a. Immune causes: Idiopathic thrombocytopenic purpura (ITP), infections (HIV, dengue, malaria), systemic lupus erythematosus, neonatal alloimmune purpura, post-transfusion purpura.
   b. Nonimmune causes: Thrombotic thrombocytopenic purpura (TTP), disseminated intravascular coagulation (DIC).
2. *Decreased production of platelets*
   a. Hereditary: Wiskott-Aldrich syndroma, Fanconi's anaemia.
   b. Acquired: Megaloblastic anaemia, aplastic anaemia, bone marrow infiltration (leukaemias, lymphomas, metastatic carcinomas), drugs (cytotoxic drugs, ethanol), radiation.
3. **Increased sequestration**: Hypersplenism
4. **Dilutional thrombocytopenia**: Massive blood transfusion.

Thrombocytosis (Thrombophilia)

It refers to increase in the platelet count above normal (4 lacs/mm^3). Thrombocytosis may be primary or reactive (secondary). Primary thrombocytosis due to myeloproliferative disorders can be distinguished from reactive (secondary) thrombocytosis by the presence of leukocytosis, immature WBCs and nucleated RBCs in peripheral blood, defective platelet function (epinephrine-induced platelet aggregation) and splenomegaly in cases of primary thrombocytosis.

Causes of thrombocytosis

i. Primary thrombocytosis: Polycythemia vera, chronic myeloid leukaemia, essential thrombocythaemia, idiopathic myelofibrosis.
ii. Secondary thrombocytosis: Infections, chronic inflammatory diseases, trauma, haemorrhage, iron deficiency, splenectomy, malignancy.

VIVA VOCE

Q1. What are the characteristics of an ideal peripheral blood smear?

Ans:
- The smear should not be too thick or too thin.
- It should occupy about central 2/3rd of the glass slide.
- The smear should be tongue shaped and it should have straight lateral borders.

Q2. What is thick smear and when is it used?

Ans: Thick smear is prepared by spreading a large drop of blood on the slide approximately 2 cm in diameter and dry it. The dried smear is dipped (2–4 times) in tap water to dehemoglobinize the RBCs and red-coloured solution comes out. The smear is fixed with methanol and stained with Romanowsky stain.

Thick smear is used for quick detection of malarial parasites and for screening of malaria.

Q3. What is fixation of smear and how is it done?

Ans: Fixation means fixation of blood cells and other things of smear to be fixed onto the slide.

So that, during subsequent staining and washing the smear do not wash off.

Usually acetone-free methyl alcohol is used for fixation. Acetone if present, it will wash away the nuclear stain and nuclear stain will be of poor quality. So, acetone-free methyl alcohol is used.

Q4. Why buffered water is used during blood smear staining? What is the ideal pH of buffered water?

Ans: Buffered water is used to maintain optimal pH during staining. If the pH of stain is acidic, it will cause poor nuclear stain and very reddish cytoplasm. On the other hand, if the pH of stain is alkaline, the stained smear will be blue due to improper staining of cytoplasm.

The ideal pH for routing blood smear is 6.8 and for malarial detection is 7 to 7.2. At pH 6.8 (with the use of diluted phosphate buffer), the stained smear imparts a reddish hue to red cells and differential staining pattern of the granules present in granulocytes. To look, malarial parasites, a pH of 7.2 is recommended in order to detect Schuffner's dots of *Plasmodium vivax, ovale* and *malariae*. (Remember Maurer's dots in *P. falciparum* and Ziemann's dots in *P. malariae*).

Q5. How platelet adequacy and platelet count are made on peripheral blood smear?

Ans: In normal healthy person, platelets are present in clumps as well as discretely. If there are platelet clumps (each clump containing ≥6 platelets), then platelet count is adequate. Usually 3–5 platelets are present per 100 RBCs. If there is <3 platelet/100 RBCs, then platelet count is low and patient is probably suffering from thrombocytopenia.

As per **Henry's clinical diagnosis and management by laboratory's methods**, in stained film from EDTA to blood, there are 7–20 platelets/oil immersion field (1000X) or one platelet per 10–30 RBCs.

For rough estimation of platelet count, take average platelet count in 10 oil immersion field on a blood film, then multiply it by 15,000 which will give reasonably good platelet count (reference WHO laboratory book).

Some advocated that under oil immersion, normal person will have 10–25 platelets per oil field (average 20). Take average platelet count under oil immersion, then multiply by 20,000 if the average is <10, multiply by 15,000 if the average is ≥10.

As per Gradwohl's clinical laboratory methods, the diagnosis is:

No. of platelets/oil immersion field	Estimated total platelet count
• Less than 1 platelet	• Decreased in number
• Several platelets with occasional clumps	• Adequate in number
• Over 25 platelets	• Increased in number

The number of platelets in 10 oil immersion fields multiplied by 2000 closely approximates the platelet count.

There are differences in opinion, but for practical reasons, take average platelet count in 10 oil immersion field on a blood film, then multiply it by 15,000 which will give reasonably good platelet count (reference WHO laboratory book).

Q6. What is platelet satellitism?

Ans: Platelet satellitism is phenomena in which platelets encircle neutrophils. It is usually seen when blood is collected in excess EDTA (though may be seen with other anticoagulants). It is caused by IgG or IgM antibodies that bind the CD16 antigen. CD16 is a low affinity F_c receptor, found on the surface of neutrophils, also present on NK cells, monocytes and macrophages. Satellitism around other leukocytes may be seen and some platelets may even be phagocytosed by neutrophils/WBCs.

Q7. What is "platelet dust"?

Ans: This was first described by Peter Wolf in 1967 which are basically microparticles and are not simply inert products of cellular debris. These microparticles are submicron vesicles shed from a variety of cells. These microparticles have roles in coagulation, cellular signaling, vascular injury and homeostasis. To date, the cell types reported to release microparticles either constitutively or when stimulated that include platelets, blood cells, endothelium, epithelium and many cancer cells.

Q8. What parasites can be identified in peripheral blood smear (PBS)?

Ans:
  i. Malaria: Most common parasite found in PBS.
  ii. Microfilaria of *Wuchereria bancrofti*
  iii. *Leishmania donovani* or LD bodies of kala-azar: Found free or inside monocytes.
  iv. *Trypanosoma cruzi*
  v. Others: Babesia, Brugia, Mansonella, etc. rarely.

Q9. What is the advantage of Leishman staining compared to Giemsa staining?

Ans: No separate fixation is needed as it contains methanol solvent within Leishman stain itself which will fix the smear. So, Leishman stain fixes and stains the smear simultaneously. Also, shorter time is required compared to Giemsa staining.

Leishman stain is a good alternative to Giemsa for malarial parasite detection. Leishman stain is superior for visualization of RBC and WBC morphology, which can be an advantage for the diagnosis of diseases involving RBCs and WBCs.

Q10. What is advantage of Giemsa stain?

Ans: Giemsa stain is most complex Romanowsky stain and it contains maximum number of azo compounds. So, Giemsa stain provides maximum intermediate shades and better toning effect. Hence, it is good for microphotography. Also, Giemsa stain is best for malarial parasite detection.

Q11. What is the use of Field's stain and modified Field's stain?

Ans: Field stain was originally used to detect malarial parasite on thick smear. But it can also detect *H. pylori* on thin sections of stomach (paraffin section, 2–4 µm thickness). Also, it can be used as a quick Romanowsky stain for thin blood film and marrow smears. Modified Field's stain is recommended for rapid staining of protozoans, such as Acanthamoeba and Trichomonas species.

Q12. How would you identify a well stained and good smear microscopically?

Ans: Ideally, the smear should be tongue shaped and after staining, a well stained blood smear will have pinkish tint at the stained portion and no staining on other portion of the slide.

Microscopically well stained smear should show following features:
- Red cells will have pinkish orange colour.
- Nuclei of white cells will be purplish blue.
- Neutrophilic granules should be violet pinkish or pale pink (neutral stain).
- Eosinophilic granules should be orange red (eosinophilic).
- Basophilic granules should be deep purple or buish black (basophilic) and granules should overlap the nuclei.
- The nuclei of the lymphocytes are dark with condensed chromatin.
- The platelets are small, round, membrane bound, pinkish granular structures.

3
Marrow Puncture Needle and Examination of Bone Marrow

Bone marrow examination is an indispensable adjunct to the study of haematological diseases and sometimes the only way for a correct diagnosis. Apart from haematological disease, many other disorders can be diagnosed by bone marrow examination. It is estimated that in adults, weight of the marrow is 1300–1500 gm.

Bone marrow or marrow can be obtained by needle aspiration, percutaneous trephine biopsy or surgical biopsy. Bone marrow aspiration (also called aspiration biopsy) is simple, safe and relatively painless. Aspiration can be performed on outdoor patients. On the contrary, trephine biopsy or surgical biopsy is not simple but can be performed on outdoor patients too.

The advantage of marrow aspiration is that, individual cells are perfectly preserved in the well-prepared marrow films and after staining subtle differences between cells can be recognized easily compared to trephine biopsy/surgical biopsy. But the disadvantage of aspiration is that the arrangement of the cells in the marrow and the relationship between different cells are more or less destroyed during aspiration. Also, in fibrosis (myelofibrosis) or in hypoplastic/aplastic anaemia, no marrow material except blood is aspirated (called dry tap).

The great advantage of trephine biopsy is that it can provide a perfect view of the structure of relatively large pieces of bone marrow (perfect alignment of different cells in marrow biopsy). Also, morphological features of individual cells can be identified by making an imprint or a smear from the marrow tissue obtained.

HISTORY OF BONE MARROW EXAMINATION

- In 1905, the Italian physician Pianese reported bone marrow (BM) infiltration by the parasite Leishmania.
- In 1927, Anirkin, a Russian physician obtained BM from the sternum using a lumbar puncture needle.
- In 1931, Arjeff, introduced needles with a guard.
- In 1935, Klima and Rosegger developed BM needles with guards.
- In 1945, Vandenberghe and Blistein were the first to use the iliac crest to obtain BM.
- In 1952, Bierman used the posterior iliac crest as the site for bone marrow aspiration and claimed to be very safe site.
- In 1958, McFarland and Dameshek described a trephination technique using the Vim-Silverman biopsy needle.

BONE MARROW ASPIRATION

The various sites for bone marrow aspiration are:

In children
- Tibia → superior medial surface of tibia, inferior to the medial to the tibial tuberosity. This site is favoured for new-born, infants and children <2 years of age.
- Posterior iliac crest and spine
- Calcaneum

In adults
- Iliac crest ⎱ Most favoured
- Anterior and posterior superior iliac spine ⎰ site nowadays
- Spinous processes of lumbar vertebra
- Sternum: It is no longer favoured though was popular in the past.

The sternum should never be attempted in children. The preferred site for children of all ages are posterior superior iliac spine or iliac crest. Upper end of tibia is also a favourite site <2 years of age but caution should be taken as the weak tibia in children is vulnerable to fractures and lacerated injury to major blood vessels may occur in inexperienced hands.

Sternum though very popular site of aspiration in the past, but now is becoming obsolete. Unless the needle is correctly inserted, there is a risk of perforating the inner cortical layer and damaging the underlying large blood vessels and right atrium leading to medical emergencies.

Aspiration from iliac spine or iliac crest has the advantage that a large amount of marrow material can be aspirated and risk of injuring major blood vessels or organs is minimal compared to sternum. Also, unlike sternum, the patient cannot see what is happening or the medical procedure as the patient is lying on his/her side or lying prone. Multiple attempts can be made be made if necessary without making patient worried.

For aspiration, different needles used are:
1. **Salah bone marrow aspiration needle:** It has three parts:
   a. Trocar
   b. Canula or stilette
   c. Adjustable side guard and screw

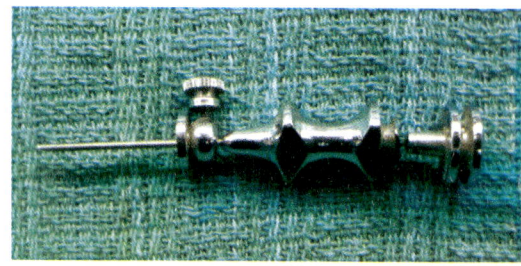

A

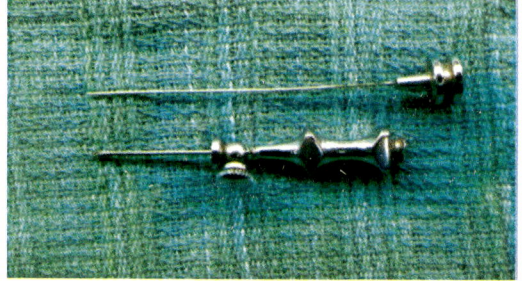

B

Fig. 3.1A and B: Salah bone marrow needle

2. **Klima bone marrow aspiration needle:** Here, there is no screw but there is a guard. But other two parts (trocar and the stilette) are there. Klima needle has the advantage as the guard has no chance of getting slipped and injuring underlying structures.

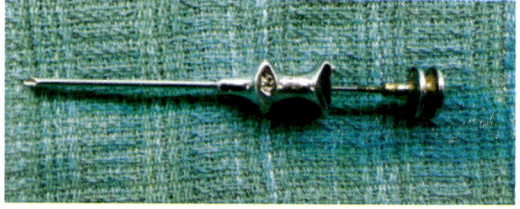

A

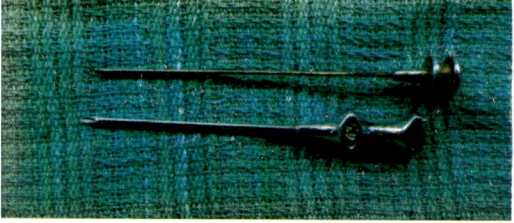

B

Fig. 3.2A and B: Klima bone marrow needle

3. **Islam's bone marrow aspiration needle**: Here dome shaped handle and T bar are intended to provide stability and control during aspiration.

Ideal bone marrow needle
- Should be stout
- 7–8 cm in length
- Adjustable guard
- Well-fitted stilette
- Edges well sharpened

Indications of Bone Marrow Aspiration

A. Diagnostic indications
1. Red cell disorders—megaloblastic anaemia, pure red cell aplasia
2. WBC disorders—leukaemia, (acute and chronic), subleukaemic leukaemia
3. Platelet disorders—idiopathic thrombocytopenic purpura (ITP)
4. Myeloproliferative disorders and myelodysplastic syndromes
5. Storage disorders—Gaucher's disease, Neimann-Pick disorders
6. Assessment of iron stares (Perls'-Prussian blue stain)
7. In evaluation of fever or pyrexia or pyrexia of unknown origin (PUO)
8. Detection of parasites—microfilaria, LD bodies of kala-azar, malaria (*Leishmania donovani*)
9. Detection of LE cell in SLE patients
10. Metastatic deposits—different carcinomas
11. Staging of lymphoma (Hodgkin and non-Hodgkin)
12. Follow-up—therapy for leukaemia and lymphoma
13. Plasma cell dyscrasia—multiple myeloma
14. Bone marrow aspirated material as a source of culture to detect infective pathogens like TB, fungus, etc.
15. Granulomas in bone marrow: TB, histoplasmosis, sarcoidosis, lymphoma
16. Cytogenetic studies, molecular genetic studies, cytochemistry and flow cytometry.

B. Therapeutic indications: Bone marrow transplant.

BONE MARROW TREPHINE BIOPSY
Three types of needles are used:
1. Jamshidi trephine needle: Most popular and most commonly used
2. Islam's trephine needle
3. Sacker-Nordin's bone marrow trephine biopsy

Indications of Bone Marrow Biopsy
- Diagnosis of leukaemia and lymphoma
- Staging of different lymphomas
- Evaluating iron stores, fibrosis, granulomas, abscesses, metastases and vascular lesions
- Detection of metastatic deposit (carcinoma)

Contraindications of Bone Marrow Examination
- Bleeding disorders or diathesis
- Haemophilia
- Infection at site of puncture

Bone Marrow Aspiration Technique

Puncture of Ilium (Superior Iliac Spine and Iliac Crest)

The usual site for bone marrow aspiration or puncture is iliac crest in adults. Only needles designed for bone marrow aspiration should be used (Salah's needle or Klima's needle). They should be stout, about 7–8 cm in length with a well-fitted stilette and preferably with a guard (Klima's needle). The point of the needle and edge of the bevel must be sharp so that it can pierce bone easily. The skin of the chosen site should be cleaned with 70% alcohol (e.g. ethanol) or 0.5% chlorhexidine. Now follow the below mentioned steps:
1. Clean the area with 70% alcohol or 0.5% chlorhexidine as stated above.
2. The skin, subcutaneous and periosteum overlying the site are infiltrated with a

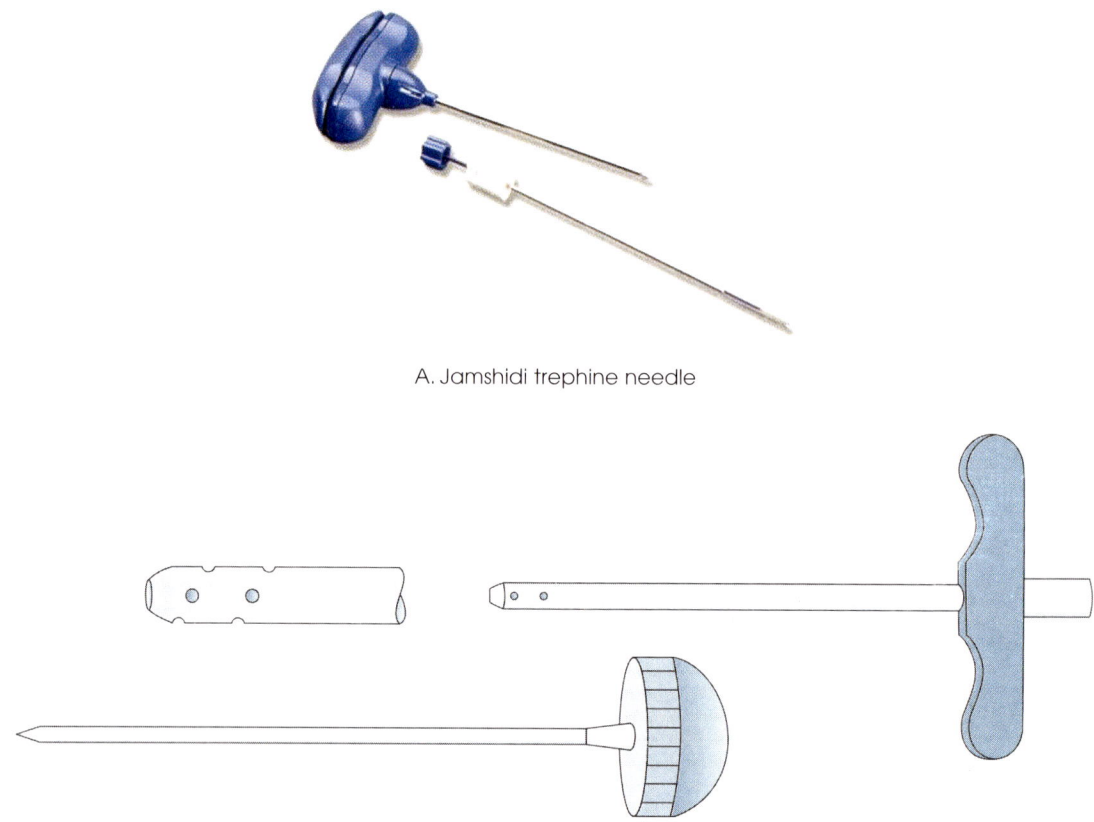

A. Jamshidi trephine needle

A modified Western of the Islam needle has multiple holes in the distal portion of the shaft in addition to the opening at the tip to overcome sampling error when the marrow is not uniformly involved in a pathological lesion.

B. Islam trephine needle

Fig. 3.3A and B: Jamshidi and Islam trephine needles

local anaesthetic (2% lignocaine) by a 2 ml syringe. Wait for 3–5 minutes.

3. With a boring movement (rotating clockwise and anticlockwise with some pressure but not full rotation). The needle is inserted to the bone. The bone is touched after passing through soft tissue (sensation of hard material as perceived by the person doing the technique). Further insertion as will give sudden release of resistance as if the needle has entered into an empty space.

4. Now the needle has entered into bone marrow space.

5. Take out the stilette.

6. With a well-fitted 2–5 ml syringe, take out 0.2–0.3 ml of marrow material.

7. Take out the needle and seal the puncture site.

8. Immediately prepare marrow films from the aspirated marrow materials.

Puncture of the Sternum

Site: Usual site in sternum is manubrium sterni or the first or second pieces of the body of sternum.

If the manubrium sterni is chosen, the puncture site should be about 1 cm above the sternomandibular angle and slightly lateral to the midline.

Marrow Puncture Needle and Examination of Bone Marrow

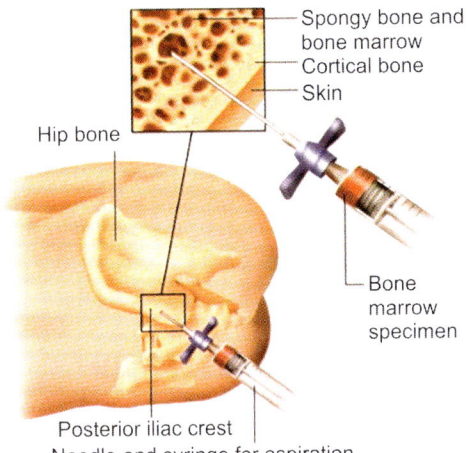

Fig. 3.4: Bone marrow aspiration

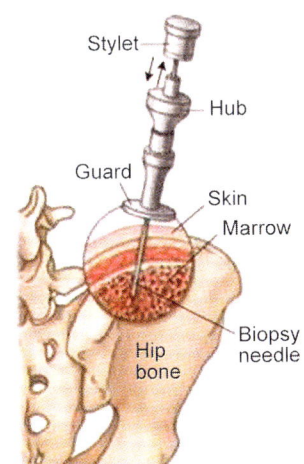

Fig. 3.5: Bone marrow aspiration by Klima's needle

If the body of sternum is chosen, the puncture site should be opposite, the second and third intercostal space slightly lateral to midline.

In case of sternal puncture, it is essential to use the guard. Clean the area as stated in puncture of ilium. Infiltrate lignocaine as stated previously. Now insert the needle with boring movement. After piercing the skin and subcutaneous tissues, when the needle touches the periosteum, adjust the guard on the needle so that the needle can be allowed to penetrate for about 5 mm further (not more than that to avoid risk of injury of blood vessels and organs). Then aspiration is done as stated in puncture of ilium.

Preparation of Marrow Films

Transfer the aspirated material without delay, as it tends to clot quickly. One drop of marrow material is delivered onto each glass slide 1 cm from one end. Get rid of extra blood by quickly sucking off with a fine Pasteur pipette leaving the greyish marrow particles behind. Some advised to tilt the slide or place the slide on a slope so that the lighter blood come down over the slide and then remove it. After removing extra blood, marrow films are prepared by pushing a spreader (glass side) or by a coverslip. The marrow particles/fragments are dragged behind the spreader and leaves a trail behind them. The marrow film should be 3–5 cm length and not more than 2 cm in width.

Bone marrow imprints: One or more visible marrow particles/fragments are picked up with a capillary pipette, or by a toothpick and immediately transferred onto a slide and made to stick to it by a gentle smearing motion. The slide is air-dried rapidly by waving it.

Crush preparations: Marrow particles in a small drop of aspirate may be placed onto a slide near one end. Another slide is carefully placed over the first slide. Now crush the bone marrow particles by giving some pressure and prepared the smear of crushed marrow particles by pulling the slides apart in a direction parallel to their surface.

Confirmation of presence of bone marrow not only blood: Presence of sand like marrow particles and irregular holes of fat in the films give assurance of marrow and not just blood has been aspirated.

Fixation of marrow films and staining: Fix the marrow films and stain them with Romanowsky stain as for peripheral blood (refer to previous chapter).

- Leishman stain is used routinely
- Prussian blue staining may be done to demonstrate iron in haemosiderin deposit or in ferritin and assessment of iron status in body. Iron in haemoglobin is not stained.
- Few slides may be stained with PAS (periodic acid–Schiff) stain or May-Grünwald stain.

Reporting of Bone Marrow Films (Myelogram)

At least 300–1000 bone marrow cells (average 500 cells) should be examined. A myelogram report should include:

i. **General cellularity of marrow**: Whether this is hypercellular or hypocellular or normocellular. As a rough guide cellularity (haemopoietic cells) occupying <25% of the particle is considered hypocellular, whereas cellularity >75–80% is hypercellular. Some follow the simple formula as regards to age → cellularity% = (100 – age)%. So, physiologically children have highest cellularity and elderly lowest cellularity.

ii. **Myeloid–erythroid ratio (M:E ratio)**: Leukocytes of all types and stages of maturation are counted together. Likewise, erythroblasts and normoblasts are counted together. A ratio is made. Normal M:E ratio is 1.2:1 to 5:1 (average 3:1). An increased M:E ratio (e.g. 6:1) may be found in erythroid hypoplasia, patients with infection or myeloproliferative disorders like CML. A decreased M:E ratio (<1.2:1) may be seen in normoblastic hyperplasia or in decreased leukopoiesis.

iii. **Type of erythropoiesis**: Whether normoblastic, megaloblastic or dyserythropoietic.

iv. **Type of leukopoiesis**: Myeloblast, promyelocyte, myelocyte, metamyelocyte, band neutrophil and mature neutrophils are present or not. Also seen up to what stage of maturation is present.

v. Number of lymphocytes, plasma cells, monocytes, etc.

vi. **Megakaryocytes**: Number of megakaryocytes is estimated better in tissue sections than in marrow films. Under low power or 100X, an average of 1–3 megakaryocytes should be found in each low power field.

vii. **Abnormal cell (if any)**: Leukaemic cells, lymphoma cells or metastatic carcinoma

viii. **Parasites**: Microfilariae, malaria, LD bodies (kala-azar)

ix. **Iron status**: done by Perls'-Prussian blue stain. It is reported as negative or 1+ to 5+, storage iron is seen in macrophages (haemosiderin or ferritin). In normal adults it is 2+, whereas 3+ is slightly increased, 4+ moderately increased and 5+ markedly increased.

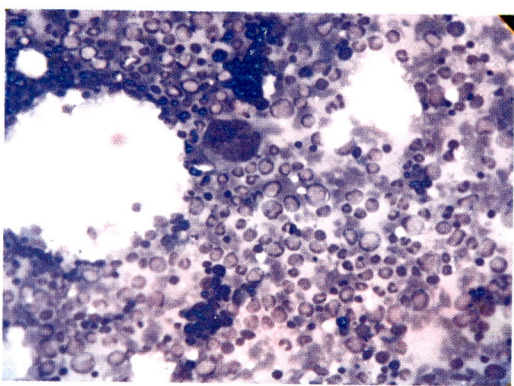

Fig. 3.6: Normal bone marrow showing trilineage haemopoietic cells (oil immersion, Leishman's stain, 1000X)

Summary of Bone Marrow Report

The report (myelogram) should include an estimate of cellularity, M:E ratio, statements about any cytological or maturation abnormalities, an estimate of the number of megakaryocytes, an estimate of the storage iron and proportion of sideroblasts and statement about any abnormal cell or other abnormal findings.

Remember, every bone marrow report (myelogram) should be interpreted along

Table 3.1: Normal ranges of differential counts in bone marrow in adults (myelogram) in aspirated material

Type of cell	Range (%)
• Reticulum	0.1–2
• Myeloblasts	0.1–3.5
• Promyelocytes	0.5–5
• Myelocytes:	
– Neutrophilic	5–20
– Eosinophilic	0.1–3
– Basophilic	0–0.5
• Metamyelocytes	10–30
• Neutrophils including bonds	7–25
• Eosinophil	0.2–3
• Basophil	0–0.5
• Monocytes	0–0.2
• Lymphocytes	5–20
• Megakaryocytes	0.1–0.5
• Plasma cells	0.1–3.5
• Proerythroblasts	0.5–5
• Early and intermediate normoblasts (basophilic and polychromatic)	2–20
• Late normoblast (pyknotic or orthochromatic)*	2–10

* The term pyknotic is preferred to orthochromatic as a description of most mature normoblasts or late normoblasts. But cells with fully haemoglobinized or mature cytoplasm (i.e. orthochromatic) is rarely seen in normal bone marrow.

with a blood smear examination of the same patient. For bone marrow at least 500 cells and for blood smear at least 200 cells should be examined as differential count.

BONE MARROW TREPHINE BIOPSY

Jamshidi Needle

This needle has the advantages than Turkel and Bethel needles or needles of Vim-Silverman type (sometimes the specimen is crushed and its architecture altered). The Jamshidi needle should be inserted by to and fro rotation through approximately 90°. It should not be continuously rotated because this tends to distort and twist the core of marrow tissue, but once the needle is inserted up to desired length, the needle is rotated clockwise (few rotations) and anticlockwise (few rotations) without any downward pressure. This is done to cut the core tissue and put the tissue within needle.

Islam's Needle

This needle has the advantage over other needles, as it can provide long uniform core of marrow-containing bone spicules and there is no distortion of bone marrow architecture. These needles are usually performed

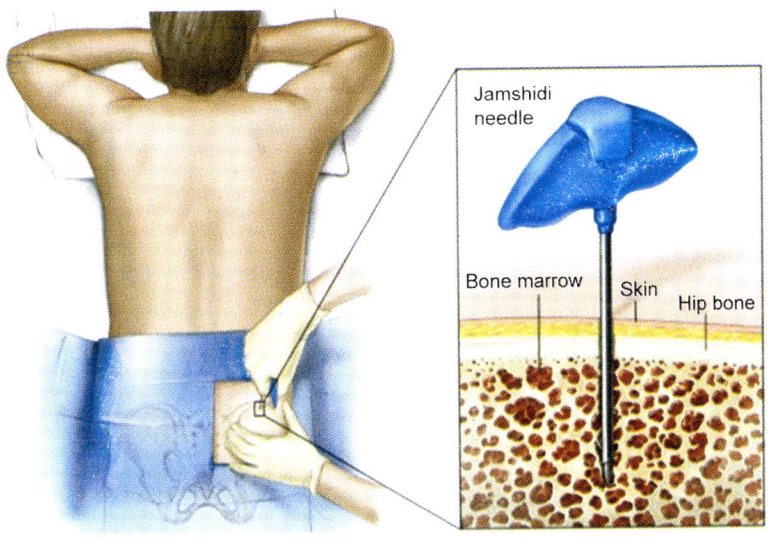

Fig. 3.7: Trephine biopsy by Jamshidi needle

at the anterior or posterior superior iliac spine. The posterior superior iliac spine provides core tissue which is longer and larger than other sites. A large trephine is sometimes of value as it provides sufficient bone marrow material for accurate diagnosis.

Other trephine biopsy needles
The other trephine biopsy needles are: Westerman Jensen, drills and disposable needles.

Bore Size of Trephine Needles
Trephines have been developed with bore size of 4–5 mm and they can be safely inserted in iliac crest (but a small skin incision and local anaesthesia is required). Bore size of 2–3 mm is also good and provides good material.

Trephine Biopsy/Histological Sections
The needle biopsy and the clotted marrow particles or fragments are fixed in Zenker's acetic solution (5% glacial acetic acid; 95% Zenker) for 6–18 hours or in B-5 fixative for 1–2 hours. Prolonged time in fixation in either fixative will make the tissue brittle. The tissue is processed routinely for embedding in paraffin, cut at 4 µm and stained routinely with haematoxylin and eosin. Giemsa and PAS stains are also frequently used. But sometimes thinner sections are needed (1–3 µm). For this, plastic or resin embeddium medium (not paraffin) is required which enables to cut sections at 1–3 µm thickness.

Examination of Stained Sections
- Haematoxylin and eosin (H and E) stain: This is excellent for demonstrating the cellularity and pattern of the marrow and for revealing pathologic changes such as fibrosis or presence of granuloma or carunoma.
- Romanowsky stain: Haemopoietic cells are better identified with this stain.
- Reticulin stain (silver impregnation stain): The bone marrow always contain a small amount of glycoprotein matrix which is actually collagen and make supporting network. This collagen or connective tissue is known as reticulin or reticulin fibers. This reticulin can be stained by reticulin stain or silver impregnation stain.
- PAS stain: To demonstrate any parasite (intracellular or extracellular), myeloblast, lymphoblast, glycogen etc.
- Myelofibrosis and myelosclerosis: Myelofibrosis refers to an increase in fine fibres, whereas myelosclerosis refers to an increase in coarse fibres. Both fibres are stained by reticulin stain. Coarse fibres predominate in myelofibrosis (chronic or idiopathic).

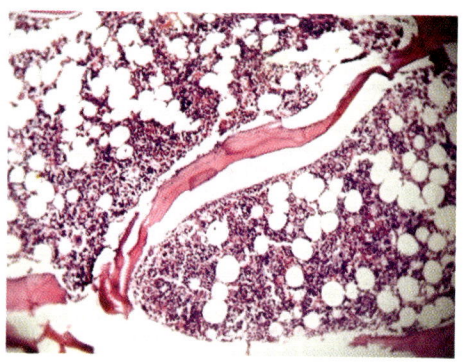

A

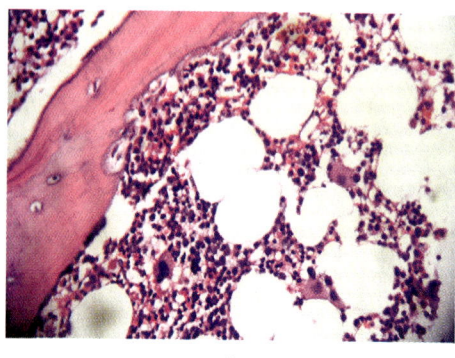

B

Fig. 3.8A and B: (A) Low power view of trephine biopsy showing marrow tissue, fat spaces and bony trabeculae; (B) High power view showing trilineage (erythroid, myeloid and megakaryocytic/thrombocytic cells) haematopoiesis including megakaryocytes

Flow chart 3.1: Pluripotent marrow stem cell and formation of haemopoietic cells

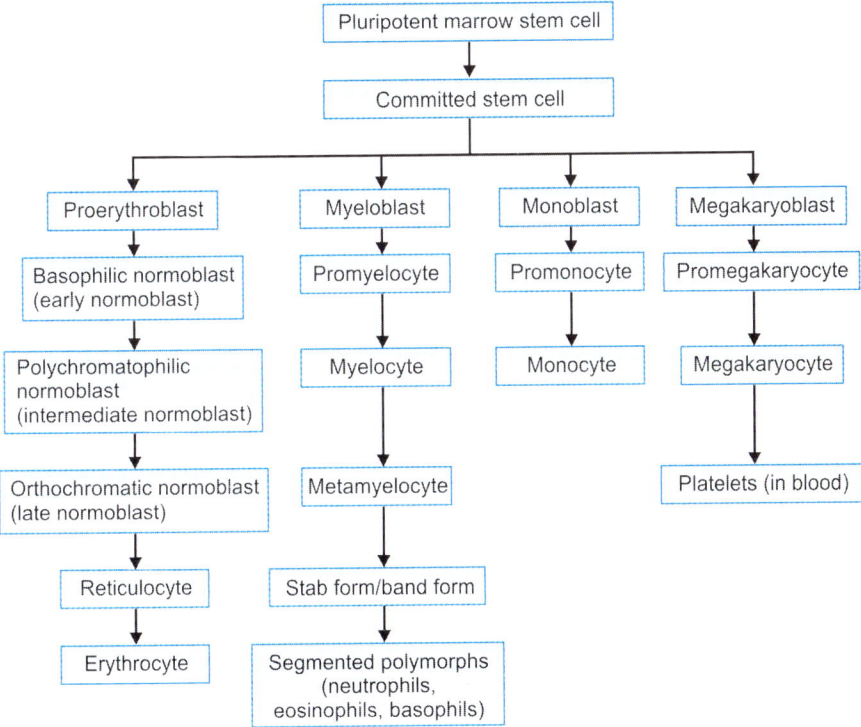

Table 3.2: Comparison of bone marrow aspiration and bone marrow biopsy

Parameter	Bone marrow aspiration	Bone marrow biopsy
1. Site	Illiac spine, sternum, tibia, spinous process of vertebra	Posterior superior iliac spine
2. Main indications	Suspected hematologic malignancies, unexplained cytopenias	Repeated dry tap, aplastic anaemia, myelofibrosis, lymphoma staging, focal lesions, hairy cell leukaemia
3. Needle used	Salah, Klima	Jamshidi
4. Information obtained	Morphology, cytochemistry, iron stain, flow cytometry (immunophenotyping), culture	Cellularity, architecture, fibrosis, focal lesions
5. Stains and special tests	Romanowsky stain, iron stain, cytochemistry, molecular genetics, flow cytometry (immunophenotyping), culture	H and E stain, reticulin stain, IHC (immunohistochemistry)
6. Reporting time	Same day	Up to 7 days

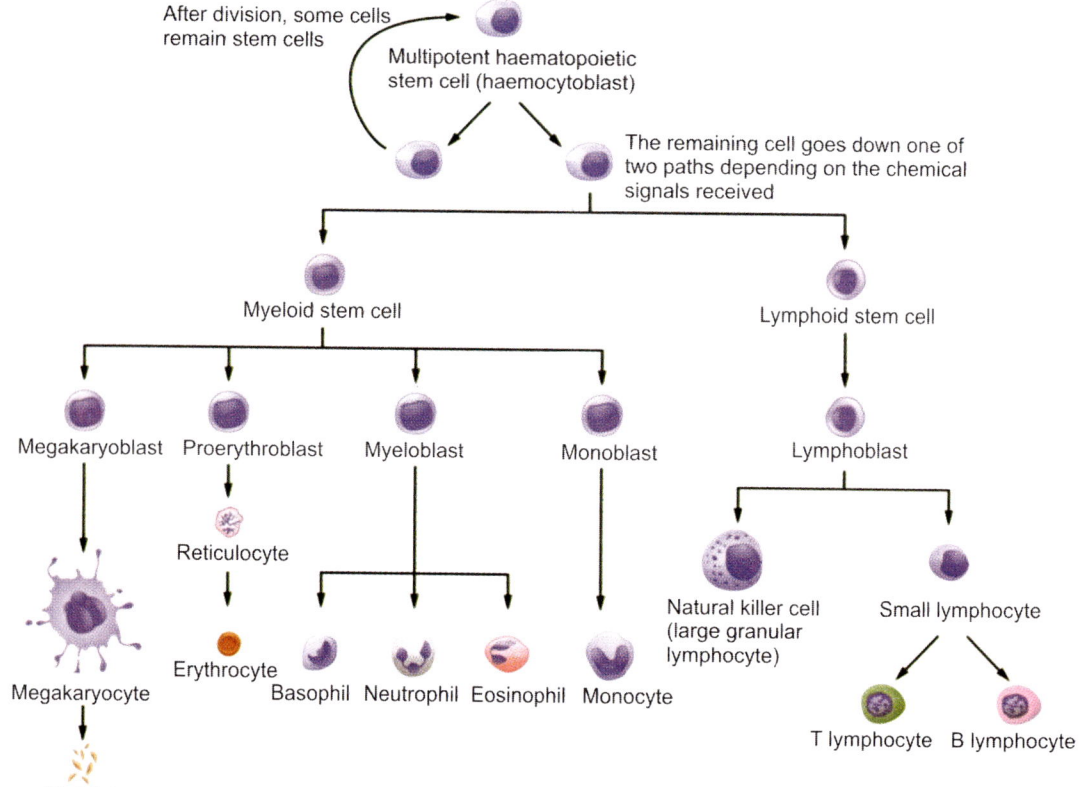

Fig. 3.9: Haematopoiesis of different blood cells in the bone marrow

- Increased reticulin fibres also occur in secondary carcinoma (metastatic deposit), osseous disorders like Paget's disease and hyperparathyroidism, in inflammatory reactions and in other myeloproliferative disorders (particulary lymphoproliferative disorders and proliferation of megakaryocytes).

VIVA VOCE

Q1. What are the parts of bone marrow needle and how to identify?
Ans: A stout wide bore needle and guard. A stillete is there within the needle which prevents blockage of the needle when it penetrates the skin, soft tissue and bone chips. The guard allows penetration of the needle up to desired length and prevents damage to the underlying tissues/organs.

Q2. What are the differences between Salah's needle and Klima's needle? Which one is better?
Ans: Salah's needle has a guard which is fixed to the needle with a side screw. Klima's needle has also a guard but unlike Salah's needle it does not has side screw and guard is fixed to the body of needle it does not has side screw and guard is fixed to the body of needle itself by a spiral thread. Klima's needle can be easily readjusted during bone marrow aspiration procedure. Klima's needle is preferable among these two as the guard is on a spiral thread and there is less chance of slipping.

Q3. Which is the best site and why?
Ans: Posterior superior iliac spine is the preferred site because:

- Patient lies prone and cannot see the procedure (patient can see sternal puncture). So, patient is less apprehensive.
- The procedure is very safe as there is no underlying important structure (like substernal aorta) and risk of damaging vital organs is minimal.

Q4. What are the absolute indications for bone marrow aspiration examination?

Ans:
- Hypoplastic/aplastic anaemia
- Sideroblastic anaemia
- Megaloblastic anaemia
- Aleukemic/subleukemic leukaemia
- Assessment of remission during chemotherapy of acute leukaemia
- Kala-azar (acute)
- ITP
- Multiple myeloma

Q5. What are the relative indications for bone marrow aspiration?

Ans:
- Chronic kala-azar
- Before starting chemotherapy for acute leukaemia
- Staging of lymphoma (Hodgkin and non-Hodgkin lymphoma)

Q6. What is dry tap and what are the causes?

Ans. When only blood and no marrow material is aspirated then it is called 'dry tap'. Common causes are aplastic anaemia, myelofibrosis, and faulty technique.

Q7. How would you confirm that marrow has been aspirated?

Ans:
i. Macroscopically, by looking at the granularily. When bone marrow smear is touched the surface is irregular and sand-like feeling due to presence of marrow particles. Marrow particles look glistening.
ii. Microscopically, by looking at the megakeryocytes and fat spaces (in-between marrow cells) under microscope. Marrow particles are dragged during smear preparation, and trail of cells is left behind.

Q8. What are the indications of trephine or bone marrow biopsy?

Ans: All the indications of bone marrow aspiration and 'dry tap' during aspirations (myelofibrosis, myelosclerosis and aplastic anaemia).

Bone marrow biopsy removes a core of bone to evaluate both bone and surrounding tissue (marrow tissue). Also associated cells, protein deposits or inflammatory processes can be assessed. It shows the relationship of the cells to each other or to the bone or the cells' precise location in relation to the bone. Bone marrow infiltration by tumour cells or cancer cells can also be examined which helps in staging in many tumours like Hodgkin and non-Hodgkin lymphomas.

Q9. What are the contraindications of bone marrow aspiration?

Ans: Haemophilia A, haemophilia B, bleeding diathesis and infection at the site of puncture.

Q10. What are the routine stains and special stains for bone marrow smear examination?

Ans: Routine stains: Leishman's stain, Giemsa stain and MGG

Special stains:

i. Perls'-Prussian blue stain: To detect iron status. Absent in iron deficiency anaemia, increased in haemochromatosis, haemosiderosis, refractory sideroblastic anaemia and decreased in aplastic anaemia and pernicious anaemia.

ii. Reticulin stain for myelofibrosis, polycythaemia vera and myeloproliferative disorders (increased in all).

iii. PAS stain, myeloperoxidase stain and Sudan black stain: Differentiate between ALL (acute lymphoblastic leukaemia) and AML (acute myeloblastic leukaemia).

4
Total Count of WBC, RBC and Platelets

For total count of blood cells (RBCs, WBCs and platelets) and haemocytometers are used. There are a number of different haemocytometers in the market and each of them has a different grid (device containing horizontal and perpendicular lines) as well as different recommended uses. Different haemocytometers are:
- Neubauer/improved or modified Neubauer chamber
- Louis-Charles Malassez device: French histologist and anatomist (1842–1909) who first invented haemocytometer.
- Burker chamber
- Thoma chamber
- Fuchs-Rosenthal counting chamber: Used mainly for total eosinophil count.

But most popular and most frequently used haemocytometer nowadays is **improved or modified Neubauer chamber**. Most haemocytometers are manufactured from crystal glass and generally measured 30 × 70 mm with a thickness of 4 mm. Two vertical lines are ground from the glass to define the cell counting area and the double cell counting chambers have a ground out 'H' shape.

OLD VS. IMPROVED NEUBAUER CHAMBER
- In the old chamber, in the central area, there are 16 large squares each having 16 small squares. But in the improved chamber there are 25 large squares, each containing 16 small squares.
- The triple lines, dividing the central area is not very close in old chamber. But in improved chamber, the triple lines are very close.
- The space occupied by the triple lines in old Neubauer chamber being used to produce extra large space.
- In old chamber, the gap between triple lines was wide and the rectangular space between them looks as similar as the

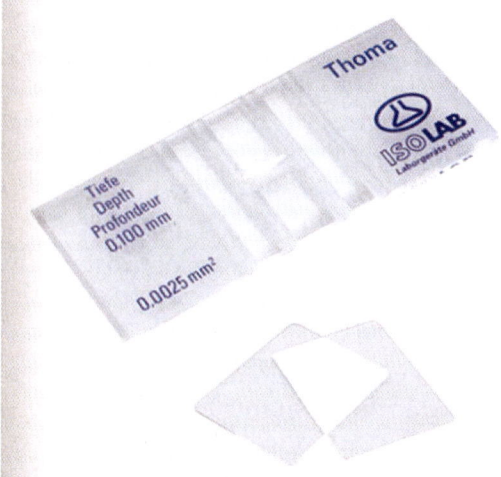

Fig. 4.1: Thoma counting chamber

Total Count of WBC, RBC and Platelets

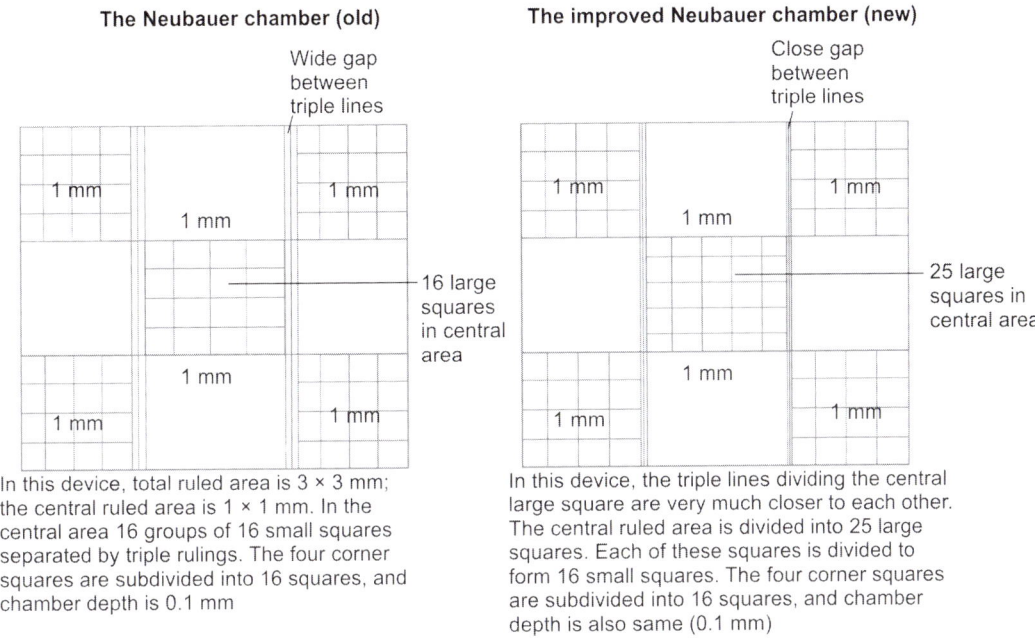

Fig. 4.2: Old and improved Neubauer chamber

squares in which the cells are to be counted. So, it makes the count very difficult and chances of error was very high.

- In old Neubauer chamber, the separating lines were very dull and some time it was very difficult to recognize them. But in the improved chamber, the separating lines are vivid and clear.
- By dividing, central space in 25 large squares, the RBC and platelet count have become easier.

Parts of Hemocytometer (Improved Neubauer's Chamber)

i. A counting chamber
ii. A WBC pipette
iii. A RBC pipette
iv. A thick coverslip

Counting Chamber

The improved Neubauer's chamber has two ruled stages separated by a small gutter (a shallow trough/channel beneath the edge of a roof). The two ruled stages again are separated from two ridges by gutters, one on each side. The surface of these two ruled stages is 0.1 mm above the surface of the stage. So, when cover glass is kept on the platform of this counting chamber, the space between the bottom of the coverslip and the base of the grooved area becomes 0.1 mm in depth.

There are two chamber stages, one above and one below, which is separated by gutter. Each stage has a ruled area measuring 3×3 mm which is divided into 9 squares. This squares measuring 1×1 mm each. The four corner squares are divided into 16 small squares ($1/4 \times 1/4$ mm each). The four corner areas (A, B, C and D are used in Fig. 4.6 for counting WBCs.

The central ruled square area (1×1 mm) is divided into 25 (5×5) small squres in the improved Neubauer's chamber. Each small square is again subdivided into 16 (4×4) smaller squares. Area of each small square is $1/5 \times 1/5$ mm or $1/25$ mm^2. For counting

Pathology Practicals

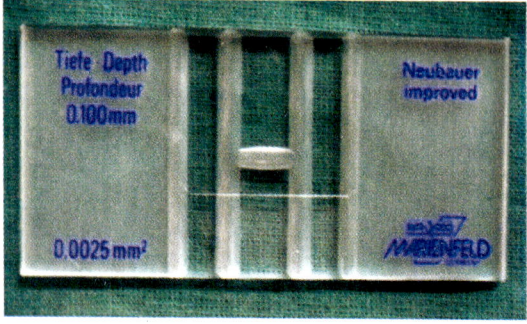

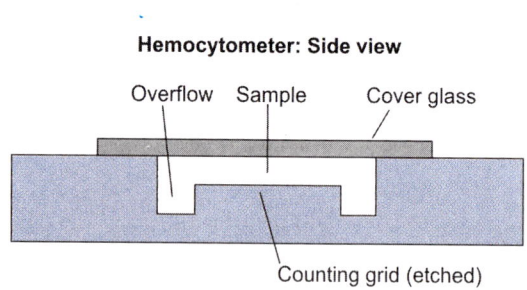

Fig. 4.3: Improved Neubauer's chamber

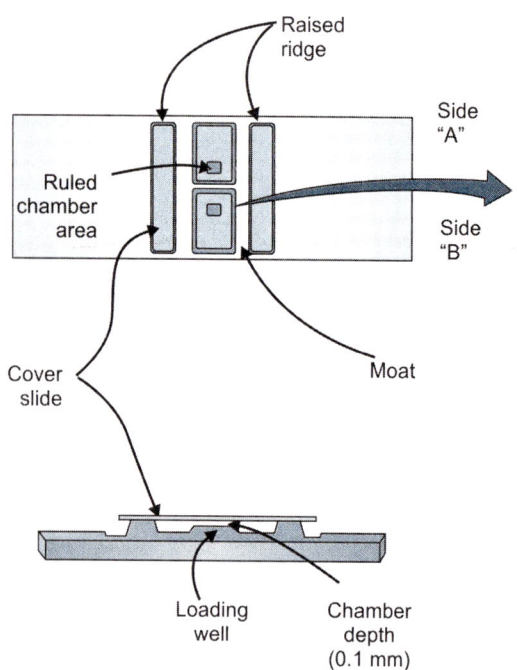

Fig. 4.4: Schematic diagram of using improved Neubauer's chamber

RBCs, this central ruled area is used. Usually four corners and one central square ruled area (blackened in picture) are used total RBC count. This area is also used for platelet count and sperm count from seminal fluid.

WBC Pipette

The pipette is marked 0.5, 1 below the bulb and 11 above the bulb. There is a white-coloured bead inside the bulb.

Uses

i. Total WBC count of blood (TLC).
ii. Total cell count from different body fluids like pleural fluid, CSF (cerebrospinal fluid, peritoneal fluid).
iii. Total platelet count, if the platelet count is very low.
iv. Total sperm count if the sperm count is low.

Blood or body fluid or seminal fluid is taken by WBC pipette and four corners of the hemocytometer are changed for cell counting.

RBC Pipette

The pipette is marked 0.5, 1 below the bulb and 101 above the bulb. There is a red-coloured bead inside the bulb.

Uses

i. Total RBC count of blood
ii. Total platelet count of blood
iii. Total sperm count from seminal fluid
iv. Total WBC count in case of leukemias when there is very high WBC count and counting in the four corners may be problematic.

Blood or body fluid or seminal fluid is taken by RBC pipette and central ruled area of the hemocytometer is charged for cell counting.

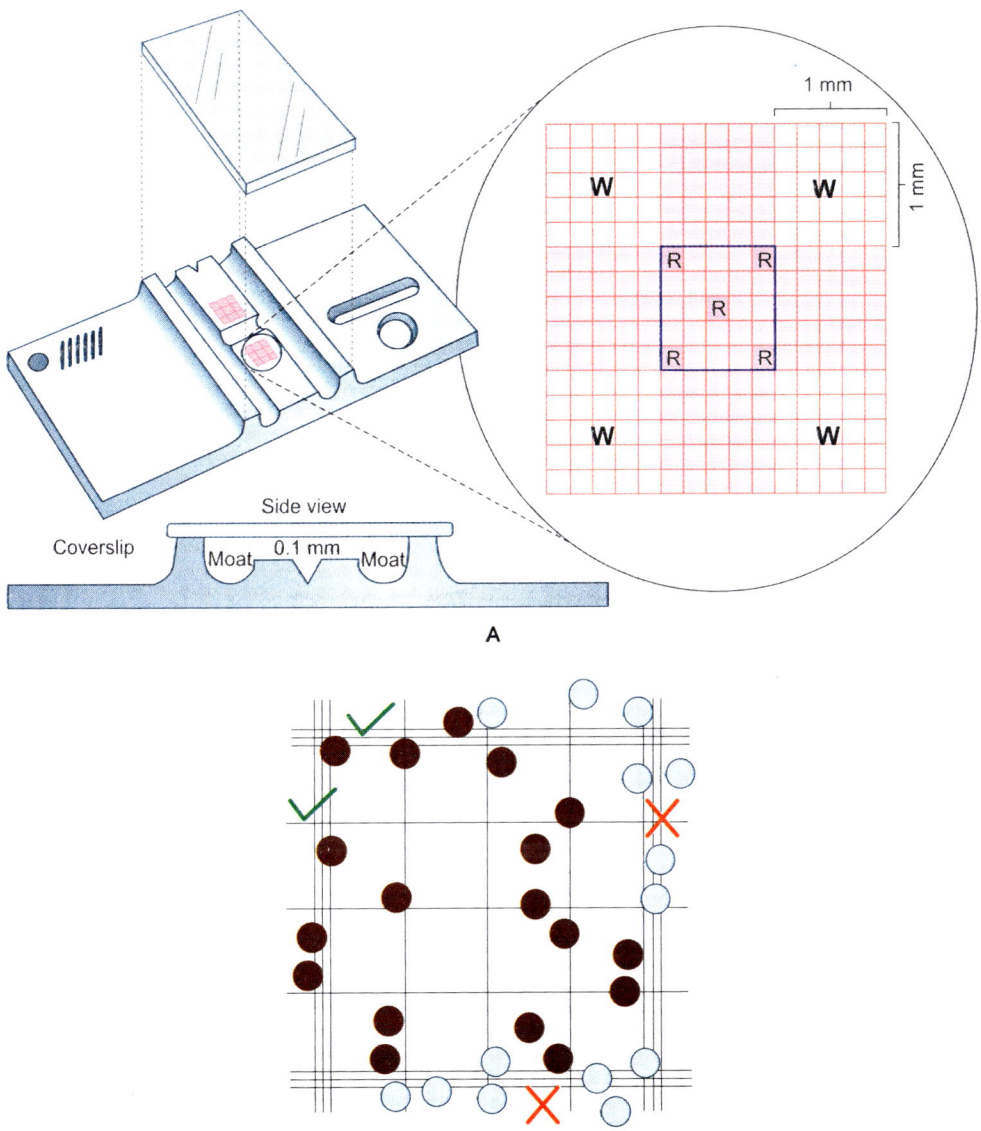

Fig. 4.5A and B: (A) Counting of WBC and RBC in the chamber; (B) Right way of counting cells. Cells on the upper and left triple lines are counted (black-coloured circles) while on right and lower triple lines are not counted (white-coloured circles)

Thick Coverslip

A specially made coverslip which has very smooth surface and even thickness of 0.3 mm or 0.4 mm or 0.5 mm is used. Commonly, coverslip with a thickness of 0.4 mm is used. Two sizes of coverslip are available in the market. One is 16 × 22 mm coverslip which is used for single ruled hemocytometer. The other coverslip is 22 × 23 mm which is used for double-ruled counting chamber.

Differences between RBC pipette and WBC pipette are given in Table 4.1.

White Blood Cell Count (Manual Method)

Blood is collected up to mark 0.5 of WBC pipette, either from EDTA or oxalate mixed

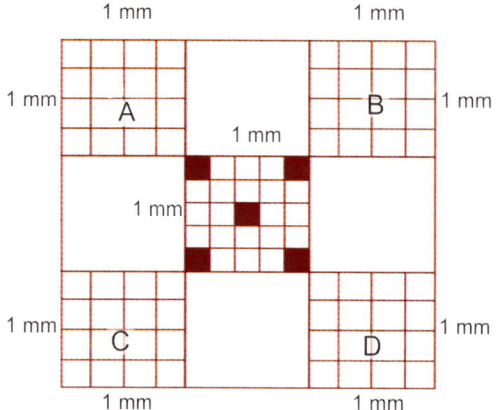

Fig. 4.6: Counting chamber in improved Neubauer's chamber

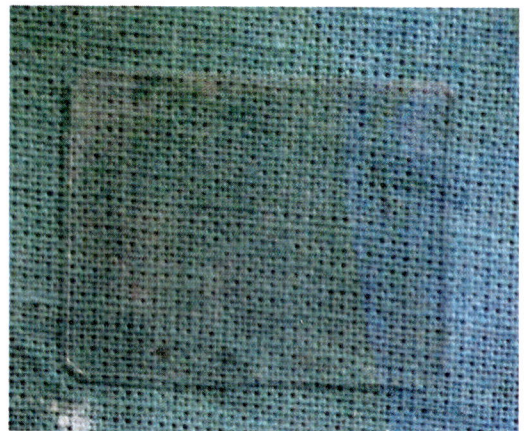

Fig. 4.9: Thick coverslip

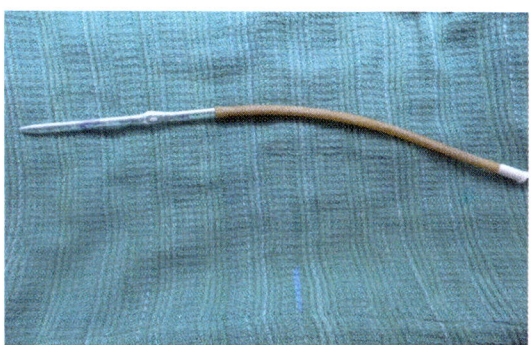

Fig. 4.7: WBC pipette

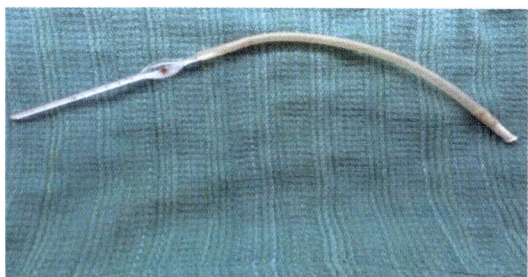

Fig. 4.8: RBC pipette

Table 4.1: Differences between RBC pipette and WBC pipette

1.	It has a red bead	It has a white bead
2.	It has graduations up to mark 101	It has graduations up to mark 11
3.	Size of bulb is larger	Size of bulb is smaller
4.	Size of lumen is smaller	Size of lumen is larger

(anticoagulated) venous blood or after finger prick (fresh blood without anticoagulant). WBC diluting fluid is then sucked up to the mark 11 above in the WBC pipette. Well mixed the blood and WBC fluid in the pipette by rotating the pipette between fingers by rotation. Then keep it over the table for few minutes (5–10 minutes). The red cells are lysed by the diluting fluid (acetic acid) but the leukocytes remain intact. Nuclei of the WBCs stain deep violet black by methylene blue or gentian violet stains.

Composition of WBC Diluting Fluid

- Glacial acetic acid: 2 ml
- Distilled water: 100 ml
- Aqueous methylene blue Solution (0.3%, w/v): 10 drops*

Or

1% aqueous solution of gentian violet: 1 ml

---

* Aqueous methylene blue solution is prepared by dissolving 0.3 gm of methylene blue in 100 ml of distilled water. Filter it before use. Alternatively, gentian violet (1 ml of 1% solution, w/v) can also be used instead of methylene blue (0.3%, w/v).

Dilution of Blood

If the blood is taken up to 0.5 mark, then the dilution is 1 in 20. Because the mark 11 above the bulb is to indicate the total volume of the marked portion of WBC pipette. Firstly, the blood is sucked (up to 0.5 mark), then the WBC fluid is taken. So, blood moves up and is diluted in the bulb and above up to mark 11 (from mark 1 to mark 11), whereas the long bar in the pipette contains only WBC fluid (up to mark 1). So, 10 volumes (11–1 = 10) contain 0.5 ml volume of blood. Hence, the dilution is 1 in 20 or 1:20.

Charging (Filling) the Improved Neubauer's Chamber

- Chamber and coverslip should be clean and dry.
- Hold the WBC pipette slightly inclined and pressure is released slowly with finger so that a small volume of WBC fluid mixed blood is allowed in the chamber under coverslip. This will be accomplished by the capillary action. Blood outside the pipette is wiped with tissue paper or cotton.
- The WBCs are allowed to settle for 2–3 minutes, so that they can be seen in the same plane of focus.

Counting of Leukocytes

WBC count is made under high power (40X) objective; but low power (10X) objective is used to focus them. The WBCs in each of the four large (1 × 1 mm) corner squares (ruled area) are counted, each of this large square has 16 small squares or division. Only WBCs within the squares are counted and cells lying on lines of any two adjacent sides (top and right, or bottom and left) are included in total WBC count.

The volume of each large square = $1 \times 1 \times 1/10$ mm (depth)

So, the volume of four large squares = $1 \times 1 \times 1/10 \times 4$ mm^3 or cu mm = $2/5$ mm^3

Let the leukocyte count (WBC) in four large squares is N.

Then, $2/5$ mm^3 of volume of blood contains leukocytes = N × dilution factor

Or, $2/5$ mm^3 blood contains leukocytes = N × 20

Or 1 mm^3 blood contains leukocytes = N × 20 × 5/2 = N × 50.

Note

i. As many leukocytes as possible should be counted; a reasonable and practical figure is to count 100 cells. If 400 cells are counted then chances of error will as low as 5%.

ii. Causes of error: These include mistaking clumped red cell debris or debris or dirt for leukocytes or clumped leukocytes. Clumped leukocytes are usually seen in blood with several hours storage or in heparinized blood (>25 IU/ml of blood).

iii. Filing or charging defects leading to error:
   a. Chamber area incompletely filled
   b. Air bubble anywhere in the chamber area
   c. Any dirt or debris in the chamber (unclean or moist chamber).
   d. Overflow of the counting and ruled area.

iv. Nowadays, bulb pipettes are not recommended because they are easily broken. The volumes of blood used are unnecessarily small and the WBC pipette is difficult to handle. Particularly charging the chamber with pipette is very difficult and needs experience. So, 20 μl micropipette (or Pasteur pipette) is used which is easy to handle.

Red Blood Cell Count (Manual Method)

Blood is collected up to the mark 0.5 in the RBC pipette, either from EDTA or oxalated mixed (anticoagulated) venous blood or after finger prick capillary blood. Wipe tip clean. RBC diluting fluid is then sucked up to the mark 101 in the RBC pipette. Clean the tip of pipette again. It is well mixed and shaken for 2–3 minutes. First few drops are discarded and then counting chamber (central ruled area) is charged. It is then kept in a most chamber or in a Petri dish with wet filter paper and allowed to settle the RBCs for 10–15 minutes; so that they can be seen in the same plane of focus.

Composition of RBC Fluid

- Formalin (40% formaldehyde): 1 ml
- Trisodium citrate: 3.13 gm
- Distilled water: 100 ml
- Tinge of eosin (optional)

Formalin acts as a preservative and prevents undesirable growth of microorganism/fungus in the diluting fluid. Eosin tinge is added to distinct the RBCs quickly but not to stain RBCs.

Alternatively, Hayem's fluid may be used (costlier than previous diluting fluid).

Composition of Hayem's fluid

- Sodium chloride (NaCl): 1 gm
- Sodium sulphate: 5 gm
- Mercuric chloride: 0.5 gm
- Distilled water: 100 ml

Remember the RBC diluting fluid should be isotonic so that RBCs are not lysed. Normal saline can be used if there is no diluting fluid available RBCs and in emergency. But normal saline cause crenation of RBCs and may form rouleax. Hence, not recommended for use.

Counting of RBCs

Red cells are counted in the central ruled are of the improved Neubauer chamber. In the central large square (1 × 1 mm) there are 25 small squares (1/5 × 1/5 mm). Four corners and central small squares are counted for RBCs. Let the RBC count in 5 small squares is N.

Volume of 5 small squares = $1/5 \times 1/5 \times 1/10 \times 5$
(depth is 0.1 mm or 1/10 mm)
= $1/50$ cu mm or mm^3

So, 1/50 mm^3 blood contains RBCs =
$N \times$ dilution factor
= $N \times 200$ (dilution of blood in RBC diluting fluid)

Then, 1 mm^3 blood contains RBCs =
$N \times 200 \times 50/1 = N \times 10,000$

Note

i. Like WBC pipette, RBC pipettes are also not used nowadays. Instead micropipette or Pasteur pipettes are used.
ii. Error in counting RBC may be due to filing or charging defects (vide WBC count).
iii. Errors may also be due to inaccurate apparatus or due to technical errors (bad technique in collecting blood, insufficient mixing of blood specimen).

Platelet Count (Manual Method)

The diluent consists of 1% ammonium oxalate. Not more than 500 ml should be made at a time. The solution should be filtered through a micropipette filter (0.22 μm) and kept at 4°C.

Method: Use venous blood preferably for platelet counts. Finger pricks may cause clumping of platelets. Fill the blood and diluent as described for RBC count and using RBC pipette. Charge the chamber (central ruled area). Keep the hemocytometer in a moist chamber. Wait for 20–30 minutes to settle down the small platelets.

Using high power (40X) objective with reduced condenser aperture, count the platelets in the same squares as indicated the RBC counting (five small squares). Suppose total platelet count is N. Then as for RBC counting.

So, 1/50 mm^3 blood contains platelets
= $N \times$ dilution factor
= $N \times 200$
Then, 1 mm^3 blood contains platelets
= $N \times 200 \times 50/1 = N \times 10,000$

Note

- If platelet count is low, then WBC pipette may be used (dilution 1:20) and four large corner squares are counted for platelets like WBCs (N × 50).
- Charged hemocytometer is kept inside a moist chamber or it can be put in a Petri dish with a moistened or wet filter paper. The moist environment does not allow evaporation of platelet fluid. Adequate time (20–30 minutes) is given to settle down the platelets.
- Platelets under high power objective (light microscope), are small (but not minute) highly refractile particles. Platelets appear bluish and must be distinguished from debris.

ELECTRONIC METHOD FOR BLOOD CELL COUNT

Total WBC count along with other routine haematologic investigations are often done by using electronic instrument like 'Coulter counter'

The coulter analyzers utilize the electrical impedance with low-frequency electromagnetic current, high frequency electromagnetic current, laser light scattering, light scattering and absorbance depending on the device used. The compact semiautomated coulter system provides only the basic WBC count, RBC count, haemoglobin level, haematocrit value. On the other hand, the coulter MAXM, ONYX, STKR and STKS use positive identification bar code system and close vial sampling. Eighteen to twenty parameters may be assessed, including WBC count, RBC count, platelet count, haemoglobin level, haematocrit value, MCV, MCH, RDW (red cell distribution width) and MPV (mean platelet volume).

Rapid performance, minimal or no technical error, elimination of visual error and biasness, more accurate and precise results are advantages of electronic system over manual or hemocytometer method. In many laboratories, use of manual methods by hemocytometer has become obsolete. Only if the result is very very low or very very high, then it is used (with more dilution for very very high count) as it may be outside the range of the electronic machine.

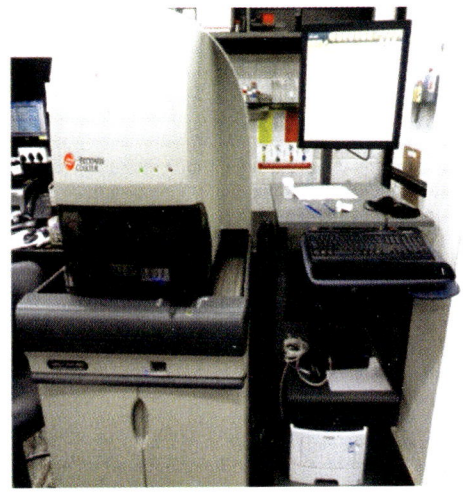

A

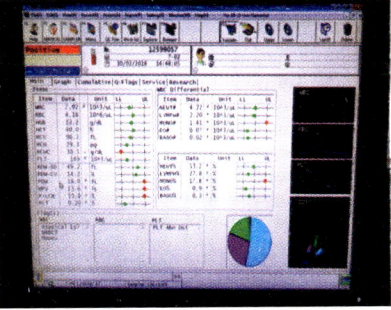

B

Fig. 4.10A and B: Automated blood cell counters

VIVA VOCE

Q1. How to identify WBC pipette?
Ans: By marks 0.5 and 1 below the bulb and mark 11 above the bulb. Also, a white bead inside the bulb.

Q2. What is the use of WBC pipette?
Ans:
- Used for total WBC count
- Sperm count in semen

- Eosinophil count
- Also may be used to count cells in any fluid where the count is more (>1000/µl), like cell count in CSF, pleural/ascitic fluid.
- RBC count in severe anaemia where RBC count is low.

Q3. How to identify RBC pipette?

Ans: By marks 0.5 and 1 below the bulb and mark 101 above the bulb. Also, a red-coloured bead inside the bulb.

Q4. What is the use of RBC pipette?

Ans:
- Used for total RBC count
- For total platelet count
- For sperm count in semen
- High TLC count

Q5. What is the electronic method for counting WBC? What are the advantages and disadvantages?

Ans: Electronic counter is based on aperture impedance method, or light scattering technology, or both. In this method, particles (WBCs) passing through a chamber in single file scatter the light and convert by a chamber in single file scatter the light and convert by a detector into pulses proportionate to the size of the cells, which are counted electronically. During counting of WBCs, a lysate is used to lyse RBCs.

Advantages
- Easy and rapid method
- High level of precision
- Very large number of cells is counted quickly
- Time saving method

Disadvantages
- The instrument is costly, so beyond the scope of small size laboratory.
- Calibration to be done at regular interval, otherwise there will be error.
- Normoblasts (nucleated RBCs) are counted as leukocytes
- Clumps of platelets are also falsely counted as WBCs.

Q6. What is electronic method of counting platelets? Is it advantageous or disadvantageous?

Ans: The principal is electrical impedance like counting RBCs.

Platelet counting by electronic method is disadvantageous.

Disadvantageous are:
- Debris and fragments of blood cells (small size) are counted as platelets.
- Howell-Jolly bodies and Heinz bodies are also counted as platelets.
- Equipment is costly and calibration error may occur.

Q7. How do you differentiate between platelets and dust particles?

Ans
- Platelets are stained light blue when stained by brilliant cresyl blue. Dust particles cannot be stained.
- Platelets have brownian movements but dust particles lack it.

Q8. Which is the best method for absolute eosinophil count (AEC)? What is the composition of diluting fluid for eosinophil count?

Ans: The best method is the automated counter which detects eosiniphil peroxidase during counting. Other methods are Fuchs-Rosenthal counting chamber or hemocytometer or using Dunger's solution. Other dilution fluids are Randolph's diluting fluid, Pilot's stain.

i. Dunger's solution:
  - Acid dye, e.g. eosin or phloxine, 0.1% aqueous solution
  - Water to lyse RBCs and rupture leukocytes

ii. Randolph's fluid:
  - Stock solution A (methylene blue, propylene glycol, distilled water)
  - Stock solution B (phloxine, propylene glycol, distilled water)

- Wrong solution is prepared from above stocks 1:1 volume

iii. Pilot's stain:
- Propylene glycol (50 ml), distilled water 40 ml, phloxine 0.1 aqueous solution, 10 ml; sodium carbonate 1% aqueous solution, 1 ml.

Q9. Why special coverslip not the ordinary one is used while doing various counts by Neubauer chamber?

Ans: Neubauer chamber and its coverslip (thicker than the ordinary coverslip) are so designed that after charging the chamber a fixed/desired amount of fluid is present in-between the ruled chamber and overlying coverslip. And the depth of fluid 0.1 mm (prerequisite for calculation). The ordinary coverslip is thin and light. Fluid depth is not 0.1 mm, so cell counts become erroneous. Moreover, coverslip of Neubauer chamber is uniformly flat while ordinary cover glass is not.

Q10. How do you clean Hb, WBC and RBC pipettes?

Ans: These pipettes are filled with distilled water and cleaned by blowing it out twice. Then, acetone is sucked into the pipette and blown it out. Acetone removes residual water within pipette and dries it completely. When pipette is completely dry, the bead with the bulb moves/rolls freely but if it is wet, bead does not rolls freely.

Q11. How sperm count is done in Neubauer chamber?

Ans: Semen diluting fluid (sodium bicarbonate 5 gm, neutral formalin 1 ml, and distilled water to make 100 ml). Semen may be diluted in a test tube (0.1 ml semen +1.9 ml diluting fluid) or in a WBC pipette (draw semen to the mark 0.5 and diluting fluid to the mark 11) and mix well. After charging improved Neubauer chamber, wait for 2–3 minutes to settle down the sperms.

Calculation: Count spermatozoa in 2 mm^3 (two large squares at two corners) and multiply by 100,000 or 1 lakh. It gives the number of spermatozoa per ml of semen (unlike in terms of per mm^3 of WBC count).

Normal range: 60–150 millions/ml. Count below 20 millions/ml is considered abnormal.

5
Erythrocyte Sedimentation Rate (ESR) and Packed Cell Volume (PCV)

ERYTHROCYTE SEDIMENTATION RATE

The erythrocyte sedimentation rate (ESR) is the rate at which red blood cells sediment in a period of one hour.

It is also known as sedimentation rate (sed rate).

Brief History of ESR

This test was invented by the Polish pathologist Edmund Biernacki in 1897. In some regions of the world, the test continues to be referred to as Biernacki's reaction. In the year 1918, the Swedish pathologist Robert Sanno Fahraeus along with Alf Vilhelm Albertsson Westergren described the same and is eponymously remembered as Fahraeus-Westergren test. But in the UK, it is usually termed Westergren test which became popular throughout world.

Mechanism of Erythrocyte Sedimentation

The ESR or rate of fall of red cells is governed by the balance between pro-sedimentation factors, mainly fibrinogen and those factors resisting sedimentation, e.g. the negative charge of the erythrocyte (zeta potential). The decreased zeta potential promotes rouleaux formation and hence raised ESR.

ESR depends upon the difference in specific gravity between red cells and plasma. Also, it is greatly influenced by the extent to which RBCs form rouleaux, which sediment stacks of RBCs than single cell. Many other factors are also responsible which include the ratio of RBCs to plasma (i.e. PCV), the plasma viscosity, the bore of the tube, dilution, if any of the blood, the verticality of ESR tube, etc.

The very important factor is rouleaux formation and red cell clumping. This is mainly controlled by the plasma concentration of fibrinogen and other acute phase protein/reactants, e.g. haptoglobin, ceruloplasmin, α_1-antitrypsin and C reactive protein (CRP). Rouleaux formation is also enhanced by increased concentration of plasma immunoglobulin. On the contrary, it is retarded by higher concentration of albumin and test done with defibrinated blood (≤1 mm/hr), which removes fibrinogen. In anaemia, there may be quantitative deficiency of RBCs, so ratio of RBCs to plasma is altered which results more rouleaux formation and increased ESR.

Methods of ESR Estimation

i. Westergren method
ii. Wintrobe method
iii. Landau method: Not accurate, used in the past in children with limited supply of blood. The method uses capillary blood from heel, toe or fingertip.

iv. Electronic method by automated analyzers.

The first two methods are commonly used methods which are done by manual technique. Of these two, Westergren method is most popular and commonly used method.

Westergren Method using Westergren Pipette

Though the equipment is sometimes called Westergren tube, it should be called pipette (more scientific term) as it is open at both ends.

Westergren pipette is a slender, thick-walled pipette. It is 300 mm long (i.e. 30 cm or 12 inches) of which lower 200 mm is graduated (markings) and upper 100 mm part is ungraduated. The pipette has an inner diameter of 2.5 mm.

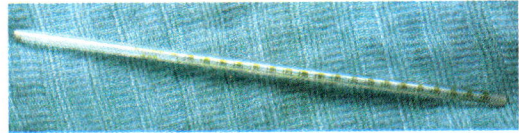

Fig. 5.1: Westergren pipette

Anticoagulant used: 3.8% trisodium citrate solution (no other anticoagulant with this method), 109 mmol/L (32 gm/L, $Na_3Ca_6H_5O_7.2H_2O$). EDTA mixed blood is used in modified Westergren method.

Blood and anticoagulant ratio: For this test 2 ml of venous blood is mixed with 0.5 ml of sodium citrate anticoagulant. So, the blood and anticoagulant ratio is 4:1.

Method or procedure: 0.5 ml of 3.8% sodium citrate solution is taken in a test tube. Then, 2 ml of venous blood (usually from antecubical vein) is mixed with the anticoagulant immediately with the help of a syringe. The sample is well mixed.

The anticoagulated blood is drawn up in to Westergren pipette up to 200 mm mark with the help of a teat or mechanical device (mouth suction is avoided). The pipette is now set exactly vertical in a Westergren stand. A spring clip, pressing on the top and rubber piece at the lower end hold the pipette in the Westergren stand or rack. Now the pipette in the rack which is vertically placed is kept at room temperature without vibration and exposure to sunlight.

Modified Westergren method: It produces the same results but uses EDTA blood rather than citrate as an anticoagulant. In this method, 2 ml of EDTA blood is diluted with 0.5 ml of 0.85% sodium chloride or with 0.5 ml of 3.8% sodium citrate. Precision is poor when EDTA blood is undiluted.

This method has the advantage that same EDTA-mixed blood may be used for other haematologic studies.

Recording result: The RBCs begin to settle down and a clear plasma zone is formed above the settled RBCs. The upper level of the RBC column is read (zero mark is upside and 200 mark is downside) at the end of one hour.

The measurement in mm is ESR (Westergren, 1 hour).

Previously it was thought that mean average ESR per hour (total duration 2 hours) is more accurate.

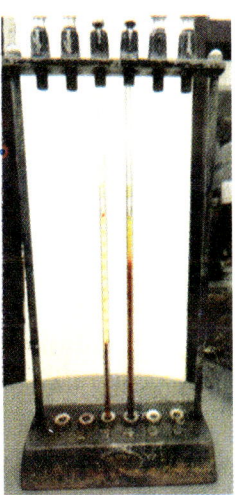

Fig. 5.2: Westergren or ESR stand (rack)

Mean ESR = (1st hour result + ½ of 2 hours result) ÷ 2

But later on, concept of mean ESR disregarded because result after 1 hour gives more accurate result.

Normal range of ESR: The ESR gradually increases with age. Westergren's original upper limit of normal (10 mm/hour for men and 20 mm/hour for women) seems to be low. According to studies by scientists, upper limits of reference values in this method should be as follows:

	Men	Women
i. Below age 50 years	15 mm/hr	20 mm/hr
ii. Above age 50 years	20 mm/hr	30 mm/hr
iii. Above age 85 years	30 mm/hr	42 mm/hr

But in Indian context, acceptable normal range for ESR is
- Men: 4–14 mm/hr
- Women: 6–20 mm/hr
- Newborn: 0–2 mm/hr
- Newborn to puberty: 3–13 mm/hr

Wintrobe's Method

Instrument: Wintrobe's tube is a special, thick-walled glass tube 11 cm long with an internal diameter of 2.5 mm and the bottom 10 cm are graduated. It has flat inner base. It is calibrated at 1 mm intervals to 100 mm and holds about 1 ml of blood. Graduations are from zero (top) to hundred (bottom) for ESR and zero (bottom) to hundred (top) for PCV.

Anticoagulant: Venous blood is mixed with EDTA (preferred), or double oxalate or heparin.

Methods

1. 2 ml venous blood is collected and mixed with anticoagulant (EDTA) in the vial immediately.
2. Wintrobe tube is filled with this blood till zero mark on top with the help of a Pasteur pipette.
3. The tube is now kept vertically over stand for one hour and is noted by measuring the free plasmatic zone above (descending orders, 0 marks on top and 100 marks on bottom).

Normal range: Men 0–9 mm/hr, women 2–20/hr.

Stages of Sedimentation (ESR)

Stage 1. Rouleaux formation: In this stage (first 15 minutes) red cells form rouleaux and minimum sedimentation occurs.

Stage 2. Formation of fine threads by proteins: During this stage (second 15 minutes) fibrinogen and globulin in plasma form network by forming fine threads. The rouleaux of red cells are trapped within this network and becomes heavier. So, they begin to fall (settling) rapidly.

Stage 3. Rapid fall of protein network: In this phase (third 15 minutes), red cell mass and protein network fall rapidly.

Stage 4. Packing of red cells: In the last 15 minutes, the sedimented red cell mass–protein undergoes packing at the bottom of pipette.

Use of ESR

1. Diagnosis
   a. **Marked elevation:** Multiple myeloma, macroglobulinaemia, tuberculosis, hyperfibrinogenemia, myocardial infarction, temporal arthritis, rheumatoid arthritis, chronic kidney disease, SLE, inflammatory bowel disease, polymyalgia rheumatica.
   b. **Moderate evaluation:** Chronic infection (chronic osteomyelitis, chronic lung abscess, chronic bronchiectasis), rheumatoid arthritis, neoplasms (Hodgkin lymphoma, carcinomatosis,

leukaemia), infective endocarditis, physiological (pregnancy), drugs (oral contraceptives, methyldopa, dextran, vitamin A, theophylline).
2. **Disease severity assessment:** ESR is a component of PCDAI (Paediatric Crohn's Disease Activity Index), an index for assessment of severity of inflammatory bowel disease in children.
3. **Monitoring response to therapy:** ESR has limited role to monitor the response to therapy in certain inflammatory disease such as rheumatoid arthritis, polymyalgia rheumatica and temporal arthritis. In Hodgkin lymphoma, ESR can be used as a crude measure to response. Also, it is used to define one of the several possible adverse prognostic factors in staging of Hodgkin lymphoma.

Causes of Slow or Decreased ESR

- Polycythemia vera
- Sickle cell anaemia, spherocytosis, poikilocytosis
- Congestive heart failure
- Stages of severe dehydration like cholera, acute gastroenteritis.
- Infections: Typhoid and undulant fever, trichinosis, malarial paroxysm, pertusis.
- Allergic states
- Drugs: Aspirin, cortisone, quinine.

In case of sickle cell anaemia, spherocytosis or poikilocytosis, there are abnormal red cells. These abnormalities of RBCs prevent rouleaux formation. Hence, decreased ESR.

Sources of Error and other Interfering Factors

- If the concentration of anticoagulant is higher than recommend the ESR may be elevated.
- Heparin alters the membrane zeta potential of RBCs and cannot be used as an anticoagulant.
- Tilting the pipette accelerates the ESR. The RBCs aggregate along the lower side, whereas the plasma rises along the upper side. Subsequently, the retarding of influence of the rising plasma becomes less effective. An angle of 3° from vertical position, may accelerate the ESR by as much as 30%.
- Plasma factors: An accelerated ESR is seen in elevated levels of fibrinogen and to a lesser extent of globulins. Albumin retards ESR. High rise of plasma viscosity also retards ESR. Cholesterol increases and lecithin decreases ESR.
- The test should be done within two hours. If the blood is stored for more than two hours, ESR will increase.
- If blood is kept in refrigerator, ESR is highly increased. So, refrigerated blood should be allowed to return to normal room temperature before the test started.
- Temperature of the environment: The ideal temperature for the test is 20–25°C. Increase in temperature is directly proportional to increased ESR.
- Bubbles left in the pipette, when the blood is filled, will affect ESR. The cleanliness of pipette is also important.
- Haemolysis may modify ESR.

Different Automated Methods of ESR

- Ves-Matic
- ESR STAT-PLUS
- SEDIMAT
- Zeta Sedimentation

Advantages of automated methods

- Provide more rapid results
- Use small sample volumes
- Save technician time
- Provide increased safety because the need for sample manipulation is decreased.

Zeta Sedimentation Rate (ZSR)

EDTA mixed blood (0.2 ml) is filled in a special capillary tube and is centrifuged in

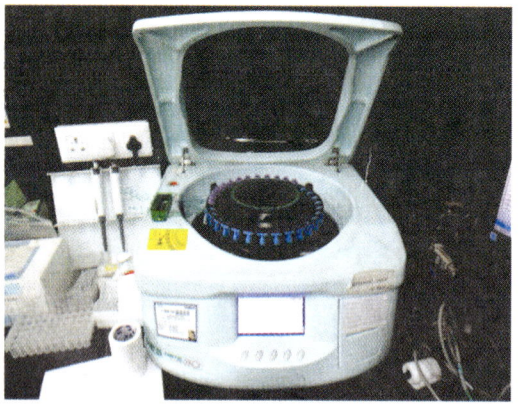 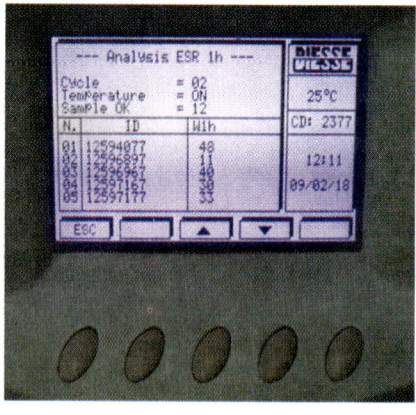

Fig. 5.3A and B: (A) Automated ESR machine; (B) Recording of ESR result

special apparatus (zeta fuge, Coulter Electronics) for four times, each for 45 seconds. The capillary tube is mechanically rotated at 180° and centrifugation is done in reverse direction at every 45 seconds for four times. The red cell rouleaux develops better and travel down the capillary tube by alternate compaction and dispersion.

Result of ZSR: ZSR is expressed in terms of percentage.

Normal range in adults 40–50%. Rise in ZSR indicates rise in ESR.

Zeta crit: It is the ratio of the height of red cells to the total height of blood column.

Advantages of ZSR
- Requires small amount of blood (0.2 ml)
- No dilution is required.
- Eliminates the effect of anaemia.
- It is more sensitive than Westergren's method of ESR estimation.
- It requires minimum time.

Micro-ESR Method

Barrett (1980) described this micro-ESR method using 0.2 ml of blood to fill a plastic disposable tube 230 mm long with 1 mm inner diameter or internal bore. Both venous and capillary blood are suitable for this method. The tube filled with blood is kept vertically on a stand and the result is read after one hour.

This method has more utility in paediatric patients.

WINTROBE'S HAEMATOCRIT (PACKED CELL VOLUME)

The term 'haematocrit' theoretically means blood separation. Wintrobe haematocrit tube is mainly used for measurement of packed cell volume (PCV).

Definition of PCV

It is defined as the volume of packed red blood cells in a given sample of blood which is expressed as a percentage of the total volume of the blood sample.

Two methods are employed for measurement of PCV.
1. Macro-method using Wintrobe tube.
2. Micro-method using capillary tube.

1. Macro-method—Wintrobe's Tube

It is a spherical, thick-walled glass tube 11cm long and has an internal diameter of 2.5 mm with flat inner base. The tube is calibrated at 1 to 100 mm intervals and holds about 1 ml of blood. The markings on the tube are in

Erythrocyte Sedimentation Rate (ESR) and Packed Cell Volume (PCV)

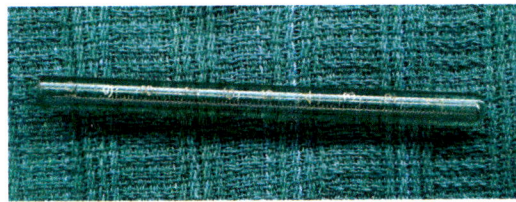

Fig. 5.4: Wintrobe's Tube

reversed directions. Ascending marking is used for determination of PCV and descending marking is used for determination of ESR.

Uses

1. Wintrobe's tube is primarily used for determination of packed red cell volume (PCV) of blood.
2. Also it can be used for determination of ESR especially for anaemia correction with the help of correction curve.
3. Buffy coat smear preparation for demonstration of LE cell and staining with Leishman stain in diagnosis of SLE.
4. Abnormal or blast cells in aleukaemic leukaemia.

Blood and anticoagulant: Venous blood anticoagulated with double oxalate powder, EDTA powder or heparin.

Method of PCV Determination (Wintrobe Tube)

1. 2 ml venous blood is taken and immediately mixed with anticoagulant. Mix well by shaking.
2. The Wintrobe tube is filled with anticoagulated blood with the help of a long Pasteur pipette from the bottom up to mark '0' or '10' above.
3. The tube is then centrifuged at 3000 r.p.m. for 30 minutes.
4. The packed cell volume (PCV) is measured by noting the upper level of column of packed red cells by the markings in ascending order. PCV is expressed as percentage of the total volume of blood.

Zones Separated after Centrifugation

1. The layer of packed red cells or PCV is lower most which is usually 45 to 50%.
2. An intermediate thin layer comprises WBCs and platelets. It is above the lower most layer (red cells). The grey-coloured layer is known as buffy coat. Normally this layer is 2 to 3%. Buffy coat layer is increased in leukaemia and severe degree of leukocytosis.
3. Upper most layer of plasma: This straw-coloured layer is above buffy coat layer and composed of free plasma. This layer may be pink in haemolysis, yellow in jaundice, and colourless in iron deficiency anaemia.

Normal Range of PCV

- Men: 45 ± 5%, i.e 40 to 50%
- Women: 41± 5%, i.e 36 to 46%
- At birth: 44 to 62%
- One year infant: 35% (approximate)
- 10 years: 37.5% (approximate)

Increased PCV: Polycythaemia, severe degree of dehydration, cholera, acute gastroenteritis.

Decreased PCV: Anaemia (usually less than 30%)

Sources of Error of PCV

- Inadequate duration and speed of centrifugation.
- Inadequate mixing of blood.
- Excess anticoagulant.
- Irregularity of the bore of Wintrobe tube.
- Trapping of leukocyte—platelet clumps in the tube will result defective red cell packing.

2. Micro-method—Capillary Tube Method for PCV

Non-graduated capillary tube (75 mm in length and about 1 mm internal diameter) is rinsed with heparin solution (1:2000 heparin or 1 in 1000 dilution). Well dry this heparinised capillary tubes at 56°C and stored.

When the test is done a capillary tube (haematocrit) is filled up with blood (finger prick or EDTA mixed venus blood) and the empty end is sealed with a micro burner. The tube is filled up ½ to 2/3 of its length (not the entire length). The tube is then fitted on the micro haematocrit centrifuge and centrifuged at 12000 r.p.m. for 5 minutes with the sealed end away from the centre.

Calculation of result: Then the capillary tube is taken out and PCB is calculated with the help of a millimetre rule commercially available.

Normal range of PCV
- Male: 47 ± 7%
- Female: 43 ± 5%

Advantages of micromethod
- Time requirement for centrifugation is short.
- Small amount of blood is required to fill the capillary tube.
- Cost effective and easy to work.

Table 5.1: Normal levels of packed cell volume (PVC) and haemoglobin

Age and sex	Packed cell volume (PCV)%	Haemoglobin (g/dl)
Adult male	40–50	13–17
Adult female (nonpregnant)	38–45	12–15
Adult female (pregnant)	36–42	11–14
Children, 6–12 years	37–46	11.5–15.5
Children, 6 months to 6 years	36–42	11–14
Infants, 2–6 months	32–42	9.5–14
Newborns	44–60	13.6–19.6

Generally, PCV% is three times that of Hb g/dl or Hb%. So, if a person has haemoglobin of 15 g/dl, his PCV will be 15 × 3 = 45% (approx).

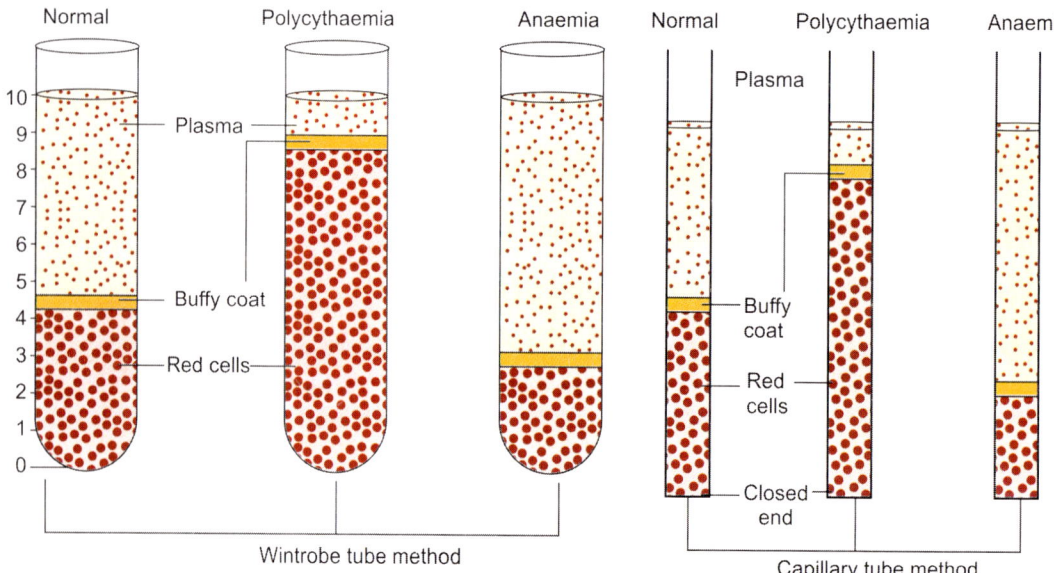

Fig. 5.5: Packed cell volume (PCV) showing comparison of normal, polycythaemia and anaemic blood samples by two different methods (Wintrobe and capillary tube)

VIVA VOCE

Q1. Why ESR is raised in anaemia?
Ans:
i. In anaemia there is low erythrocyte mass compared to plasma. This change in the ratio of erythrocyte to plasma favours rouleaux formation and quicker sedimentation.
ii. Microcytes sediment more slowly and macrocytes somewhat more quickly compared to normocytes. The sedimentation of RBCs is directly proportional of RBC aggregates and inversely proportional to the RBC surface area. The microcytes have lower surface area to volume ratio.

Q2. Why ESR is low in sickle cell anaemia and spherocytosis?
Ans: Red cells with abnormal or irregular shape (poikilocytosis) hamper rouleaux formation. In sickle cell anaemia, the RBCs are abnormal in shape (sickle or crescentic in shape). So, ESR become low because of slower rouleaux formation.

In spherocytosis, because of the spherical shape (normal biconcave shape) RBCs have more surface area. As ESR is inversely proportional to the RBC surface, this increase in surface area causes decreased ESR.

Q3. How ESR can be used to monitor prognosis of disease?
Ans: ESR can be used to see the response to treatment in some diseases like tuberculosis, rheumatoid arthritis, polymyalgia rheumatica and temporal arteritis. If these diseases respond to treatment, the ESR tends to be lower over time.

In Hodgkin's disease, ESR, of less than 10 mm in first hour indicates good prognosis while ESR of more than 60 mm in first hour indicates poor prognosis.

Q4. Compare Westergren and Wintrobe methods of ESR as far as advantages and disadvantages are concerned.
Ans: Westergren method is more sensitive when ESR is high. Because ESR in this method has three phases with a longer second phase, so sinking of RBCs occurs better in a larger tube add longer second phase gives more accurate result when ESR is high.

But in Wintrobe's tube sinking of RBCs occurs quickly and packing is fast because it has a shorter tube length. So, Wintrobe's method is more sensitive when ESR is low.

Q5. Why Westergren's method is preferred to Wintrobe's method? While estimating ESR.
Ans:
i. When ESR becomes high Westergren method gives more accurate result.
ii. It is more sensitive because the pipette is longer and there are more markings (graduations).

Q6. What are advantages of Wintrobe's method?
Ans: In this method, ESR is estimated first and then the Wintrobe tube is centrifuged to get PCV. Moreover, the colour of plasma gives clues to certain diseases. Yellow plasma indicates jaundice, red-coloured plasma indicates haemoglobinaemia (intravascular haemolysis) and white in hyperlipidaemia (chyle).

Q7. What is automated ESR method?
Ans: The blood was drawn into special MONOSED vacutainers of Monitor 100® (1.6 ml, 120 mm long, 6 mm diameter) with 1.28 ml of automatic draw containing 0.32 ml of 3.2% sodium citrate. The blood citrate mix reaches up to a maximum length of 60 mm from the bottom of the tube. After proper mixing, the samples were immediately transferred to the analyzer. The ESR reading is taken through a 45 mm high window, 2 mm above the maximum sample level. The Monitor 100® has the advantage of giving the result of 100 samples in 30 minutes (equivalent to 1 hour Westergren reading) and 60 minutes (equivalent to 2 hours Westergren reading). The machine Monitor 100® supplied by Electra Lab, Italy.

Marked discrepancy in the ESR result was noted for high ESR values when compared between manual and automated methods. But it was not seen for normal ESR values. So, a correction factor to be applied when ERS is very high for this automated method.

Q8. What are the length and diameter of Wintrobe's tube? What amount of blood it can hold?

Ans: The tube has length of 110 mm and internal diameter of 3 mm. It is graduated at 1 mm intervals and marked 0 to 100 mm from above downward and also from below upwards.

The tube can hold about 1 ml of blood.

Q9. How PCV is used to determine red cell indices?

Ans:
i. **Mean corpuscular volume (MCV)**
   It is the average volume of RBC and is calculated from red cell count and haematocrit volume

   MCV = PCV in L/L ÷ RBC count/L (normal value is either 85 + 8 fl or 77–93 fl.)

ii. **Mean corpuscular haemoglobin (MCH)**
   It is the content by weight of haemoglobin of average red cell.

   MCH = Hb/L ÷ RBC count/L (normal range is either 29.5 + 2.5 pg or 27–32 pg)

iii. **Mean corpuscular haemoglobin concentration (MCHC)**
   It is the average of haemoglobin concentration and haematocrit value which is expressed in terms of PCV (0.45 deciliter normally).

   MCHC = Hb/dl ÷ PCV in L/L (normal range is either 32.5 + 2.5 g/dl or 30–35 g/dl)

As MCHC is independent of RBC count and size, it is considered to have greater clinical significance as compared to other red cell indices. It is low in iron deficiency anaemia but usually normal in macrocytic anaemia.

Clinical significance of red cell indices

- In iron deficiency anaemia and thalassaemia, MCV, MCH and MCHC are reduced.

- In anaemia due to acute blood loss and haemolytic anaemias, MCV and MCH are usually within normal limits.

- In megaloblastic anaemia, MCV and MCH are high but MCHC is usually normal. This is because the amount of haemoglobin increases proportionately with the increase in cell size. Hence, MCHC remains normal though MCV and MCH are high.

Q10. What are the values of red cell indices (absolute values) when there is both iron and folate deficiencies?

Ans: Anaemia is macrocytic and hypochromic. So, MCV is high, MCH is low or normal and MCHC is low.

6

Haemoglobin Estimation

INTRODUCTION

Hemoglobin (American) or haemoglobin (British); abbreviated as Hb or Hgb, is the iron-containing oxygen-transporting **metalloprotein** in the red blood cells of all vertebrate anaemias as well as the tissue of some invertebrates. It carries oxygen in the blood from respiratory organs (lungs) to other parts of the body or tissues. In the tissues, Hb releases oxygen to permit aerobic respiration which provides energy by metabolic process.

In mammals including humans, the protein component in red blood cell is about 96% by dry weight and approximately 35% when water is included. Hb has an oxygen carrying capacity of 1.34 ml O_2 per gram. The mammalian Hb can bind up to four oxygen molecules. Hb also transports other gases like carbon dioxide (CO_2) in respiratory system, some of which form carbaminohaemoglobin in which CO_2 is bound to globin protein thiol group. It can also bind nitric oxide (NO) to a globin protein thiol group.

Apart from red cells, Hb is also found in the A9 dopaminergic neurons of the substantia nigra, macrophages, alveolar cells and mesangial cells of kidney. In these tissues, haemoglobin does not act as oxygen carrier rather it acts as an anti-oxidant and a regulator of iron-metabolism.

SYNTHESIS OF HAEMOGLOBIN

It is synthesized in a complex series of steps. The heme part is synthesized in mitochondria and in the cytosol of immature RBCs. The globin protein is synthesized by ribosomes in the cytosol of RBC. Production of Hb continues in the cells (RBCs) throughout its early development from the proerythroblast to the reticulocyte in bone marrow. At this stage, the nucleus of mammalian red cells is lost but not in birds and in some other species. Even after losing the nucleus in mammalian RBCs, residual ribosomal RNA allows further synthesis of haemoglobin until the recticulocytes loses its RNA as soon it enters the vasculature. This haemoglobin-synthetic RNA has reticulated appearance and hence it is named **reticulocyte**.

HAEMOGLOBIN DERIVATIVES

Methaemoglobin (Hi)

Methaemoglobin is a derivative of haemoglobin in which the ferrous iron of haemoglobin is oxidized to the ferric state which results in the inability of Hi to combine reversibly with oxygen. The polypeptide chains are not altered.

Up to 1.5% of total haemoglobin may be methaemoglobin in normal person.

Increased in the Hi the blood will cause cyanosis and functional anaemia. Cyanosis becomes evident when the methaemoglobin concentration is 1.5 g Hi/dl or 10% of total haemoglobin in blood. Five abnormal haemoglobins have been identified in humans, whose principal consequence is asymptomatic cyanosis as a result of methaemoglobinemia. These are known as haemoglobin M (HbM) disease.

But most cases of methaemoglobinemia are secondary or acquired mainly due to drugs. These drugs are nitrates, nitrites, quinones, chlorates, sulfonamides, phenacetin, aniline dyes, etc.

Sulfhaemoglobin (SHb)

Sulfhaemoglobin is a mixture of oxidized, partially denatured forms of haemoglobin which is formed during oxidative haemolysis. During oxidation of haemoglobin, sulphur from source is incorporated into the heme rings of haemoglobin. It results in the formation of green-coloured hemochrome, known as sulfhaemoglobin (SHb). Further oxidation of this sulfhaemoglobin will result in the denaturation and precipitation of haemoglobin known as **Heinz bodies**. Unlike methaemoglobin, sulfhaemoglobin cannot be reduced back to haemoglobin (irreversible) and it remains within the cells until they break down.

Sulfhaemoglobin (SHb) has been reported after receiving drugs like sulfonamide, phenacetin, acetanilid, in patients with severe constipation or bacteremia due to *Clostridium perfringes*. Normal person may have <1% sulfhaemoglobin. Sulfhaemoglobinemia results in cyanosis but is usually asymptomatic.

Carboxyhaemoglobin (HbCO)

Haemoglobin can bind with carbon monoxide (CO) with an affinity 210 times greater than that for oxygen. Carbon monoxide can bind with Hb even its concentration in the air is very low (0.02–0.04%). In this situation, HbCO or carboxyhaemoglobin will be formed.

Endogenous CO is produced during degradation of heme to bilirubin, usually accounts for 0.5% of carboxyhaemoglobin.

Carboxyhaemoglobin cannot bind to and carry oxygen. Also increased concentration of HbCO, shifts the Hb–oxygen dissociation curve towards left resulting in tissue anoxia.

Increased carboxyhaemoglobin is fomed due to acute carbon monoxide posisoning. The chief sources of CO are illuminating gas, gasoline motors, gas heaters and tobacco smoking. Chronic exposure through tobacco/cigarette smoking may lead to chronic increase of HbCO and left shift of oxygen dissociation curve. Hence, smokers tend to have higher haematocrit/PCV (increased red cell mass) and may have polycythemia too.

NORMAL HAEMOGLOBIN TYPES IN HUMAN

Human haemoglobin is formed of two pairs of globin chains to each of which is attached one molecule of haem. There are six different types of globin chains, designated by the Greek letters α, β, γ, δ, ε, and ζ. The composition of a haemoglobin is specified by a formula such as $\alpha_2 \beta_2$ (adult haemoglobin) which indicates a tetramer containing two α chains (one pair) and two β chains (one pair). The α chain is directed by two α genes, α_1 and α_2 which are present on chromosome 11. The γ chain is directed by two genes like α chains, these are $^G\gamma$ and $^A\gamma$, which are also present on chromosome 11.

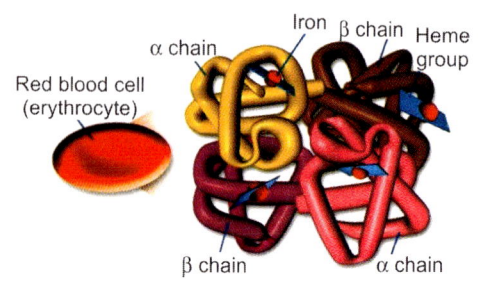

Fig. 6.1: Structure of haemoglobin

Haemoglobin Estimation

In the first three months of embryonic development, when blood cells are produced in the yolk sac, embryonic haemoglobins such as Hb Gower 1 ($\zeta_2 \epsilon_2$), Hb Gower 2 ($\alpha_2 \epsilon_2$) and Hb Portland ($\zeta_2 \gamma_2$) are produced. As erythropoiesis shifts to the liver and spleen, the fetal haemogloblin, (HbF) ($\alpha_2 \gamma_2$) appears. When erythropoiesis shifts to the bone marrow during the first year of life, the adult haemoglobins (HbA) ($\alpha_2 \beta_2$) and HbA$_2$ ($\alpha_2 \delta_2$) begin to be produced.

In the embryo
- Gower 1 ($\zeta_2 \epsilon_2$)
- Gower 2 ($\alpha_2 \epsilon_2$)
- Haemoglobin Portland 1 ($\zeta_2 \gamma_2$)
- Haemoglobin Portland 2 ($\zeta_2 \beta_2$)

In the foetus
Haemoglobin F ($\alpha_2 \gamma_2$)

After birth
- **Haemoglobin A ($\alpha_2 \beta_2$)**, the most common Hb (95%)
- **Haemoglobin A$_2$ ($\alpha_2 \delta_2$)**: δ chain synthesis begins late in the third trimester and in adults, it has normal range of 1–3.5%.
- **Haemoglobin F ($\alpha_2 \gamma_2$)**: It is present in large amount at birth (65–95%) but in adults, it is trace in amount (<1%).

Hb Variants in Different Diseases

- **Haemoglobin H (β_4)**: A variant form of haemoglobin, formed by tetramer of β chains, which may be present in variants of α thalassaemia.
- **Haemoglobin Bart (γ_4)**: A variant of haemoglobin, formed by tetramer of γ chains, which may be present in α thalassaemia.
- **Haemoglobin S ($\alpha_2 \beta_2^S$)**: Hb found in sickle cell disease, here glutamine is replaced by valine in β_6 position.
- **Haemoglobin C ($\alpha_2 \beta_2^C$)**: Here, there is substitution of glutamic acid by lysine molecule in β_6 position.
- **Haemoglobin SC disease**: A compound heterozygous form with one sickle gene and another encoding haemoglobin C.
- **Haemoglobin AS disease**: A heterozygous form causing sickle cell trait with one adult gene and one sicke cell disease gene.
- **Haemoglobin D—Punjab ($\alpha_2 \beta_2^D$)**: The disease produces mild anaemia.
- **Haemoglobin E ($\alpha_2 \beta_2^E$)**: Another variant due to a variation in the β chain gene. This variant causes a mild chronic haemolytic anaemia.
- **β Thalassaemia major**: Moderate to high increase of HbF and normal to slight increase of HbA$_2$.
- **β Thalassaemia minor**: Moderate to high rise of HbA$_2$, normal or slight increase in HbF.
- **Hb Bart—hydrops faetalis (α thalassaemia)**: Haemoglobin Bart (γ_4) is 80–90%, some HbH and Hb Portland. Usually HbA, HbA$_2$ or HbF absent.

DIFFERENT METHODS OF HAEMOGLOBIN ESTIMATION

1. Photocoloroimetric method: Cyanomethaemoglobin method or Drabkin's method
2. Acid haematin method or Sahli method
3. Alkaline-haematin method
4. Oxyhaemoglobin (HbO$_2$) method
5. Tallqvist method
6. Copper sulphate method
7. Lovibond comparator method
8. HemoCue method
9. Chemical (iron content) method
10. Van Slyke's oxygen capacity method or gasometric method
11. Automated analyzer method
12. Spectroscopic method
13. Haemoglobin colour scale method

Of these methods, cyanomethaemoglobin (HiCN) method or Drabkin method is most widely used and reliable method. Acid haematin method or Sahli's method used in the past mainly in the small laboratories, now become obsolete as it is less accurate. With the invent of automated analyzer, other methods are being replaced in modern laboratories as it is accurate, reliable and fast.

Table 6.1: Nature of method used and principle of the method

Method	Principle of the method

1. Colorimetric method
  A. *Visual colorimetric method*
    i. Sahli's method or acid haematin method
    ii. Alkaline haematin method
  B. *Photocolorimetric or photoelectric method*
    i. Cyanomethaemoglobin (HiCN) method
    ii. Automated analyzer
    iii. Haldane method
    iv. Oxyhaemoglobin method
    v. HemoCue method
	These methods are based on measuring the colour of haemoglobin of the test compared to standard. This is done either by **naked eye (visually) or by photocolorimetry**. The optical density of a coloured solution is directly proportional to the concentration of the coloured material in the solution

2. Physical method	Specific gravity
3. Gasometric method	Oxygen combining capacity of haemoglobin
4. Chemical method	Iron content of the haemoglobin

Acid Haematin or Sahli Method

This method of Hb estimation is not very accurate because different forms of haemoglobins are not converted to acid haematin, and the brown colour which develops is unstable and begins to fade almost immediately after it has its peak. Also, there is subjective biasness of colour matching. It is done in some rural areas where colorimeter is not available.

Principle

Haemoglobin is converted into acid haematin by adding N/10 hydrochloric acid. The acid haematin solution is further diluted with the acid until its colour (brown) matches exactly that of the permanent standard (brown glass reference block) of the comparator block.

But the acid haematin formed in this method is a colloidal suspension and it can not be read in colorimeter which requires optically clear solution.

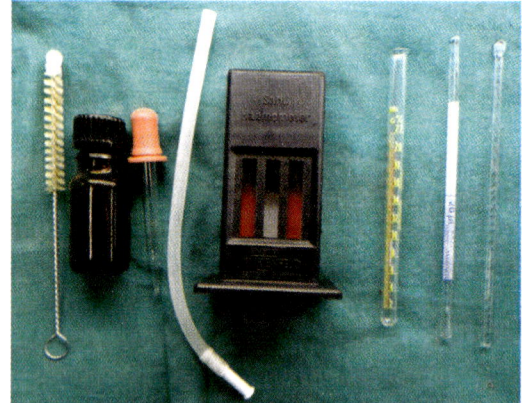

Fig. 6.2: Reagents and equipment for Sahli's method

Reagents and Equipment

1. Hydrochloric acid solution (N/10 or 0.1 N)
2. **Haemoglobinometer pipette or Sahli's pipette:** This is a slender special pipette with a single mark of 0.02 ml or 20 cu mm.
3. **Haemoglobinometer tube (calibrated tube):** This tube has markings on ascending order on both sides. On one side it shows grams per 100 ml (left side) and other side it shows percentage (right side). Presently used Hellige's tubes are square shaped, it has 14.5 gm as 100%.
4. **Sahli's haemoglobinometer or comparator box:** It is used to match the colour

of acid haematin formed in the haemoglobinometer tube with that of colour standard in the comparator box.
5. **Glass rod (stirrer)**: For mixing the blood in the square/round tube.
6. **Distilled water**

Procedure

The graduated haemoglobinometer tube is filled to the lowest mark, i.e. till 20 mark with N/10 HCl (0.1 N). Now, with the help of haemoglobinometer piptte or Sahli's pipette draw 20 cu mm of blood. This blood can be EDTA or double oxalate mixed or it can be from finger prick (capillary blood). This blood is immediately mixed with the N/10 HCl present in the haemoglobinometer tube. Mix them well by shaking the tube well. The tube is then allowed to stand with in the comparator box and keep it for 10–30 minutes (at least 10 minutes) for full conversion of the haemoglobin into acid haematin (development of brown colour).

Distilled water is then added drop by drop and stirred with a stirrer (glass rod) till the colour matches well with the fixed colour (reference) in the comparator box. The matching or comparison should be done only in natural day light.

Reading: The mark matching with the upper level of diluted acid haematin indicates the level of haemoglobin and is expressed in terms of gm/dl.

Note
- After 10 minutes, 95% colour develops (conversion of haemoglobin to acid haematin) and after 20 minutes 98% colour develops.
- This method does not estimate caboxyhaemoglobin, methaemoglobin, fetal haemoglobin and sulfhaemoglobin.
- Non-haemoglobin substances like protein, lipid or cell stroma may affect the colour of blood diluted with N/10 HCl. They may interfere with the converted acid haematin and hence the result.

Advantage of the method: It is easy, simple and cheap method.

Disadvantages of the method
i. It is not an accurate method.
ii. It cannot measures all type of haemoglobins like caboxyhaemoglobin, methaemoglobin, foetal haemoglobin and sulfhaemoglobin as it cannot convert these haemoglobins into acid haematin.
iii. As it is a visual method chances of error is high because of subjective variation.

Sources of errors
i. Improper collection of blood (venipuncture technique, finger prick).
ii. Improper mixing of blood with anticoagulant (EDTA).
iii. Delay in taking results. The brown colour of acid haematin is unstable and the colour fades away with time.

Cyanomethaemoglobin Method (by Colorimetric or Spectrophotometric Method)

As already described, this is the most widely used method of haemoglobin estimation in the world. Also, as a best quality control this method is internationally recommended.

Principle of this Method

Blood is mixed with potassium cyanide and potassium ferricyanide mixture. Potassium ferricyanide oxidises haemoglobin to methaemoglobin (Hi). Then potassium cyanide provides cyanide ions (CN^-) to it, and it is converted to cyanomethaemoglobin (HiCN). This cyanomethaemoglobin has a broad absorption, maximum at a wavelength of 540 nm. The absorption of the solution is measured in a photoelectric colorimeter or spectrophotometer using 540 nm wavelength or yellow-green filter with that of a standard HiCN solution.

Remember, in this **method haemoglobin, methaemoglobin and carboxyhaemoglobin can be measured but not the**

sulfhaemoglobin (sulfhaemoglobin can be measured by spectroscopic method or photoelectric method at 620 nm wavelength and alkaline haematin method).

Original Drabkin's solution
- Potassium cyanide (KCN): 50 mg
- Potassium ferricyanide [$K_3Fe(CN)_6$]: 200 mg
- Sodium bicarbonate ($NaHCO_3$): 1 gm
- Distilled water: 1000 ml

Modified Drabkin's solution (as recommended by International Committee for Standardization in Haeatology or ICSH)
- Potassium cyanide: 50 mg
- Potassium ferricyanide: 200 mg
- Potassium dihydrogen phosphate: 140 mg
- Non-ionic detergent: 1 ml (like Nonidet P40 from Sigma, Triton X-100 or Saponic 218)
- Distilled water: 1000 ml

The original Drabkin's solution had a pH of 8.6. But the modified Drabkin's solution has a pH of 9.6. This modified solution is less likely to cause turbidity from precipitation of plasma proteins. Also it takes shorter conversion time (3–5 minutes) compared to original Drabkin's solution (15–25 minutes).

Reference solution: It can forms to the international specifications and is available commercially. It contains 550–850 mg of haemoglobin/Litre and it is dispensed in 10 ml sealed ampoules.

Procedure

20 cu mm (20 µl) of blood is collected (EDTA or oxalate mixed venous blood or capillary blood after finger prick) with the help of haemoglobinometer pipette. This blood is then mixed with 4 ml of Drabkin's solution in a test tube. Invert the test tubes several times for proper mixing. So, dilution of blood is 201 times (dilution factor is 201).

Allow the mixture to stand at room temperature for 15–25 minutes (minimum 15 minutes) for complete development of cyanomethaemoglobin (HiCN). Test solution is compared with the standard and reagent blank in a colorimeter or spectrophotometer.

Calculation

Hb concentration of the test
= optical density of test solution/optical density of standard solution × **concentration standard (mg/100 ml) × dilution factor/1000**

Note

If 20 cu mm (0.02 ml) of blood is mixed with 4 ml of Drabkin's solution, then dilution factor is 200, whereas if 20 cu mm (0.02 ml) of blood is mixed with 5 ml of Drabkin's solution, then dilution factor is 250.

Advantages of Cyanomethaemoglobin Method

1. The test result is accurate, so, ICSH recommends it.
2. It measures different forms of haemoglobin (except sulfhaemoglobin)
3. The standard solution is commercially available as per international specification (International Committee for Standardization in Hematology or ICSH). So, the test can be easily standardized.
4. Cyanomethaemoglobin reagent (also called Drabkin's solution) is very stable.

Disadvantages of Cyanomethaemoglobin Method

1. The use potassium cyanide (KiCN) in the preparation of Drabkin's solution is a potential health hazard. However, Drabkin solution contains only 50 mg of KCN/litre, so it is relatively safe. To produce serious health problem/poisoning, someone has to swallow 600–1000 mg of it (12–20 liters of solution).
2. It takes longer time (15–25 minutes) for complete conversion of cyanome-

thaemoglobin (HiCN). Modified Drabkin solution takes shorter time (3–5 minutes).
3. If the blood contains carboxyhaemoglobin (HbCO), this rate of conversion is more slower.

Note

To avoid cyanide (KiCN), lauryl sulphate has been proposed as it has similar properties to HiCN.

Other Methods of Hb Estimation

1. **Oxyhaemoglobin method:** This is the quickest and simplest method for use with a photoelectric colorimeter. The haemoglobin is converted to oxyhaemoglobin (HbO_2) with the help of liquor ammonia (ammonium hydroxide) solution and is read in 540 nm wavelength or with yellow-green filter. The reliability of this method is not affected by a moderate rise in plasma bilirubin. But the result is not satisfactory in presence of carboxyhaemoglobin, methaemoglobin or sulfhaemoglobin.

2. **Alkaline haematin method:** There are two methods which follows alkaline haematin method: (a) The standard method using Gibson and Harrison's standard, (b) The acid alkali method.

    It is a useful ancillary method under special circumstances as it gives a true estimate of total haemoglobin even if methaemoglobin, carboxyhaemoglobin or sulfhaemoglobin is present. Plasma proteins and lipids have a little effects on the development of colour. Fetal haemoglobin (HbF) and Bart haemoglobin (γ_4) cannot be estimated by this method as they are resistant to alkali denaturation normally. But this problem can be overcomed by heating the solution containing HbF or γ_4 in a boiling water for 4–5 minutes.

3. **Spectroscopic method:** For qualitative and quantitative estimation of methaemoglobin and sulfhaemoglobin; spectroscopic examination of blood is very reliable.

4. **Chemical (iron content) method:** Normally iron content of haemoglobin is 0.347%. Hb estimation of blood can be done by estimating total blood iron and dividing it by 3.47. This method is no longer in use.

5. **van Slyke's oxygen capacity method or Gasometric method:** It is an indirect method which estimates the amount of haemoglobin from the amount of oxygen it absorbs with the use of van Slyke's apparatus. This method is very complicated.

- Oxygen carrying capacity measured by van Slyke apparatus
- Based on formula, 1 gm of Hb carries 1.34 ml of oxygen
- It does not measure carboxyhemoglobin
- Sulfhemoglobin
- Methemoglobin
- Time-consuming and expensive
- Result is 2% less than other methods

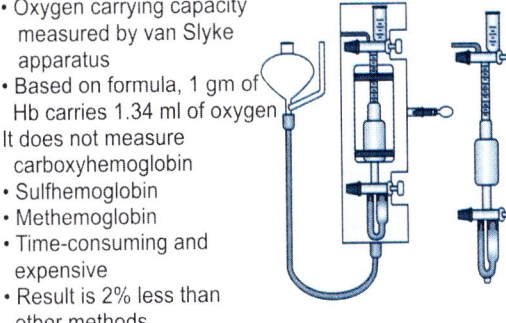

Fig. 6.3: Gasometric method

6. **Specific gravity method:** Normal specific gravity of human average in men is 1.057 and in women is 1.053. By calculating specific gravity of an unknown sample, its haemoglobin content is estimated. This method is very rapid and uncomplicated. It is used to screen the potential blood donors for anaemia.

7. **WHO haemoglobin colour scale method:** The haemoglobin colour scale (HCS) is a simple, rapid and cheap method for Hb estimation with a finger prick sample. It has been developed for use in resource—poor settings when there is no laboratory. The method relies on comparing the colour of a drop of blood sample absorbed onto a filter paper with standard colour on a laminated card, varying from pink to

dark red. These colours correspond to haemoglobin levels of 4, 6, 8, 10, 12, and 14 g/dl. Intermediate shades can be identified, allowing haemoglobin levels to be judged to 1 g/dl. This test is used for mass screening of anaemia and has been adopted by World Health Organization (WHO).

8. **HemoCue method:** In this method, the reaction in the microcuvette is a modified azide methaemoglobin reaction. The microcuvette contains three reagents in dried forms (sodium deoxycholate, sodium nitrite, sodium azide) which convert Hb into azide methaemoglobin (HiCN). Single purpose derived photometer (colorimeter) uses double wavelength filters (570 nm and 880 nm) and measures Hb.

It is WHO approved method for Hb estimation among blood donors.

Normal/Reference Range of Haemoglobin

- Adult males: 13–17 g/dl
- Adult females (nonpregnant): 12.0–15.0 g/dl
- Adult females (pregnant): 11.0–14.0 g/dl
- Child: 6 months–12 years: 11.5–15.5 g/dl
- Chidren: 6 months–6 years: 11.0–14.0 g/dl
- Infants: 2–6 months: 9.5–14.0 g/dl
- Newborns: 13.6–19.6 g/dl

Decreased in Hb concentration: Hb is decreased in all anaemias, in most causes as a consequence of another disease or a deficiency (folate, vit B_{12}, iron).

Increased in Hb concentration

- Hb is increased as a physiologic response to high altitude due to low oxygen tension or in advanced lung or cardiac disease.
- Certain myeloproliferative neoplasms, especially polycythaemia vera (when Hb in men is >18 gm/dl and in women is 16.5 gm/dl).

Limitations of Accurate Hb Estimation

- Errors arise from improper venipuncture or finger prick that may induce haemoconcentration.
- During sample preparation in manual methods, dilution mistakes may occur, or there may be sample turbidity due to improperly lysed RBCs during processing by automated counters which affect the accuracy of the results.

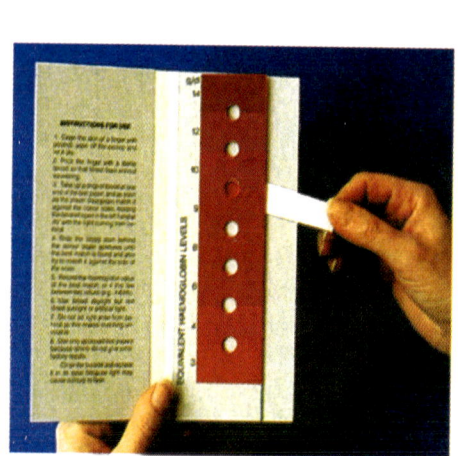
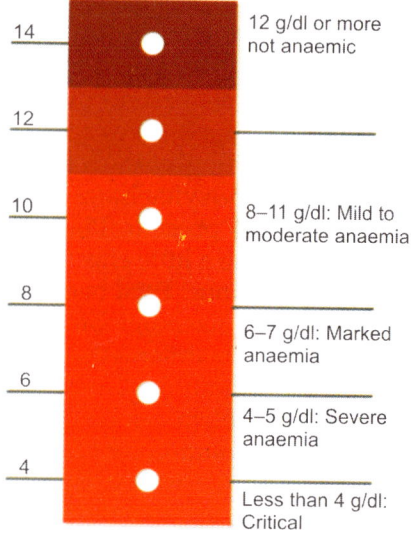

Fig. 6.4: Haemoglobin colour scale (HCS)

- Hyperlipidaemia, dehydration, marked leukocytosis or high plasma protein result in erroneous result.

Haemoglobin Colour Scale (HCS) Method

The haemoglobin colour scale is a simple, rapid and cheap method for Hb estimation with a finger prick sample. It has been developed for use in resource-poor settings when there is no laboratory. The method relies on comparing the colour of a drop of blood sample, absorbed onto a filter paper with standard colours on a laminated card, varying from pink to dark red. These colours correspond to haemoglobin levels of 4, 6, 8, 10, 12 and 14 g/dl. Intermediate shades can be identified, allowing haemoglobin levels to be judged to 1 g/dl. This test has been adopted by World Health Organization (WHO).

Table 6.2: Advantages and disadvantages of different methods of haemoglobin estimation

Name of the method	Advantages	Disadvantages
1. Sahli method	• Simple • Cheap	• Inaccurate results • Inter-observer variability • Colour developed (acid haematin) is unstable • No international standard
2. Cyanomethaemoglobin method	• Stable compound (HiCN) gives accurate measurement • International standard available	• Turbidity due to other factors may cause inaccurate results • Time consuming • Reagent cyanide is toxic
3. Tallqvist method	• Simple and rapid • Inexpensive and portable • Reagents and electricity not required	• Results affected by size, thickness of blood spot, temperature, lighting and humidity • Only supplied filter paper can be used which is limited quantity.
4. Copper sulphate method	• Inexpensive • Simple and rapid • Electricity not required	• Inaccurate • Requires fresh solutions • Only ranges of Hb levels are obtained not exact figure • Proper disposal of standard solutions
5. Haemoglobin colour scale method adapted by WHO	• Simple and portable • Cheap • Electricity not required	• Inter-observer biasness
6. Lovibond comparator method	• Rapid and simple • Useful for routine screening • Electricity not required	• Expensive • Requires precise dilution • Requires large drop of blood • Subjective interpretation
7. HemoCue	• Simple and portable • Rapid and immediate result • Accurate and reliable • Easy to perform • Battery operated	• Expensive as it uses disposable cuvettes
8. Automated analyzer	• Accurate • Reliable	• Expensive • Small laboratories or rural setups cannot afford

VIVA VOCE

Q1. Which is better and practical method for haemoglobin estimation and why?
Ans: In laboratories, where there is no autoanalyzer, cyanomethaemoglobin estimation is most widely used method for haemoglobin estimation. Because it has several advantages over other methods:
i. Cyanomethaemoglobin is a stable compound and colour does not fade easily. But in other methods like Sahli's (acid haematin) method, colour begins to fade after ten minutes. So, in acid haematin method, lower haemoglobin level will be obtained if reading is delayed.
ii. Almost all haemoglobin except sulfhaemoglobin is converted to cyanomethaemoglobin. So, this method can calculate almost all haemoglobins.
iii. This is a colorimetric method, so personal error like matching colour as in Sahli's method is absent.
iv. A stable reference standard is available.
v. The test result is accurate, hence, ICSH (International Committee for Standardization in Haematology) recommends it.

However, automated analyzer method is best as it is reliable, accurate and fastest.

Q2. What are the different uses of haemoglobin (Hb) pipette?
Ans: It uses 0.02 ml (20 mm^3) of blood (or fluid). So, Hb pipette can be used wherever different dilutions are required:

i. For RBC count: 4 ml RBC fluid + 0.02 ml blood (dilution 1:200).
ii. For total WBC count: 0.4 ml Türk's/WBC fluid + 0.02 ml blood in a small test tube to mix it (dilution 1:20).
iii. For platelet count: 0.4 ml platelet count fluid + 0.02 ml blood (dilution 1:20).
iv. For eosinophil count: 0.2 ml of Dunger's fluid + 0.02 ml blood (dilutions 1:20).
v. It can be used for body fluid cell count, sperm count, etc. also.

Q3. Why is N/10 HCl used in Sahli's method, not N/5 or N/15 HCl?
Ans: The Sahli's method (acid haematin method) has been standardized by using N/10 HCl. Brown colour of the comparator glass is equivalent to the colour of acid haematin produced by using N/10 HCl in a standard blood sample which contains 14.8 gm% Hb. Test sample is compared against this standard sample.

Q4. In automated cell counter, what chemical regent is used to detect Hb?
Ans: Sodium lauryl sulphate (SLS) is used which converts all Hb into detectable chromogen rapidly.

Q 5. What are the physiological variations of Hb concentration?
Ans:
i. Splenic contractions may occur after strenuous exercise which pumps more blood in the circulation as spleen is a reservoir of blood. So, hemoconcentration and falsely raised Hb occurs. Even anticipation of venipuncture (blood) collection may cause splenic contraction as observed by Brown A et al.
ii. Hb raises as increase with altitude.
iii. Hb value highest in the morning and lowest in the evening.

Q6. What are the conditions where Hb is falsely raised?
Ans:
i. When blood is drawn for Hb estimation during intravenous blood transfusion or iron containing drugs.
ii. After burns, acute diarrhoea, severe dehydration due to hemoconcentration.

Q7. In which diseases, Hb level is raised?
Ans:
- Polycythaemia vera
- COPD (chronic obstructive pulmonary disease)
- Emphysema.
- Renal cell carcinoma due to ectopic productions of erythropoietin

- Congenital heart disease in adults
- Smoking for long duration may cause smoker's polycythemia due to formation of carboxyhaemoglobin.

Q8. What are the conditions where Hb is falsely decreased or spurious/pseudo anaemia?
Ans:
i. In 3rd trimester of pregnancy, due to increase in plasma volume, Hb concentration falls (1–2 gm/dl).
ii. Splenomegaly due to pooling of red cells in spleen
iii. Congestive heart failure due to fluid retention
iv. Multiple myeloma/paraproteinemia
v. During hypervolaemia (intravenous fluid infusion), Hb level falls.

Q9. Why should the stirrer not taken out of Haemoglobin meter tube?
Ans: If stirrer is taken out of tube immediately small amount of acid haematin (formed during reaction) sticking to the stirrer (glass rod) is lost which will give lower Hb result. So, the stirrer should be lifted from the solution in the upper part of the tube when reading is taken.

Q10. In Sahli's method, why are flat comparator glasses and square tube are preferred?
Ans: It is easier to compare flat surface rather curvature or round surfaces. So, square tube containing acid haematin can be easily compared with flat brown surface of comparator box. Error due to curvature can be avoided.

7. Bleeding Time (BT), Clotting Time (CT), Prothrombin Time (PT) and APTT Time

BLEEDING TIME

Definition: The time required for complete stoppage of free flow blood from a deep puncture wound on the skin is known as bleeding time.

Principle: A standard incision is made on the skin and the total time the incision bleeds (starting of bleeding to end of bleeding) is measured. Cessation of bleeding indicates the formation of hemostatic plugs which are dependent on an adequate number of platelets and on the ability of the platelets to adhere to the subendothelium and to form aggregates.

Standardized Template Method for BT

Materials
- Sphygmomanometer
- Cleansing swabs
- Template bleeding time device (commercially available)
- Filter paper (1 mm thick)
- Stopwatch

Method: Place a sphygmomanometer cuff around the patient's arm above the elbow. Inflate the cuff to 40 mm Hg pressure and keep this pressure throughout the entire test. Clean the ventral (volar) aspect of the forearm with 70% ethanol. Choose an area of forearm skin (cleaned) that is devoid of visible superficial veins. Press a sterile metal template with a linear slit 7–8 mm long firmly against the skin aligned along the long axis of the arm and use a scalpel blade with a guard (the tip of the blade should protrudes 1 mm through the template slit). Then make an incision 6 mm long and 1 mm deep.

Modifications of the template and blade which make two simultaneous cuts with a spring mechanism are also available commercially.

Now, blot off the blood exuding from the cut with filter paper at 15 seconds interval. Do not contact the wound during this procedure. When bleeding has ceased, carefully oppose the edges of the incision and apply an adhesive strip to lessen the rise of keloid formation and an ugly scar.

Normal range: 2.5–9.5 minutes.

Ivy's Method for BT

This test is almost similar to the previous standardized template method. But instead of a standardized incision, two punctures, 5–10 cm apart are made in quick succession using a disposable (or No. 11 surgical blade). The punctures should have cutting depth of 2.5 mm and width of just 1 mm is suitable. When the bleeding has ceased, a sterile adhesive strip is placed on the wounds.

Normal range: 2–7 minutes.

Duke Method for BT

The ear lobule (or heel of an infant) is cleaned with 70% alcohol and allowed to dry. A 3 mm deep stab wound is made with the help of disposable lancet in the margin of ear lobe (or heel). Stopwatch is started when the wound starts to bleed. The flowing blood is soaked by a filter paper lightly and gently at 15 seconds interval. When the wound stops to bleed, the stopwatch is pressed to stop. The time is noted as bleeding time.

Normal range: 2–5 minutes

Interpretation of the Test (BT)

- Bleeding time 1–9 minutes: Normal
- Bleeding time 9–15 minutes: Platelet dysfunction
- Bleeding time >15 minutes: Critical, test must be discontinued and pressure should be applied to the wound to stop bleeding.
- Bleeding time may be prolonged due to low platelet count or thrombocytopenia ($<100,000/mm^3$). When platelet counts are low, expected bleeding time can be predicted with the following formula:

$$\text{Bleeding time (BT)} = \frac{30.5 \times \text{platelet count}/mm^3}{3850}$$

A bleeding time longer than that expected calculated time from number of platelet alone (using above formula), may be due to defective platelet function in addition to platelet number.

- The Ivy's method and standardized template method are better to evaluate bleeding time.

Causes of Prolonged Bleeding Time

1. **Thrombocytopenia (platelet count $<100,000/mm^3$):** It may be primary (essential) or secondary. When the platelet count is $<50,000/mm^3$, patient may have very long bleeding time and the bleeding may be difficult to arrest. So, bleeding time is contraindicated in this situation.
2. **Defective or qualitative abnormality of platelets:** They may be congenital such as thrombasthenia, storage pool defects or acquired; due to drugs, the presence of paraprotein (multiple myeloma) or platelet abnormalities as in myelodysplastic syndromes (MDS).
3. **von Willebrand's disease:** There is defective platelet adherence to the sub-endeothelium as there is absence/defective von Willebrand factor.
4. **Vascular abnormalities:** As found in Ehlers-Danlos syndrome, or in pseudo-xanthoma elasticum.
5. **Deficiency of clotting factors:** Occasionally sever deficiency or factor V or XI or afibrinogenaemia may cause prolonged bleeding time.
6. **Others:** Severe liver disease, leukaemia, DIC, aplastic anaemia.

Interfering Factors

- The normal range may vary if the puncture wound is not of standard depth and width.
- Ingestion of certain drug before the test will cause prolonged BT. Examples: aspirin, dextran, streptokinase, mithramycin.
- Heavy alcohol consumption may cause prolonged BT.
- Touching the incision, during the test will break of haemostatic plugs or fibrin strands that will lead to prolonged BT.

CLOTTING TIME OR COAGULATION TIME

Definition: Coagulation time is the time required for a whole blood sample to coagulate *in vitro* under standard conditions.

Principle of the test: Coagulation or clotting time (CT) measures all three stages of coagulation (intrinsic pathway, extrinsic pathway and common pathway) as a whole but it is more sensitive to intrinsic pathway defects. Utmost care should be taken so that thromboplastin (tissue factor) does not enter

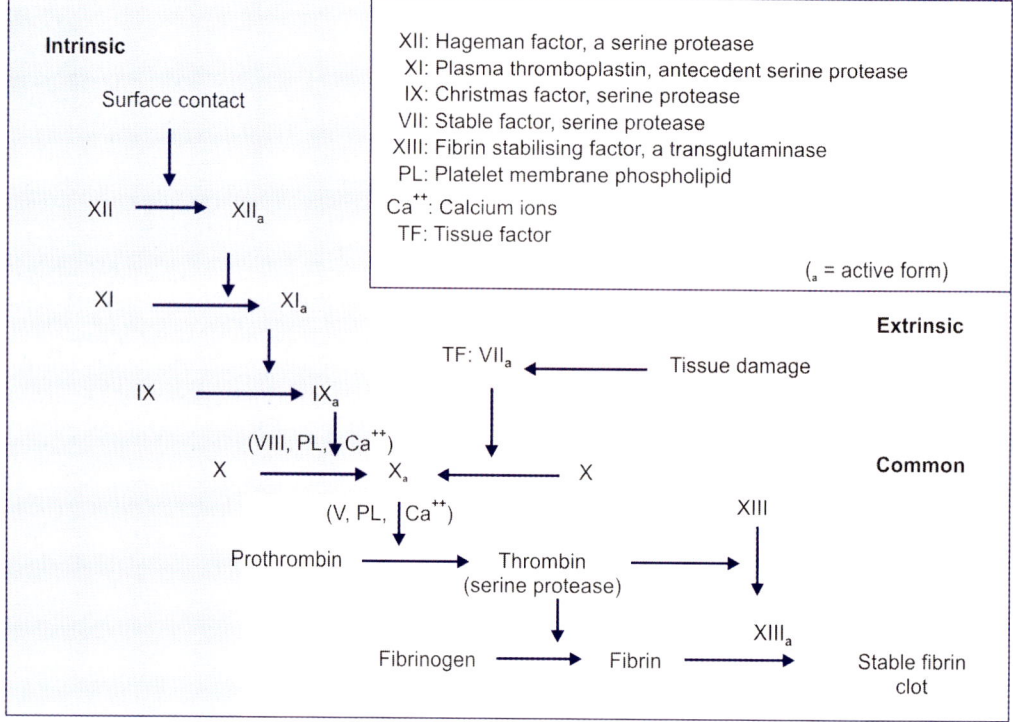

Fig. 7.1: The three pathways that makeup the classical blood coagulation pathway

into the blood sample as a very small amount will cause shortened CT. It is usually not affected by mild to moderate deficiency of platelets, because for normal coagulation (clotting) only very small number of platelets are required.

Two methods are done for CT:
1. Lee and White method
2. Capillary tube method of Wright

Lee and White Method

Requirements
- Stopwatch
- Equipment for collection of blood
- Clean, dry glass test tubes (10 × 75 mm), three in number
- Water bath (37°C), preferable

Methods
- Make a clear venipuncture with as little trauma to the connective tissue between skin and vein as possible.
- Draw 3–5 ml of blood by a disposable plastic syringe or siliconized dry glass syringe.
- After detaching the needle, deliver 1 ml of blood in each of the three test tubes (10 × 75 mm).
- Place all the 3 test tubes containing blood in a stand so that they remain upright and undisturbed at room temperature. If water bath is available, then place the tubes at 37°C.
- Check the coagulation by tilting the test tubes or by gentle tipping. The first test tube is gently tilted every minute while other test tubes are examined every 30 seconds. When the blood samples are clotted (test tubes can be inverted without blood running down the edge of the tubes).
- The average of the clotting time in three test tubes gives the result.

Normal range: 5–11 minutes at 37°C

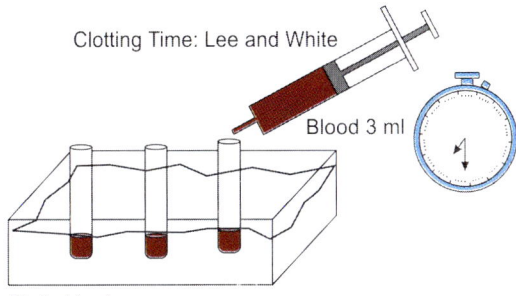

Fig. 7.2: Lee and White method of clotting time

N: 5–11 min

Note

i. Rise of temperature will speed up the coagulation process, so the test should be done at a particular temperature.
ii. If the test is done at room temperature (without water bath) then the time will vary with regard to temperature and time of tipping. If someone waits for 10 minutes before starting to tip, then normal CT value may go as high as 20–25 minutes. Whereas if someone waits for 5 minutes before starting to tip, range will be 8–18 minutes.
iii. Vigorous agitation of the test tubes will significantly shorten coagulation time (CT). So, one should tip the tubes very gently to see if the blood has clotted (no movement of blood).

Capillary Tube Methods of Wrights

Blood is collected from a clean finger prick (aseptic precautions) in 4–5 fine capillary tubes. The tubes are sealed at both ends by flame (alternatively by chemical plasticine) and the capillary tubes are kept in a water bath at 37°C.

After one minute, one end of the tube is broken gently and the breakage of tube is repeated every 30 seconds until a thin line of unbroken coagulum is stretched between the two broken ends.

Normal range: 6–10 minutes (if test is done in room temperature the CT will be longer; not recommended).

Prolonged Coagulation Time

1. **Haemophilia A** (deficiency of factor VIII. and **haemophilia B** or Christmas disease (deficiency of factor IX).
2. **Anticoagulant therapy** (hyperheparinemia or warfarin therapy).
3. **Hypoprothrombinaemia:** Seen in cirrhosis of liver, obstructive jaundice, vit K deficiency, malignancy of liver.
4. **Fibrinogen deficiency:** When fibrinogen level falls below 50 mg/dl in blood.
5. **von Willebrand's disease:**

PROTHROMBIN TIME (PT)

Definition: Prothrombin time is the time required for clotting of citrated plasma (platelet poor) in a glass test tube after the addition of calcium chloride and thromboplastin (tissue factor).

Reagents

i. **Patients control plasma samples:** Patients control plasma samples (preferably platelet poor) are prepared from whole blood and citrate anticoagulant in a ratio of 9:1.
   - Sodium citrate (3.8%) solution: 0.5 ml
   - Whole blood: 4.5 ml

   Whole blood and sodium citrate (3.8%) are mixed well gently. Then **platelet-poor plasma (PPP)** is prepared by centrifugation at 2000 gm for 15 minutes at 4°C (approximately 4000 r.p.m./minute). It should be kept at room temperature for prothrombin time assay. The test should be done within 2 hours of collection.

ii. **Thromboplastins:** Thromboplastins are tissue extracts obtained from different species and different organs. Majority of thromboplastins now in use are extracts of rabbit brain or lung. It is now commercially available as powder.

iii. **Calcium chloride ($CaCl_2$):** 0.025 mol/litre. The test reagent is prepared fresh before use.

Points to Remember
- Tissue thromboplastin serves two functions. It activates extrinsic pathway and provides phospholipid surface for certain coagulation reactions.
- Calcium chloride ($CaCl_2$) supplies calcium ions or Ca^{2+} which bind vitamin K dependent factors (II, VII, IX and X) to phospholipid.

Methods
1. Put 0.1 ml of plasma into a glass test tube placed in a water bath and add 0.1 ml of thromboplastin.
2. Wait for 1–3 minutes to allow the mixture to warm at 37°C.
3. Then add 0.1 ml of warmed $CaCl_2$ (previously kept at water bath in a separate test tube) to that mixture in the glass test tube.
   Mix well the contents and start the stop watch.
4. The test tube is continuously tilted within the water bath and look for clot formation.
5. As soon as the fibrin clot is formed, the watch is stopped and the time is recorded.

Normal values: 11–16 seconds (when rabbit thromboplastin is used)

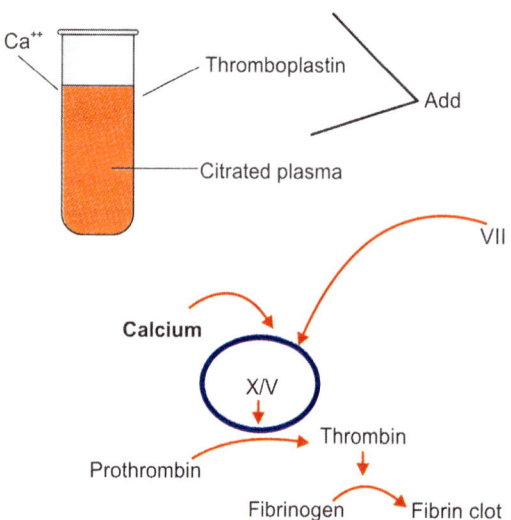

Fig. 7.3: Schematic diagram of prothrombin time (PT)

International Normalized Ratio (INR)

The result of prothrombin time (PT) in seconds which is performed on a normal individual will vary according to the type of analytical system employed. This is due to the variations between different types and batches of manufacture's tissue factor used in the reagent to perform the test. The **international normalized ratio (INR)** was devised to standardize the test results. Each manufacturer assigns an **ISI value (international sensitivity index)** for any tissue factor they manufacture. The ISI value is usually between 0.94–1.4 for more sensitive and 2.0–3.0 for less sensitive thromboplastins.

The INR is the ratio of a patient's prothrombin time to a normal (control) sample, raised to the power of the ISI value for the analytical system being used.

For example, a ratio of 2.5 (patient's PT to control PT) using a thromboplastin with ISI of 1.4, then INR be calculated using this formula:

$$INR = 2.5^{(1.4)} = 3.61 \text{ (normal INR} = 1.0 \text{ ratio)}.$$

Prothrombin index =
$$\frac{\text{PT of control plasma}}{\text{PT of patient's plasma}} \times 100\%$$

Suppose PT of control plasma and patient's plasma are 12 second and 16 seconds respectively, then prothrombin index would be $12/16 \times 100\% = 75\%$.

Cause of Prolonged Prothrombin Time (PT)

1. **Oral anticoagulant therapy:** Oral anticoagulants like warfarin interfere with the carboxylation of vitamin K-dependent factors. PT is the standard test for monitoring oral anticoagulant therapy.
   But INR is preferred to monitor patients on anticoagulant therapy. For all other uses, the use of PT is encouraged over INR. The recommended range for INR during most indications for oral

anticoagulants is 2–3, or 2.5–3.5 for patients with mechanical heart valves.

2. **Vitamin K deficiency:** PT is useful test to detect vitamin K deficiency. It measures three vitamin K-dependent factors (II, VII and X) out of four (II, VII, IX and X).
3. **Liver disease,** particularly obstructive jaundice, cirrhosis, malignancy of liver.
4. **Inherited deficiency of extrinsic or common pathway coagulation factor(s):** Deficiency of VII, X, V, II or I.
5. **Others:** Post-partum hypofibrinogenaemia, DIC.

ACTIVATED PARTIAL THROMBOPLASTIN TIME (APTT)

Synonym: Partial thromboplastin time with kaolin (PTTK) and kaolin cephalin clotting time (KCCT). Also known as partial thromboplastin time (PTT).

Principle: This test measures the clotting time of plasma after the activation of contact factors but without added tissue thromboplastin, and so it evaluates the overall efficiency of the intrinsic pathway. To standardize the activation of contact factors, the plasma is first pre-incubated with kaolin. A standardized phospholipid is provided to allow the test to be performed on platelet-poor plasma.

Reagents

1. **Platelet-poor plasma:** Both from the patient and control as described in PT.
2. **Kaolin:** 5 g/litre or 0.5 gm% in barbitone buffered saline pH is 7.4. A few glass beads are added to aid resuspension. This suspension is stable at room temperature. In place of kaolin, other insoluble surface active substances such as elagic acid or celite can also be used.
3. **Phospholipid:** Commercially available lyophilised reagent and working solution is prepared as per direction. This reagent must be sensitive to detect deficiencies of factors VII, C, IX and XI, at concentration of 20–25 IU/dl.
4. **Calcium chloride (CaCl$_2$):** 0.025 mol/litre

Methods

1. Mix equal volume of the phospholipid reagent and the kaolin suspension (0.5 ml each) and leave in a glass tube in water bath at 37°C.
2. Place 0.1 ml of control and patient's (test) plasma in two separate glass tubes. Add 0.2 ml of prewarmed kaolin phospholipid solution to these tubes. Mix the contents well and gently. Start the stopwatch immediately.
3. Keep it in the water bath at 37°C and wait for 10 minutes, with occasional shaking.
4. At exactly 10 minutes, add 0.1 ml of prewarmed CaCl$_2$ and start a second stopwatch.
5. The tubes are tilted back and forth in front of a good light source and watch for appearance of fibrin clot. The watch is stopped when the clot forms and the time is recorded. The time taken by the mixture to clot is the APTT.

Normal range: 30–40 seconds.

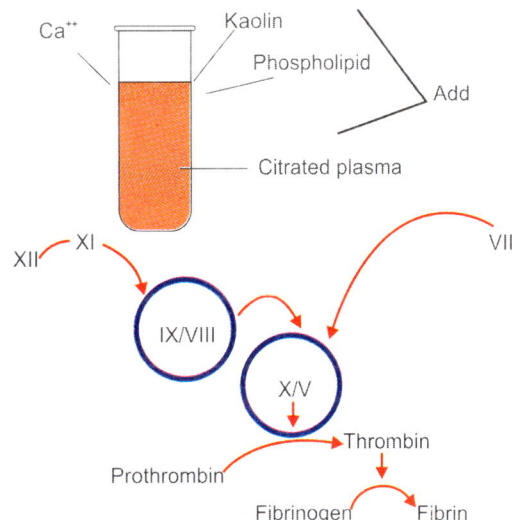

Fig. 7.4: Schematic diagram of activated partial thromboplastin time (APTT)

Causes of Prolonged APTT

- **Inherited deficiency**: of factor VIII and factor IX. Also prolonged in inherited deficiencies of other coagulation factors in intrinsic pathway and common pathway.
- **Circulating inhibitors**: Inhibitors may be of two types—specific and nonspecific. **Specific inhibitors** are directed against specific coagulation factors. The most common specific inhibitor is antibody against factor VII. **Non-specific inhibitors** are antibodies that are not directed against specific coagulation factors but block the interaction of clotting factors, e.g. lupus inhibitors.
- Liver disease
- Disseminated intravascular coagulation (DIC)
- Heparin administration: Heparin accelerates the action of antithrombin and inhibits thrombin and factors Xa, XIa and IXa.
- Massive transfusion with stored blood
- A circulating anticoagulant

Causes of Shortened APTT

- Thrombosis
- Pregnancy

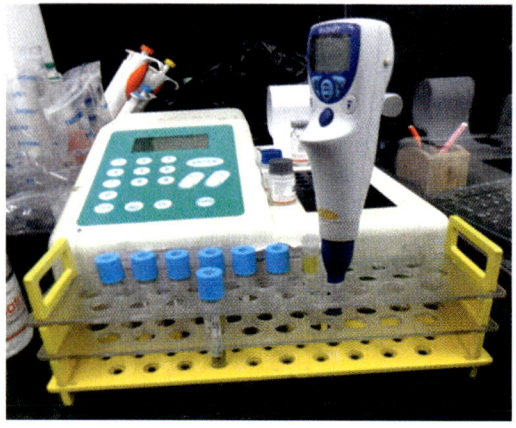

Fig. 7.5: Coagulometer (coagulation analyzer) to determine PT and APTT

Points to Remember

- **Bleeding time (BT)**
  i. It is the time taken for a standard skin puncture to stop bleeding
  ii. This test examines the ability of blood vessels to constrict and platelets to form a hemostatic plug.

- **Clotting time or coagulation time (CT)**
  i. It is the time required for a whole blood sample to coagulate *in vitro* under standard conditions.
  ii. It measures all three stages of coagulation (intrinsic pathway, extrinsic pathway and common pathway).

- **Prothrombin time (PT)**
  i. It is the time required for clotting of platelet-poor citrated plasma in a glass tube after the addition of thromboplastin (tissue factor) and calcium chloride.
  ii. The prothrombin time along with its derived measures of prothrombin ratio (PR) and international normalized ratio (INR) are assays evaluating the extrinsic pathway of coagulation.
  iii. The PT may used along with APTT as the starting points for investigating excessive bleeding or clotting disorders.

- **Activated partial thromboplastin time (APTT)**
  i. It is used to monitor the functioning of the intrinsic and the common coagulation pathways.
  ii. A relatively rare cause of prolonged APTT is presence of antibodies against coagulation plasma factors/proteins. These are known as inhibitors. Some of the cause are: Autoimmune diseases, pregnancy, dermatologic conditions, malignancies (prostate cancer, lymphoma), haemophilia A and B, patients receiving clotting factors to control their bleeding disorders.

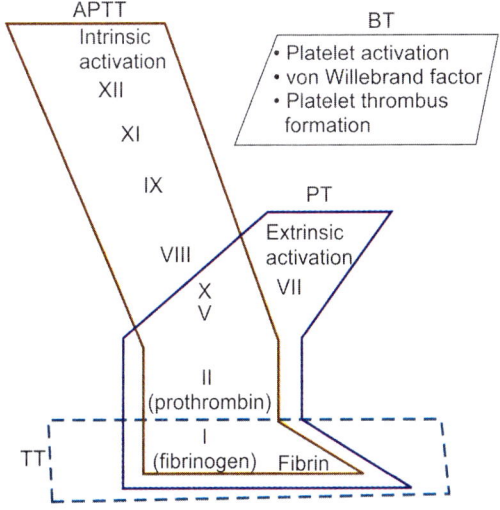

Fig. 7.6: Basic test for haemostasis

BT: Bleeding time, APTT: Activated partial thromboplastin time, PT: Prothrombin time, TT: Thrombin time

VIVA VOCE

Q1. What are intrinsic and extrinsic pathways of coagulation and why are they named so?

Ans: The clotting system can be activated by two pathways—either by intrinsic pathway or by extrinsic pathway. The intrinsic pathway is activated by exposing factor XII to any thrombogenic surface (as for example, glass surfaces or other negatively charged surfaces). On the other hand, extrinsic pathway requires exogenous triggering agent (which was originally provided by tissue extract or tissue thromboplastin prepared from animal tissue rich in tissue factor like rabbit brain). Later on, kaolin or kaolin-cephalin become available commercially which is used nowadays as tissue factor.

But this division is somewhat confusing as intrinsic pathway is relevant *in vitro* (outside body), whereas extrinsic pathway is relevant *in vivo* (within body), after vascular injury/damage.

Q2. Why kaolin and phospholipids are added for doing APTT?

Ans: Kaolin leads to surface contact activation. So, initiating the intrinsic system of coagulation from factor XII onwards. Hence, it is called activated PTT or APTT.

On the other hand, exogenous phospholipids (platelet factor 3) act as alternative to blood platelets and are necessary for coagulation. Within body, platelets are source of phospholipids. This exogenous phospholipids also known as partial thromboplastin. Hence, APTT is also known as partial thromboplastin time.

Q3. Why is incision made parallel to antecubital fossa during template method of bleeding time (BT) estimation?

Ans: Incision is made parallel to antecubital fossa so that no wound is formed as there will be absence of retraction of skin. But if incision is made right angle or obliquely to the antecubital fossa, the skin edges will be retracted and a spindle-shaped wound/scar will be formed.

Q4. What are the effects of circulating anticoagulants in blood?

Ans: Circulating anticoagulants are inhibitors of coagulation like heparin and other anticoagulants present in blood. Presence of circulating anticoagulants cause prolonged PT and APTT.

Q5. If a patient has normal PT but prolonged APTT, then what are the possibilities?

Ans:
i. Defect in intrinsic pathway or congenital deficiency of factors require for intrinsic pathway. As for example, haemophilia A, haemophilia B, deficiency of factor XI, factor XII, prekallikrein and HMWK (high molecular weight kininogen).
ii. Deficiency of von Willebrand factor (vWF) in von Willebrand's disease (also prolonged bleeding time).
iii. Presence of heparin and other anticoagulants in blood (circulating anticoagulants).

Q6. If a patient has prolonged PT and normal APTT, then what are the possibilities?

Ans:

i. Congenital deficiency of factor VII, which is very rare.
ii. Initiation of oral anticoagulant therapy (warfarin).

Q7. In above scenario (question No. 6), how would you ascertain the exact cause?

Ans: When a patient has prolonged PT and normal APTT, then prothrombin (PT) is repeated with 1:1 mixture of patient's plasma and normal plasma (control) as substrate. If the prolongation is corrected, then the cause is factor VII deficiency.

The normal plasma present in 1:1 mixture supplies factor VII required for normal prothrombin time.

If it is not corrected, then the cause is presence of an inhibitor in blood.

Q8. If a patient has prolongation of both PT and APTT, then what are the possibilities?

Ans: In this case, both tests are repeated with 1:1 mixture of patient's plasma and normal plasma (control) as substrate. If both PT and APTT now become normal, then the patient has deficiency of one or many of these factors; factors I, II, V, and X (common for PT and APPTT).

After that, individual specific assay is done to find out deficiency of particular factor.

Q9. What is thrombin time (TT)? What are the causes of prolonged TT?

Ans: This is time required for testing the conversion of fibrinogen into fibrin. It depends on aqequate fibrinogen levels.

Prolonged thrombin time (TT) is seen in afibrinogenaemia, dysfibrinogenaemia, DIC (disseminated intravascular coagulation) and heparin like inhibitors.

Q10. What is clot retraction study?

Ans: A clot forms at the end of blood coagulation. In normal circumstances, the clot undergoes contraction. When serum is expressed from the clot, the clot becomes denser. The platelets release one substance (called thromboplastin) which is responsible for clot retraction. Normal clot retraction begins within 30 seconds after the blood has clotted, and at 1 hour it is about 30% normally.

Clot retraction test is done when there is suspicion of haemorrhagic disorders related to platelets. Poor clot retraction is seen if platelet count is low (thrombocytopenia) or in poor platelet function with normal platelet count (thrombasthenia).

Blood Grouping and Rh Typing

The **term blood group** refers not only to erythrocyte antigen system but also to the immunologic diversity expressed by other blood constituents including leukocytes, platelets and plasma.

International Society of Blood Transfusion (ISBT) Working Party recognizes 35 significant blood group systems though there are about 200 red cell antigens. Landsteiner first discovered **ABO system** in 1901. After that, **MNS system** in 1927, **Psystem** in 1927, **rhesus** or **Rh system** in 1939, **Lutheran system** in 1945, **Kell system** in 1946, **Lewis system** in 1946, **Duffy system** in 1950, **Kidd system** in 1951 were discovered.

Other significant systems of those 35 systems (recognized by ISBT) are Diego, Yt, Xg, Scianna, Dombrock, Colton, Landsteiner – Wiener, Chido/Rodgers, Hh, Kx, Gerbich, Cromer, Knobs, Indian, Ok, Raph, John Mitton Hagen, I, Globoside, GIL, RHAG.

Most blood group genes (with a few exceptions) are located on the autosomal chromosomes and are inherited following Mendelian rules of inheritance. These blood group genes are expressed equally when inherited in a co-dominant manner (i.e. two allelic forms are expressed equally when inherited in a heterozygous state. The specific alleles at a particular locus of gene in an individual constitute the genotype. Outward expression of this genotype is known as phenotype.

With regard to blood transfusion practice, most important blood group systems are ABO and Rh systems. Because, A, B and Rh D antigens are most immunogenic (they are capable of eliciting a strong antibody response on stimulation) and their alloantibodies can cause destruction of transfused RBCs or they may induce hemolytic diseases of newborn (HDN). ABO antigens are also important for organ transplantation (graft rejection).

Apart from A, B, RhD antigens other important antigens in transfusion medicine as per their strong immunogenicity are D, K, C, FY^a, c, E, k, e, JK^a, S and s.

Almost always, an individual has the same blood group for life, but very rarely an individual's blood type changes through addition or suppression of an antigen in infections, autoimmune diseases or malignancies. Another rare cause in blood group change is bone marrow transplant.

ANTIBODIES TO RED CELL ANTIGENS

Mainly there are two main types: Naturally occurring and immune or acquired antibodies.

1. **Naturally occurring antibodies:** These antibodies are formed without any

antigenic stimulus (RBC antigens). These are present in the serum of persons who lack that particular antigen(s) in the RBC, e.g. isoagglutinnins (antibodies) of ABO blood grouping system. These antibodies are IgM in nature and react to corresponding antigen at a temperature below 37°C. These antibodies very rarely may be seen in other blood group systems.

It is presumed that these antibodies develop due to antigenic stimulus from the similar type of antigens present in the intestinal bacteria or foods consumed by newborns. The infant regards these antigens as foreign and develops antoibodies to those foreign antigens which are not present in their own cells/RBCs. Hence, blood group A persons develop anti-B antibodies, blood group B persons develop anti-A antibodies, blood group O persons develop both anti-A and anti-B antibodies while blood group AB persons do not have any antibody.

2. **Immune or acquired antibody**: These antibodies develop when different antigens either in RBC or body fluids are introduced in a person who do not have these antigens. The person consider those antigens foreign and immune or acquired antibodies (agglutinins) are formed. Example: Mismatched blood transfusion or after pregnancy. Most of these antibodies are IgG in nature and react best at 37°C.

ABO SYSTEM

There are four main types of blood groups: A, B, AB and O. Blood group A again can be subdivided into A_1 and A_2. The much rarer A subgroups are A_3, A_x and A_m. But the A_1 and A_2 subgroups are important only. So, ABO system increases to six: A_1, A_2, B, A_1B, A_2B and O. About 80% of blood group A and blood group AB belong to A_1 or A_1B respectively. ABO antigens are found predominantly on erythrocyte membrane protein band 3 and 4.5, membrane glycophorin and structural glycolipids. In addition to red cells, these antigens are also expressed on platelets, white blood cells and various body tissues. As ABO antigens are found on most tissues of the body, they are often referred to as "histo-blood group" antigens. They may be found in soluble form in various body secretions (in secretors).

Although ABO antigens have been detected on erythrocytes in a six-week old foetus but these antigens are poorly expressed at birth. Antigenicity increases gradually and becomes fully expressed around one year of age (some believe full expression needs three years of age).

The blood groups A, B, AB and O are determined by presence or absence of A and B antigens on the red cell membrane. There is another antigen called O antigen which remains silent.

Actually, these A, B or O antigens on red cells are controlled by three allelic genes on the long arm of chromosome 9. The A and B genes are co-dominant but the O antigen is amorph or silent (it has no effect on antigenic structure).

The cellular expression of A and B antigens is determined by another gene, called H gene. The H gene (genotype HH or Hh) produces a transferase enzyme, which changes precursor or substance present on RBCs into **H substance**. The A and B genes produce specific transferase enzymes that convert H substance into A and B antigens respectively. But the O gene produces an inactive transferase so that H antigen persists unchanged on red cells.

In the absence of H genes (designated as hh), the precursor substance remains unconverted and H substance is not synthesized. So, A and B genes, if present cannot be expressed and **Bombay blood group (Oh)** type results. Their red cell type is group O. But unlike group O individuals, Bombay blood group persons (Oh) have no H antigen on RBC. As there is no expression of A, B antigens and absence of H antigen, their plasma contain antibodies against all of them, i.e. anti-A, anti-B and anti-H. These

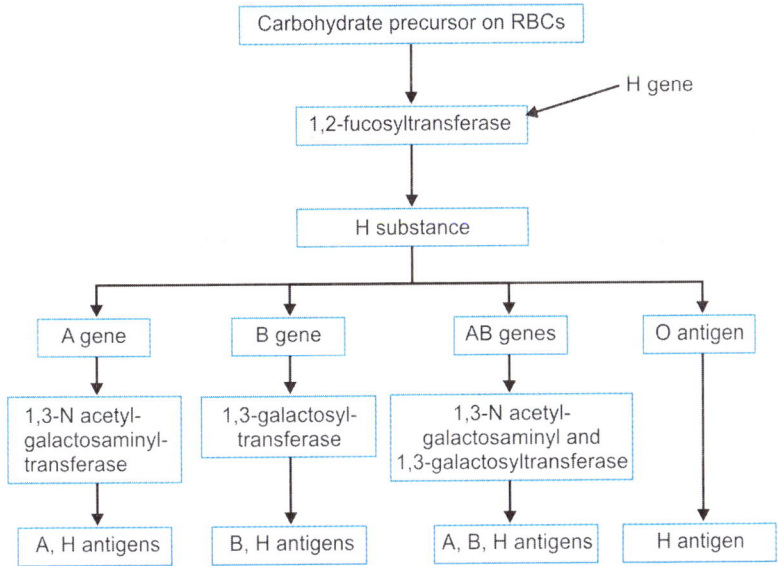

Fig. 8.1: Formation of A, B and H antigens on RBCs

antibodies are active at 37°C. Therefore, Bombay blood group persons should be transfused only with Oh blood.

Secretors and Nonsecretors

Secretors are persons who secrete A, B, and H antigen (called ABH substances) into body fluids (such as plasma, saliva, sweat, tears, semen, milk, etc.). These ABH substances are secreted in water-soluble form of glycoprotein. The ability of secretion is dependent on presence of a dominant secretor gene (Se). About 80% of Caucasian persons are secretors (genotype Sese or SeSe) and remaining are nonsecretors (sese). Both secretors and nonsecretors express ABO antigens on red cells.

Differences between A_1 and A_2 Subgroups of Blood Group A and AB

Subgroups of A are distinguished by their lack of agglutination with anti-A_1 lectin prepared from *Dolichos biflorus* or with anti-A_1 reagent derived from serum of group O or B persons that has been absorbed with A_2 cells.

Features	A_1	A_2
Quantitative differences		
• Reaction with diluted anti-A	+ + + +	+ +
• Antigenic sites:		
a. In adults	1,000,000	250,000
b. In newborns	310,000	140,000
Qualitative differences		
• Reaction with *Dolichos biflorus* (Anti-A_1) lectin	+ + + +	0
• Anti-A_1 in serum	Absent	1–8%
• N-acetylgalactosaminyl-transferase activity	Normal activity (optimal at pH 6)	Decreased activity (optimal at pH 7)

Table 8.1: Antigens, antibodies and other features in ABO blood grouping system

	ABO blood groups			
Antigen (on RBC)	Antigen A	Antigen B	Antigens A + B	Neither A nor B
Antibody (in plasma)	Anti-B antibody	Anti-A antibody	Neither antibody	Both antibodies
Blood type	Type A Cannot have B or AB blood Can have A or O blood	Type B Cannot have A or AB blood Can have B or O blood	Type AB Can have any type of blood Is the universal recipient?	Type O Can only have O blood Is the universal donor?

In India, frequency of blood group A is 22.88%, blood group B is 32.26%, blood group AB is 7.44% and blood group O is 37.12%.

Method of ABO Blood Grouping

It can be done by slide or tube method or by microplate method. Slide method is satisfactory but not as sensitive as tube method because slide method cannot detect weak anti-A or anti-B reverse serum grouping. Monoclonal anti-A and anti-B reagents are used for blood grouping.

Again, ABO blood grouping can be of two: Forward grouping and reverse grouping.

Forward grouping: Here, one drop of 2–5% red cell suspension is tested with one drop each of commercially prepared anti-A and anti-B.

Reverse grouping: Here, two drops of patient or donor serum are tested against one drop of reagent erythrocytes of known A (usually A_1) and B phenotype. But this is not done in infants under 4 months of age as the corresponding antibodies are normally absent.

Preparing red cell suspension

Depending upon the specific technique employed 2, 5, 10, 20, or 50% red cell suspensions are required. These can be prepared by suspending in saline the packed red cell obtained from citrate or oxalate blood or from a skin puncture into saline.

Preparation of 2% red cell suspension:
1. Take 5 ml of normal saline in a test tube. To it, add several drops of anticoagulated or fresh blood.
2. Centrifuge in order to get packed red cells (3000 r.p.m. for 10–20 minutes)
3. Withdraw the supernatant fluid as completely as possible.
4. Add 0.1 ml of this packed red cells to a test tube which contains 4.9 ml of normal saline. Mix them well. This represents 2% red cell suspension (as 0.1 ml of packed red cell in total 5 ml of suspension).

For preparation of 5% red cell suspension, add 0.25 ml of packed red cell to 4.75 ml of saline. For preparation of 10% red cell suspension add 0.5 ml of packed red cells to 4.5 ml of saline in the last step (step 4) of the above procedure.

Blood Grouping and Rh Typing

Blood group	Antigen + antibody(ies) present		As donor	As recipient
A	Antigen A	Makes anti-B	Compatible with: A and AB. Incompatible with: B and O, because both make anti-A antibodies that will react with A antigens	Compatible with: A and O. Incompatible with: B and AB, because type A makes anti-B antibodies that will react with B antigens
B	Antigen B	Makes anti-A	Compatible with: B and AB. Incompatible with: A and O, because both make anti-B antibodies that will react with B antigens	Compatible with: B and O. Incompatible with: A and AB, because type B makes anti-A antibodies that will react with A antigens
AB	Antigens A and B	Makes neither anti-A nor anti-B	Compatible with: AB only. Incompatible with: A, B and O, because All three make antibodies that will react with AB antigens	Compatible with all groups universal recipient. AB makes no antibodies and therefore will not react with any type of donated blood
O	Neither A nor B antigen	Makes both anti-A and anti-B	Compatible with all groups universal donor. O red cells have no antigens, and will therefore not stimulate anti-A or anti-B antibodies	Compatible with: O only. Incompatible with: A AB and B, because type O makes anti-A and anti-B antibodies

Red Blood Cell Compatibility Table

Recipient	Donor							
	O–	O+	A–	A+	B–	B+	AB–	AB+
O–	✓	✗	✗	✗	✗	✗	✗	✗
O+	✓	✓	✗	✗	✗	✗	✗	✗
A–	✓	✗	✓	✗	✗	✗	✗	✗
A+	✓	✓	✓	✓	✗	✗	✗	✗
B–	✓	✗	✗	✗	✓	✗	✗	✗
B+	✓	✓	✗	✗	✓	✓	✗	✗
AB–	✓	✗	✓	✗	✓	✗	✓	✗
AB+	✓	✓	✓	✓	✓	✓	✓	✓

Slide Method (ABO Grouping)

This method is satisfactory but less preferable compared to tube method. However, in small laboratories, resource poor set ups, in emergency situations or during mass blood group screening this can be done.

Sample: A 20% red cell suspension is used. Alternatively, fresh blood by finger prick or cells from clotted blood may be used.

Reagent: Monoclonal anti-A and anti-B reagents (commercially available) blue-coloured vial: Anti-A, yellow-coloured vial: Anti-B. Monoclonal anti-AB is also available.

Test procedure
1. Take a clean glass slide. Mark anti-A on left side corner and anti-B on middle and control on right side corner of that slide.
2. Two drops of blood or 20–40% red cell suspension are placed by a Pasteur pipette at each three demarcated areas.
3. On the left side a drop of anti-serum, on the middle a drop of anti-B serum and on the right a drop of normal saline are added separately.
4. The serum cell suspensions are mixed separately with the help of glass rod or by the corners of another clean slide. Alternatively, wooden swabstick breaking off can also be used.
5. The slide is then tilted with hands gently and carefully for 2–3 minutes.

Test result: Results are read within 2–5 minutes depending on the appearance of agglutination of red cells (positive or negative) as follows:
  i. Blood group A: Agglutination with anti-A serum (left corner) but not with anti-B serum (middle).
 ii. Blood group B: Agglutination with anti-B (middle) but not with anti-A (left corner).
iii. Blood group AB: Agglutination on both left and middle portions.
 iv. Blood group O: No agglutination on left and middle portions.

Control should be negative. If there is agglutination in the control that means either the method or technique is faulty or the reagents are of expired/poor quality.

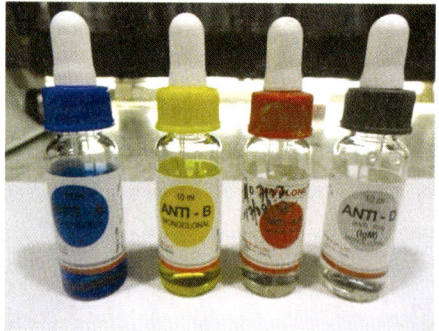

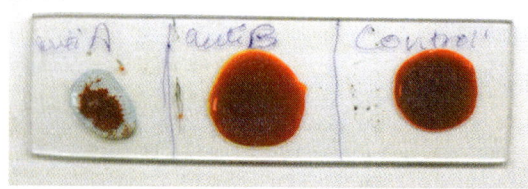

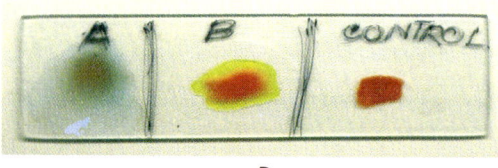

Fig. 8.2A to D: ABO blood grouping. (A) Monoclonal anti-A (green coloured), anti-B (yellow coloured) and anti-AB (colourless) serum. Also anti-D serum (colourless) on rightmost side **(upper left)**; (B) Blood group A **(upper right)**; (C) Blood group B **(lower left)**; (D) Blood group O **(lower right)**

Tube Method (ABO Grouping)

i. Take 3 glasses or plastic tubes (75 × 12 mm) and add one drop each grouping reagent to 3 tubes to labelled anti-A, anti-B and anti-AB respectively.
ii. Put 1 drop of 2–5% of red cell suspension to each tube.
iii. Mix the suspension by tapping the tubes and leave them undisturbed for 15–30 minutes. Check agglutination.

Test result: Agglutination is judged by the macroscopic appearance of agglutination in round bottom tubes. If positive it will show "graininess", whereas in the absence of agglutination the sedimented cells appear as a smooth round bottom. This agglutination is better visualized under microscope. A scoring system depending upon agglutination pattern can be employed.

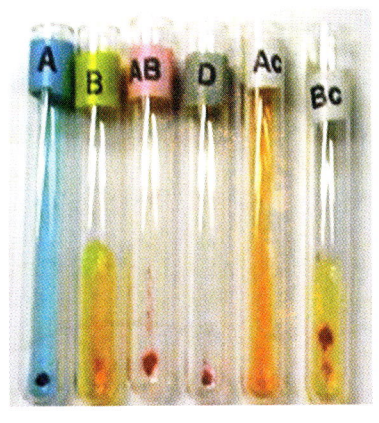
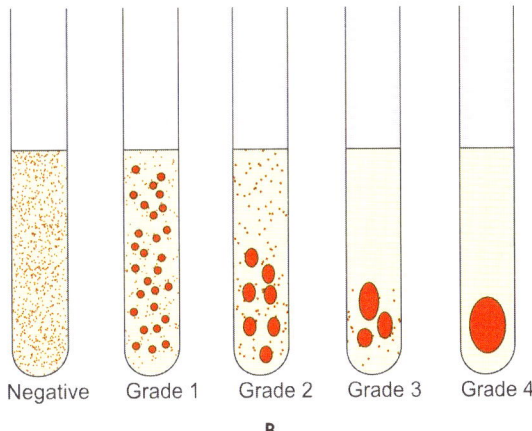

Fig. 8.3A and B: (A) Test tube methods for blood grouping; (B) Scoring system (grades 1 to 4) in test tube method of blood grouping

Table 8.2: Scoring of results in red agglutination tests

Description	Symbol	Agglutination score*
a. Negative result: All cell-free and evenly distributed	–	0
b. Cell button dislodges into fine granules, only visible microscopically	+ or weak (W)	3
c. Cell button dislodges into finely granular clumps, just visible macroscopically	1 +	5
d. Cell button dislodges into many small clumps, macroscopically visible	2 +	8
e. Cell button dislodges into several large clumps, macroscopically visible	3 +	10
f. Cell button remains in one clump, macroscopically visible	4 + or complete (C)	12

*__Agglutination score__: Further classification depending upon the number of red cells present in the clump. Hence, clumping of average 12 cells (score 4+), average 10 cells (score 3+), average 5 cells (score 1+).

For determining the particular blood group following the agglutination pattern in the slide method described early.

Serum Grouping (Reverse Grouping)

In the serum grouping or reverse grouping, patient's serum is tested against known red cell antigens on RBCs. If the patient's serum contains anti-A, anti-B or both it will agglutinate known antigen A, antigen B or both antigens in red cells. Red cells form blood group A contains antigen A, blood group B contains antigen B, blood group AB contains both antigens and blood group O contains no antigen (serves as control) on their red cells. For A antigen, A_1 subtype is commonly used. A_2 cells should be used if there is suspected presence of anti-A_1

Microplate Method

ABO grouping may be carried out on one U well plate (96 wells) and monoclonal reagents (anti-A, anti-B, anti-AB) are used. Using Pasteur pipette (or commercial reagent dropper) 1 drop of monoclonal reagent or antiserum is added to each well of the U well plate. Then 1 drop of 2–5% patient's red cell suspension is added to these rows. This is done for forward grouping.

For reverse grouping at the same time 1 drop patient's serum or plasma are added to separate wells of the plate. To this known antigens 1 drop (antigen A, antigen B or antigen AB) are added to the serum/plasma. Control may be used.

Now, mix them on a microplate shaker. Leave the microplate at room temperature (20°C) for 15 minutes. Then centrifuge the plate at 700 r.p.m. for 1 minute.

The plate can be read for agglutination by one of the two methods:

1. Streaming (microplate set an angle) or agitation.
2. Automated microplate readers

False Positive Results (ABO Grouping)

- **Rouleaux formation**: Marked rouleaux formation can simulate true agglutination. In reverse grouping the two can be distinguished by repeating the test using serum diluted 1 in 2 or 1 in 1 saline. The rouleaux will disappear but agglutination will persist. If rouleaux are apparent in forward grouping test, then tests should be repeated after washing the patient's red cell thoroughly with normal saline.
- **Cold agglutinins**: Sometimes true agglutination of red cells develops due to cold agglutinins at or below 20°C. If ABO compatibility is ruled out, then the presence of cold agglutinins like anti-P_1 or anti-I antibodies may be the cause of this false positivity. In that case, patient's red cells are washed several times with warm (37°C) saline and blood grouping (ABO)

Table 8.3: Forward and reverse groupings

ABO blood group	Forward grouping		Reverse grouping	
	Anti-A	Anti-B	A_1 antigen on RBC	B antigen on RBC
1. Blood group A	+	–	–	+
2. Blood group B	–	+	+	–
3. Blood group AB	+	+	–	–
4. Blood group O	–	–	+	+

is repeated. There will no chance of false positivity.
- **Warm antibodies**: These antibodies are absorbed to red cell of patient. Agglutinin other than anti-A, anti-B or anti-D (Rh typing) which cause agglutination at 37°C are occasionally seen. Presence of antibodies like anti-Lu, anti-M, anti-K or anti-S antibodies are responsible for this.
- **Bacterial contamination**: Infection of RBCs by bacteria both in vivo and in vitro may cause polyagglutination in normal sera. Bacterial enzyme expose T receptors on red cell surface. As most human sera contain anti-T antibodies, such infected red cells get agglutinated in normal serum. Hence, blood group O may appear as blood group AB.

False Negative Results (ABO Grouping)

1. Failure of agglutination or weak reactions are usually due to improper sera. If the sera are kept at room temperature for longer time the potency is lost.
2. Failure to add grouping reagent or insufficient volume will cause false negative results.
3. In reverse grouping test, failure to recognize lysis as a positive result may end up in giving false negative reports. To avoid lysis, reagents (anti-A and anti-B) should contain EDTA to prevent complement activation in presence of fresh patient's serum as seen in tile method of grouping.
4. Miscellaneous: Wrong technique, poor quality of red cells, etc.

Rh System

The rhesus (Rh) system was so named because Landsteiner and Wiener (1940) published studies of animal experiments involving the immunization of Guinea pigs and rabbits with rhesus monkey erythrocytes. The antiserum produced agglutinated 85% of human erythrocytes, and the antigen defined was called the **Rh factor**.

Using five basic antisera anti-D, anti-C and anti-E, anti-c and anti-e, Wiener identified five different factors or antigens and named them as Rh_0, rh', $rh''hr'$, hr''. While Fisher postulated that Rh antigens (C, c, D, d, E, e) are determined by three pairs of closed linked allelomorphic genes which are located on chromosome No. 1. These three pairs are C or c, D or d and E or e. Every human carries one member of these three pairs from each parent. Each gene can control production of a specific antigen. But the antigen controlled by D locus is the strongest immunogen, called the Rh D antigen. The six Rh genes give 8 allelomorphs and 8 antigenic patterns. The nomenclature suggested by Fisher later on accepted by WHO expert by WHO Expert Committee in 1977.

Table 8.4: Comparison of Wiener, Fisher and Rosenfield nomenclature

Wiener	Fisher	Rosenfield
Rh_0	D	Rh 1
rh'	C	Rh 2
rh''	E	Rh 3
hr'	c	Rh 4
hr''	e	Rh 5

Table 8.5: The Rh genes and antigens as per Fisher's nomenclature, accepted by WHO (1977)

	Genes	Antigens
Rh positive	CDe	CDe
	cDE	cDE
	cDe	cDe
	CDE	CDE
Rh negative	Cde	Cde
	cdE	cdE
	cde	cde
	CdE	CdE

Rh D is the most strong antigen amongst those 8 antigens and other antigens (which do not have D) are much less antigenic than D and do not have clinical relevance. In clinical practice, therefore, Rh positive or Rh negative depends on the presence of D antigen on surface of red cells which can be detected by adding strong anti-D serum and noting agglutination. Nearly about 95% Indians, 90% Chinese and 85% Caucasians have this Rh D antigen and hence they are Rh positive (Rh+). Only 5–6% Indians do not have Rh D antigens and are Rh negative (Rh–).

During blood transfusion, after ABO compatibility, Rh+ blood can be safely transfused to Rh+ persons. But if the person is Rh– then not only RHD negative blood but also presence of CE antigens should be checked by adding anti-C and anti-E serum. When all these three antigens (CDE) are negative, then only it should be transfused to Rh– persons. This anti-D serum is actually IgG in nature.

There are six antisera corresponding to the Rh antigens. They are anti-C, anti-c, anti-D, anti-d, anti-E and anti-e. But in humans only five of these antisera have been detected and anti-d is absent. This may be probably because d antigen is not immunogenic or amorph to produce antibody against it.

Rh Grouping Method

Slide Methods

1. Place one drop of anti-D (commercially available) onto a slide.
2. Add two drops of red cell suspension (50%) or whole blood (citrated/oxalated/fresh).
3. Mix well and distribute over a large area of the slide.
4. Tilt it for 2–3 minutes.

Result: Clumping of cells (both macroscopic and microscopic) indicates Rh D positive and no clumps indicate Rh D negative.

Tube Methods

1. Add one drop of anti-D serum in a test tube

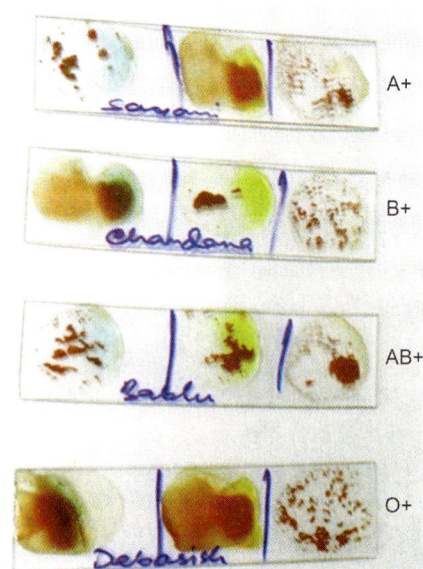

Fig. 8.4: Three compartments. First drop of blood on left side mixed with anti-A serum, middle drop of blood mixed with anti-B serum and last drop of blood on right side mixed with anti-D (Rh) serum. All are Rh group positive with ABO blood grouping of A, B, AB and O respectively

2. Add one drop of 5% red cell suspension and mix well
3. Incubate in a water bath at 37°C for 30–60 minutes.
4. Check for agglutination

Result: Agglutinations or clumps seen under the bottom of the tube indicate Rh D positive and no clumps indicate Rh D negative.

REACTIONS OR COMPLICATIONS FOLLOWING BLOOD TRANSFUSION

A. **Immediate complications**
   1. Rigor followed by pyrexia
   2. Allergic urticaria over the body and anaphylaxis
   3. Air embolism
   4. Haemolytic transfusion reactions leading to haemoglobinuria, haemolytic shock, and renal failure.
   5. Cardiac failure due to massive transfusion (volume overload).

6. Systemic infection due to contamination of blood.

B. Delayed complications
1. Infections: Hepatitis, malaria, HIV, syphilis, cytomegalovirus, Epstein-Barr virus (EBV), etc.
2. Past transfusion thrombocytopenic purpura
3. Delayed haemolytic crisis due to immune body production
4. Pulmonary microembolism.
5. Thrombophlebitis.

CONCEPT OF UNIVERSAL DONOR OR UNIVERSAL RECIPIENT

Universal donor: Blood group O person is often considered as universal donor because of absence of antigen A or antigen B on red cells. Plasma of blood group O person contains anti-A and anti-B. But these agglutinins or antibodies get diluted when blood is transfused to the recipient (patient) because of large serum in the recipient. So, these antibodies become inactive and no untoward reactions occur.

Universal recipient: Blood group AB person is often considered as universal recipient because of absence of anti-A or anti-B isoantibody in the serum. Any blood group when transfused to these persons, the red cells of donor's blood do not find any antibody to react with. Hence, there is no transfusion reaction.

The above definition is based on ABO grouping system. But when it is combined with Rh typing then persons with blood group O and Rh D negative (Rh−) are called universal donors. Likewise, persons with blood group AB and Rh D positive (Rh+) are universal recipients.

Table 8.6: Comparison of ABO and Rh blood grouping

Parameter	ABO blood group	Rh blood group
1. Antigenic locus on gene	Chromosome 9	Chromosome 1
2. Antigens	A, B, AB	D (only clinically significant)
3. Distribution of antigens	RBCs, platelets, body fluids, many tissues (called histo blood group)	RBCs only
4. Nature of antibody	Naturally occurring	Immune or acquired
5. Development of antigens	Weak expression at birth (full expression after 1 year of age)	Fully developed at birth
6. Antibody class	IgM	IgG
7. Optimal reaction temperature of antibody	4°C	37°C
8. Whether antibody can fix compliment	Yes	No
9. Optimal reaction medium	Saline	Anti-human globulin
10. Hemolysis following mismatched transfusion	Intravascular haemolysis due to complement mediated haemolysis	Extravascular and predominantly in spleen by mononuclear phagocyte (MP) or macrophage system

GEL CARD METHOD (COLUMN AGGLUTINATION OR MICROTYPING SYSTEM)

Microtyping system or column agglutination method is based on gel technology. In this test, gel (dextran acrylamide gel) is held in microtubes contained in a plastic card (hence the name gel card). This sephadex gel presents in each microtube is prepared in a buffer solution. This gel contains group specific antisera/antibody/antiglobulin (for Coombs' test) and sodium azide as preservative. These are incorporated into the gel during manufacture.

Principle of the Test

Cells are poured over the microtube first. As for example, for blood grouping RBC suspension is poured. Then the microtubes are incubated at 37°C followed by centrifugation which pulls the cells downward and react with the antibody incorporated into gel. If antigen over cells are present against particular antibody, haemagglutination will occur. Normal RBCs can pass through the gel but the agglutinated RBCs cannot because of their adherence and large size and gel matrix acts as a sieve. The agglutinated RBCs get trapped at various sites within the gel and thus formed a red line (positive test).

If the specific antigen is absent on RBCs, agglutination does not occur and RBCs easily pass through the gel and reach the bottom of the tube. No red line is formed due to absence of agglutination (negative test).

Uses

i. Blood grouping (ABO and Rh typing) and crossmatching
ii. Coombs' antiglobulin test
iii. For diagnosis of sickle cell anemia, PNH (paroxysmal nocturnal haemoglobinuria)
iv. For diagnosis of different infective organisms (diphtheria, syphilis, measles, parvovirus, etc.)
v. Antibody identification

Advantages of gel card method

i. This method is easy, accurate, standardized.
ii. It needs small sample volume and reduces exposure to biohazardous samples.
iii. This method has greater sensitivity compared to conventional methods
iv. Cell washing is not required for Coombs' test.
v. Chances of error is almost absent as this is not done manually.

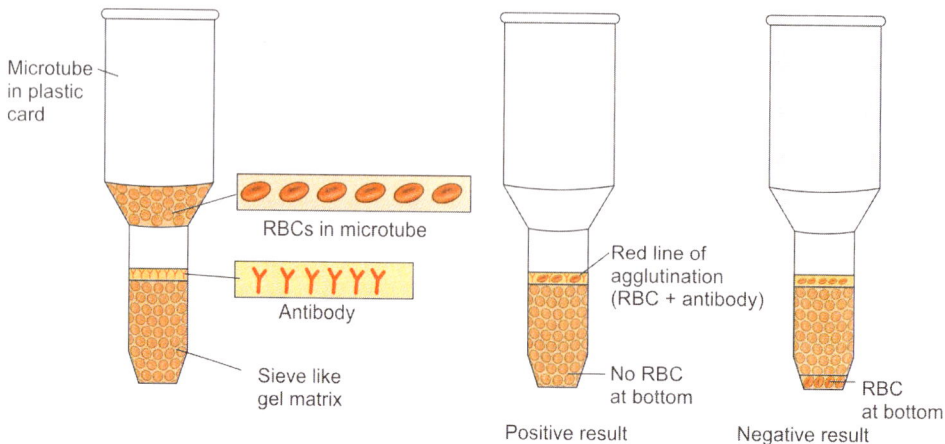

Fig. 8.5: Gel card method of blood grouping (column agglutination or microtyping system)

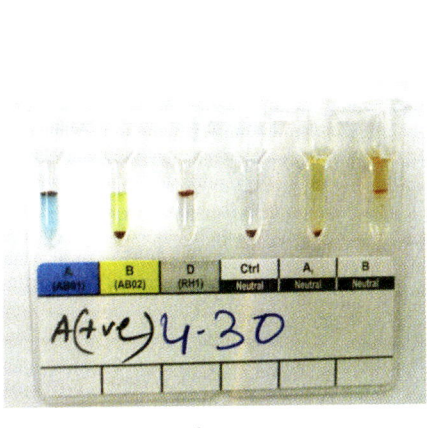

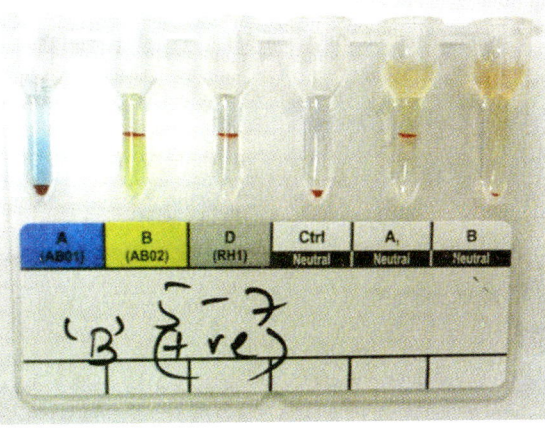

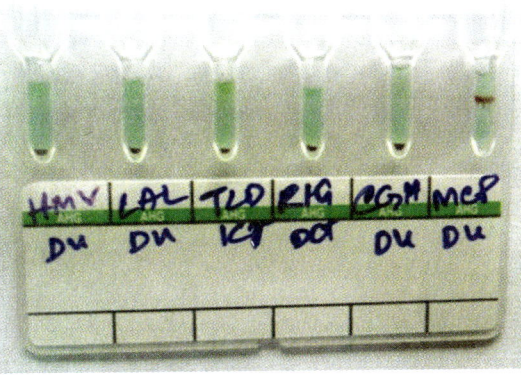

Fig. 8.6A to D: A to C showing ABO blood grouping in gel card method. (A) Blood group A+; (B) Blood group B+, (C) Blood group O+. There are six tubes. First one contains anti-A serum, second one contains ant-B serum, third tube contains anti-D serum, fourth tube is control, fifth tube contains antigen A₁, and sixth (last) tube contains antigen B. Particular agglutination is marked by a ring in the middle of that corresponding tube; (D) It shows Du blood grouping system. Among the six cases, only last case is Du positive

Disadvantage: It is expensive compared to conventional glass and tube method. Also it needs a special centrifuge.

SOLID PHASE ADHERENCE TECHNOLOGY

This method of cell grouping uses a microplate in which solid phase walls are coated with reagent RBCs or red cell stroma. Serum sample is added to it and if there is antibody in the serum it is captured by the antigen(s) over RBC surface/stroma. Then indicator RBCs (coated with monoclonal IgG) are added and the mixture is centrifuged. This indicator RBCs now attach to the antibody which was captured by coated RBCs. Agglutination occurs and is indicated by diffuse adherence of indicator red cells along the microwell (positive test). If there is no antibody in serum, then there is no agglutination (haemagglutination). This is indicated by RBCs forming a button at the bottom of the microwell (negative test).

Table 8.7: Cause of unexpected results (false positive or false negative) during blood grouping

Cell grouping (forward grouping)

Unexpected negative	Unexpected positive
i. ABO subgroup	i. Polyagglutinable RBCs
ii. Antisera stored improperly	ii. Acquired B antigens, seen in gastric or colon cancer, intestinal obstruction
iii. High levels of soluble blood group substances	iii. Foetomaternal haemorhage
iv. Antigenic suppression seen is leukaemia or cancer	iv. Wrong (out-of-group) transfusion
	v. RBCs coated by Wharton's jelly of umbilical cord
	vi. Bone marrow transplantation

Table 8.8: Serum grouping (reverse grouping)

Unexpected negative	Unexpected positive
i. ABO subgroup	i. Monoclonal antibodies (immunoglobulins)
ii. Newborn and elderly persons	ii. Transfusion of plasma components
iii. Immunosuppression	iii. Cold-reacting agglutinins
iv. Hypogammaglobulinaemia	

VIVA VOCE

Q1. What is Bombay blood group?

Ans: Both antigens A and B or RBCs are formed from H substance (H antigen). The dominant H gene is located on chromosome 19. This H gene encodes for an enzyme that converts a carbohydrate precursor substance present in red cell into H substance (H antigen). A and B genes encode for specific transferase enzymes that convert H substance into A and B red cell antigens. O gene encodes for inactive transferase enzyme that cannot convert H substance in blood group O red cells.

Rarely, persons do not inherit H gene (very rare HH genotype) and they are unable to produce H substance (H antigen). So, they cannot produce A and B blood group antigens on RBC membrane. This rare blood group is called Bombay blood group or Oh group. It was first discovered in Bombay, Maharashtra, among Marathi speaking people. Hence, it was named Bombay blood group. As, there is absence of blood group antigen A, B and H on RBC membrane, the plasma of Bombay blood group people will contain anti-A, anti-B and anti-H antibodies.

Q2. What are the subtypes of blood group A?

Ans: There are two subtypes—A_1 and A_2 in blood group A. A_1 subgroup is 80% and A_2 subgroup is 20% based on the presence of A_1 antigen or A_2 antigen on RBCs. A_1 has greater number of antigenic site than A_2 (10^6 site vs. 250,000 site). A potent anti-A_1 serum (anti-A_1) can agglutinate A_1 red cells but not A_2 red cells. There is no specific anti-A_2

serum. So, A_2 red cell does not agglutinate and pretends to be blood group O.

However, a saline extract of seeds of *Dolichos biflorus* is now routinely used in subtyping A blood cells (RBCs). It agglutinates A_1 blood cells and A_1B blood cells.

Saline extract of seeds of *Ulex europaeus* is used to agglutinate A2, A2B and O cells. It is actually an anti-H lectin.

Q3. Why reverse grouping (serum grouping) is not done before 4 months of age in infants?

Ans: There are no corresponding natural antibodies as regard to antigen(s) present on RBCs in infants below 4 months of age. So, reverse grouping (serum grouping) will give inaccurate result. It will pretend to be blood group AB as serum lacks any natural antibody.

Q4. Which method is better for blood grouping—tube method or slide method and why?

Ans: The tube method is better because the reaction between red cells and anti-serum is enhanced because of centrifugation to make red cell suspension. So, even the weaker antigen like A_2 can be detected apart from other/strong antigen(s). Tube method is recommended for both ABO and Rh blood grouping.

Q5. How would you distinguish agglutination from rouleaux formation?

Ans: When dilution with saline is done, it disperses rouleaux but cannot disperse agglutinated cells. Because agglutinated cells (antigen–antibody bonds) are firmly attached with each other.

Q6. Other than alloagglutination, what are the other causes of agglutination?

Ans:
i. Autoagglutination: It is due to presence of cold agglutinin.
ii. Psuedoagglutination: It is aggregates red cells due to non-immunological cause like excess rouleaux formation as seen in multiple myeloma, or in macroglobulinaemia (due to high level of paraproteins in blood).
iii. Polyagglutination or pan agglutination: If RBCs are contaminated by certain bacteria like *Pseudomonas aeruginosa*, then RBCs may be agglutinated by all blood group sera (antibody) or even by normal human serum. This phenomenon is known as **Thomson-Friedenreich phenomenon**. It is due to unmasking of a particular antigen (T or Tk antigen), which is present on human RBCs. Human serum contains anti-T antibody normally. So, when T antigens on RBCs are unmasked, agglutination occurs in blood groups. This is very rarely observed *in vivo*. Ex vivo (*in vitro*), it can be demonstrated by use of an anti-T lectin prepared from peanut.

Q7. What do you mean by one unit of blood?

Ans: Usually one unit of whole blood means 350 ml of whole blood mixed with 49 ml of anticoagulant CPDA-1 (citrate phosphate dextrose adenine).

Q8. How blood and blood products are stored?

Ans:
i. Whole blood and packed red cells: At 2 to 6°C in refrigerator for 35 days.
ii. Platelet concentrate: At 20 to 24°C for 3 days with continuous agitation.
iii. Fresh frozen plasma: Below –25°C for one year.
iv. Cryoprecipitate: Below –25°C for one year.

Q9. What is chimerism that can be found unexpectedly during blood grouping?

Ans: Sometimes a blood sample may contain more than one population of red cells. It may result from (i) transfusion of ABO compatible but not ABO-identical blood, (ii) foetomaternal haemorrhage and (iii) bone marrow transplantation (when blood group of donor is different from that of recipient).

Q10. What do you mean by major crossmatch and minor cross match?

Ans: The name 'crossmatch' came from the past practice of testing, the recipient's serum against donor's RBCs (major crossmatch) and donor's serum against recipient's RBCs (minor crossmatch). However, minor cross match is less important as antibodies in donor blood becomes diluted or neutralized in recipient's plasma (volume is more than donor unit). Minor crossmatch is also less important for antibody screening and identification.

Q11. What are the advantages of gel card method for blood grouping?

Ans: In gel card method, the monoclonal antibodies are used (unlike polyclonal antibodies in other methods). So, it is very sensitive and weak antigens can also be detected.

Part II

Clinical Pathology

9. Urine Examination
10. Lumbar Puncture Needle, Cerebrospinal Fluid and Other Body Fluids

9

Urine Examination

Urine examination provides a wide variety of useful information regarding the disease involving the kidney and lower urinary tract. In the evaluation of urine, many tests are done. These tests include: Chemistry, microbiology, routine urine wet analysis, and some other special tests. Some modern techniques like immunocytochemistry, DNA ploidy, cell cycle analysis and molecular genetics (PCR) are also performed on urine specimens.

At present, **three types of urinalysis** are performed. These are:
1. A screening wet urinalysis (routine examination of urine)
2. A reagent strip (dipstick or multistick paper strip)
3. Specialised urinalysis (like cytological examination of malignant cells, PCR, DNA analysis, flow cytometry, etc.).

Composition of Normal Urine

A normal healthy person excretes approximately 1500 ml of urine in 24 hours. Normal urine is clear and pale-yellow in colour which has typical aromatic odour due to presence of volatile organic acids. The yellowish colour of urine is due to presence of urochromes, which comes as breakdown product of urobilinogen. Freshly voided urine is slightly acidic (pH 6.0 to 6.8) which becomes alkaline on standing due to release of ammonia from urea decomposition. This urea decomposition occurs due to role of contaminated bacteria which initiates urease activity that splits urea.

Urine is composed predominantly of water (95%) and other soluble waste products (urea, creatinine, uric acid) and excess electrolytes (sodium, potassium, calcium, chloride, phosphate and others). Most hormones and drugs after their function in the body, are usually excreted through urine. So, urine can be ideal specimen for evaluating hormonal disorders and drug over dose.

Normal urine after standing will often crystallise certain chemicals like urates and phosphates under alkaline conditions and urine becomes turbid now. Epithelial cells, WBC, RBC are occasionally seen in normal urine. Their presence in increased number indicates a pathological condition or disease.

Urine Collection Methods

Urine specimens may be collected in a variety of methods according to type of specimen required the collection type and patient type.

- **Randomly collected specimen:** It is usually not preferred as urine may be

Table 9.1: Benefits of common tests performed with urine specimens

Type of test	Detection	Clinical Use Screening	Clinical Use Diagnostic	Clinical Use Monitoring	Clinical Use Prognostic
1. Wet urinalysis (routine examination)	Glycosuria (diabetes) Proteinuria Haematuria Leukocyturia Infections Crystalluria	++++	++	++	+
2. Reagent strip (dipstick, multistick)	Glycosuria Proteinuria Haematuria Leukocyturia Infections	+++	+/−	+	+
3. Urine microbiology (culture, etc.)	Infections	++	++++	++	+
4. Conventional urinalysis	Glomerular and renal tubular disease Lower urinary tract disorders Non-bacterial infections	+	++++	+++	++
5. Modern diagnostics (PCR, DNA analysis, flow cytometry)	Urothelial cancer	−	+	+++	++

collected soon after patient has consume water/fluid (urine is diluted).

- **First morning specimen:** It is the choice of specimen for urinalysis and microscopic analysis because the urine is generally more concentrated.
- **Midstream clean catch specimen:** This specimen is strongly recommended for microbiological culture and antibiotic susceptibility testing because of reduced incidence of cellular and microbial contamination.
- **Timed collection specimen:** It may be required for quantitative measurement of certain analytes (creatinine, urea, sodium, potassium, calcium, uric acid, catecholamines, metanephrines, vanillylmandelic acid (VMA), etc.).
- **Collection from catheters** (e.g. Foley's catheter): For patients who have difficulties to micturate and are using catheters.
- **Suprapubic aspiration:** It may be necessary when a non-ambulatory patient cannot be catheterised or where there are concerns about obtaining a sterile specimen by conventional methods.
- **Paediatric specimen:** For infants and small children, a special urine collection bag or condom may be attached to the urethral opening.
- **24 hours specimen:** It is of value to quantify 24 hours urinary protein excretion (helpful to diagnose nephritic syndrome and other cause of heavy proteinuria).

Urine Collection Recommendations (the CLSI* Guidelines)

- Primary (routine) specimen containers to have a wide base and a capacity of at least 50 ml.
- Sterile collection containers for all microbiological specimens.
- 24 hours specimen containers to have a capacity of at least 3 litres.
- Specimen containers should have secured closure to prevent specimen loss and to protect the specimen from contaminants.
- Amber-coloured container for specimen required for assay of light sensitive analytes such as urobilinogen and porphyrins.

*Clinical and Laboratories Standards Institute, USA.

Preservation of Urine

The urine should be examined within 1–2 hours after voiding. If delay is anticipated, then the specimen is best preserved in a refrigerator (but do not freeze) at an acid pH and without any preservative.

Chemical preservatives prevent decomposition and contamination of bacteria and fungi.

- **Toluene** (2 ml/100 ml urine): It is best all-round preservative. But it interferes with the protein examination by sulphosalicylic method.
- **Thymol** (one crystal): It can preserve urine for a few days. However, it may have false positive reaction for protein.
- **Boric acid** (1% or 1 gm/100 ml urine): It is used for many hormones and other substances.
- **Formalin** (1 drop/30 ml urine): It is an excellent preservative for the formed elements (erythrocytes, WBC, casts, etc.).
- **Sodium carbonate**: Rarely used for preservation of urobilinogen.
- **Sodium fluoride**

Table 9.2: Urine report of a normal adult

Physical examination

- Urine volume: 600–2000 ml/day (24 hours)
- Colour: Pale yellow or straw coloured
- Appearance: Clear (cloudy if there is phosphate)
- Odour: Faint aromatic
- Sediment: Nil
- Specific gravity: 1.016–1.025 (specific gravity of distilled water is 1, also written as 1016–1025)

Chemical examination

- pH (reaction): 4.6–8 (mean 6.1), acidic
- Protein (mainly albumin): Scant amount (<150 mg/24 hours urine)
- Reducing substance (glucose): Nil or glucose ≤130 mg/day urine
- Ketone bodies: Nil
- Bile salt and bile pigment: Nil
- Bence-Jones protein: Absent
- Urobilinogen: 0.5–2.5 mg/24 hours or 0.5–1 mg/dl
- Phosphates: Nil or trace
- Nitrites: Nil

Microscopical examination

- WBC: 0–5/hpf (usually 0–2, but up to 5/hpf in morning urine) *
- RBC: 0–2/hpf
- Cast (hyaline casts): 0–2/lpf
- Epithelial cells (squamous, cuboidal or transitional ≤15–20/hpf (usually 3–5/hpf)
- Crystals: Urates, uric acid, calcium oxalate in acid urine and phosphates, biurates in alkaline urine normally may be present
- Bacteria: None
- Yeast: None
- Parasite (Trichomonas, *Schistosoma haematobium*, microfilaria): None

hpf: High power field, lpf: Low power field, * increased number may be seen in menstruating women.

Physical Examination of Urine

Urine Volume

The 24 hours urine discharged by a healthy adult with normal water/fluid intake is about 1500 ml. Because it varies widely with fluid intake, physiological condition and diet of the human body. Urine discharged during day is about 3–4 times more than that of night. Children (6–12 years) discharge about 800–1200 ml of urine and infant about 500–600 ml of urine in 24 hours.

A urine volume >2000 ml/24 hours is termed **polyuria** and urine <400 ml/24 hours is called **oliguria**. **Anuria** is complete absence of urine formation. **Oligoanuria** when <100 ml/day.

Causes of polyuria
- Diabetes insipidus/diabetes mellitus
- Compulsive water drinking
- Intravenous saline/fluid infusion
- Chronic glomerulonephritis
- Chronic pyelonephritis
- Benign nephrosclerosis
- Hyperparathyroidism
- Addison's disease
- Drug like diuretics

Causes of oliguria
- Severe dehydration (diarrhoea, vomiting, excessive sweating)
- Acute glomerulonephritis (mainly in children)
- Renal ischaemia in a patient of shock
- Obstruction to urinary outflow
- Bilateral hydronephrosis
- Toxic or ischaemic nephrosis
- Blood transfusion reaction or following surgery.

Colour

The yellow colour of normal urine is mainly due to the pigment urochrome and to a small amounts of urobilins and uroerythrin. Urochrome excretion is believed to be proportional to the metabolic rate and it is increased in high fever, thyrotoxicosis and starvation. The uroerythrin (pink pigment) may be deposited in uric acid or urate crystals (black dust deposit) and it should not be confused with blood. Colourless or pale urine in a normal person may be seen after high fluid intake and darker urine (deep yellow or mustard coloured) when fluids are withheld.

Change in urine colour (pathologic and others)
- Red urine: Frank haematuria (gross haematuria), haemoglobinuria or methaemoglobinuria, beets and aniline dye.
- Brown black: Methaemoglobinuria, presence of melanin and homogentisic acid (alkaptonuria)
- Yellow-green: Bilirubin, biliverdin
- Milky white: Presence of chyle in urine (chyluria), plenty of neutrophils (pyuria), emulsified paraffin used in vaginal cream.
- Cloudy: Excess phosphates, carbonates, urates and uric acid in urine, prostatic fluid, radiographic dye.

Specific Gravity

Specific gravity is the density of a substance (weight per unit volume) as compared to that of the density of water which is 1.000 (also written as 1000). Specific gravity of a solution largely depends on the amount of solute present and also on temperature of the solution. It increases with increasing concentration of solute and decreases with increasing temperature as urine volume increases with temperature and density decreases.

Kidney can produce urine with specific gravity which ranges from 1.005 to 1.035. Urine of low specific gravity is called **hyposthenuric** (≤1.007). Urine of fixed specific gravity about 1.010 is known as **isosthenuric**. The specific gravity of the protein-free glomerular filtrate is about 1.010 and its osmolar concentration is about 285 mOsm.

Specific gravity of normal urine is contributed by urea (20%), sodium chloride (25%), sulfate and phosphate mainly. Normal adult with normal diets and normal fluid intake produces urine of specific gravity 1.016–1.022 during a 24-hour period. If there is no fluid intake for 12 hours or 24 hours then specific gravity becomes 1.022 or ≥1.026 respectively.

Causes of high specific gravity
- Concentrated urine: Due to excessive sweating, fever, vomiting.
- Acute nephritis
- Uncontrolled diabetes mellitus (crystalloids not the colloids are responsible)
- All causes of oliguria.

Cause of low specific gravity (specific gravity <1.010)
- Excessive fluid or water intake
- Diabetes insipidus
- Chronic nephritis
- Hypertension with renal involvement
- All causes of polyuria except diabetes mellitus

Cause of low and fixed specific gravity (1.010–1.012)
- End stage renal disease (chronic nephritis)
- Arteriosclerotic kidney
- ADH deficiency

Measurement of Specific Gravity of Urine

It can be done by following methods:

a. **Urinometer (hydrometer):** The urinometer vessel is filled with three-fourths full with urine (about 70–80 ml, minimum 15 ml urine). The urine should be foamless. The urinometer is inserted with a spinning motion to make sure that the instrument is floating freely without touching the sides or the bottom of the container. Read graduations at the lowest level of the urinary meniscus. If the urine amount is less than dilute the urine to raise the volume till 70–80 ml. Take the reading and multiply by the dilution factor (take last two digits).

Correction factor for temperature: Add or subtract 0.001 for each 3°C above or below the standardisation temperature (usually 20°C).

Correction for protein and glucose: Subtract 0.003 for every 1 gm/100 ml of protein and 0.004 for every 1 gm/100 ml of glucose.

b. **Refractometer:** The refractive index of a solution is related to the content of dissolved solids present. It is the ratio of the velocity of light in air to the velocity of light in a solution. The instrument requires only a few drops of urine (unlike the minimum 15 ml of urine necessary for urinometer).

In Goldberg refractometer, the specific gravity of urine can be read directly from the calibration. But the specific gravity reading on refractometer is usually slightly lower than a urinometer reading on the same urine by about 0.002.

c. **Reagent strips/dipsticks:** This is basically colorimetric method. The principle of the specific gravity area is based on a pKa change of certain penetrated polyelectrolytes in relation to ionic concentration. The reagent is sensitive to the number of ions in the urine specimen. An indicator changes colour in relation to ionic concentration and is translated to specific gravity values.

Chemical Examination of Urine

The pH

The pH (reaction) of urine can be measured by:
- Litmus paper or other pH indicator papers: It can detect broad range of pH 1 to 12. Note the colour change. If red = acidic, orange = normal, yellow = alkaline.
- Reagent strip: Indicators like methyl red and bromothymol blue give a range of orange, green and blue as the pH rises.

The test permits differentiation of pH values to half a unit within the range of 5 to 9.
- pH electrode: pH can be measured by pH meter with a closed glass electrode.
- **Titration method:** The pH of the urine is largely dependent on the amount of mono- and di-basic phosphate present. Titratable acidity is measured by titratating an aliquot of 24 hour urine (collected on ice) with 1/10 (N) NaOH with pH 7.4 as an endpoint.

Causes of acidic urine
- Ketosis: Diabetes, starvation, fever in children.
- Systemic acidosis: Metabolic acidosis, respiratory acidosis
- Acidification therapy: Acidification therapy when used to treat urinary tract infection.
- Others: Diet containing high protein, some fruits like cranberries.

Causes of alkaline urine
- Alkaline tide: The urine becomes less acid after a meal as a result of secretion of acid into the stomach. On the contrary, at night during the mild respiratory acidosis of sleep, a more acid urine may be formed.
- Systemic alkalosis: Severe vomiting, excess alkali ingestion, hyperventilation.
- Urinary tract infection: Caused by Proteus and Pseudomonas. They split urea to bicarbonate and ammonia.
- Alkalinization therapy: It is used to prevent crystallization of uric acid, oxalate, cystine, streptomycin and sulphonamides.
- Others: Diet high certain fruits and vegetables, especially citrus fruits.

Test for Reducing Substance (Glucose)

Glucose and other reducing substances in urine can be detected by:
a. **Copper reduction test**
   i. Benedict's test
   ii. Fehling's test
   iii. Copper reduction tablet test
b. **Reagent strip method:** Glucostix, clinistix, multistix, chemstrip (glucose oxidase-peroxidase method)
c. **Osazone test:** In this test, glucose osazone crystals are formed which are detected microscopically.

In the past, the two tests which had been most commonly used to show the presence of reducing substances in urine are those of Benedict and Fehling (more commonly Benedict's test). In these two tests alkaline cupric copper solutions are reduced to cuprous oxide.

Benedict's test and Fehling's test are mainly used to detect whether glucose is present in the urine or not. Other reducing substances that give positive results are:

- Other sugars: Pentoses, fructoses, galactose and lactose (but not sucrose)
- Salicylic acid
- Ascorbic acid (vit C)
- Homogentisic acid
- Creatinine
- Uric acid
- Formaldehyde

Benedict's Qualitative (Semiquantitative) Test

Benedict's reagent (qualitative)
- Tri-sodium citrate: 173 gm
- Sodium carbonate (anhydrous): 100 gm
- Copper sulphate: 17.3 gm
- Distilled water, add up to: 1000 ml

Dissolve tri-sodium citrate and sodium carbonate in 500 ml of distilled water. Dissolve copper sulphate in 500 ml of distilled water with gentle heat in another container. Mix the two solutions.

Principle of the test: All monosaccharides and disaccharides (glucose, galactose, lactose, pentose, levulose) reduce cupric sulphate in alkaline environment into insoluble cuprous oxide of yellow or red colour.

Cu^{++} $\xrightarrow{\text{hot alkaline solution}}$ Cu^{+}
(cupric ion) (cuprous ion)

$Cu^{+} + OH \longrightarrow CuOH$ (yellow)

$2\,CuOH \xrightarrow{\text{heat}} Cu_2O + H_2O$ (red)

Method: To 5 ml of Benedict's qualitative reagent (blue in colour) add 8 drops of urine (0.05 ml). Boil it over a flame for 3–5 minutes or set in a boiling water bath for 5 minutes. Cool it. Notice the change in colour.

- Negative: No change in colour (blue)
- Trace: Pale green with slight cloudiness
- 1+ (<0.5% glucose): Green or yellow-green deposit
- 2+ (0.5–1% glucose): Yellow deposit
- 3+ (1–2% glucose): Orange or orange-red deposit
- 4+ (>2% glucose): Brick red precipitate

Sensitivity of the test: ≥50 mg%

Fehling's Test

Fehling's reagent

1. *Solution A*
   - Copper sulphate: 34.65 gm
   - Distilled water: 500 ml

2. *Solution B*
   - Sodium hydroxide: 125 gm
   - Sodium potassium tartarate: 173 gm
   - Distilled water: 500 ml

Method: In a test tube take 2.5 ml each of solution A and solution B of Fehling's reagent. Mix well and boil. Add 8 drops (0.5 ml) of urine and boil again for 3–5 minutes. Cool it. Notice the change in colour and get the result (as in Benedict's test).

Benedict's Quantitative Test for Sugar

Quantitative reagents

- Sodium carbonate (anhydrous): 100 gm
- Sodium/potassium citrate: 200 gm
- Potassium thiocyanate: 125 gm
- Copper sulphate: 18 gm
- Potassium ferrocyanide (5%): 5 ml
- Distilled water up to: 1000 ml

Method: If the Benedict's qualitative test for urine is positive, then this quantitative test can be done to ascertain exact amount of sugar present in urine. If strongly positive, then urine may be diluted (1:10). In a conical flask, take 25 ml of Benedict's quantitative reagent. To it, add 15 gm of crystalline sodium carbonate and boil. When it is boiling then add urine sample drop by drop from a graduated burette until the blue colour completely disappeared and a chalky white colour develops.

At this point, all cupric ion originally in solution is reduced. *It is know that 0.05 gm of sugar is needed for complete reduction of this 25 ml of Benedict's quantitative reagent.*

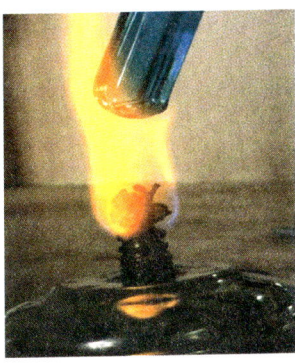

A

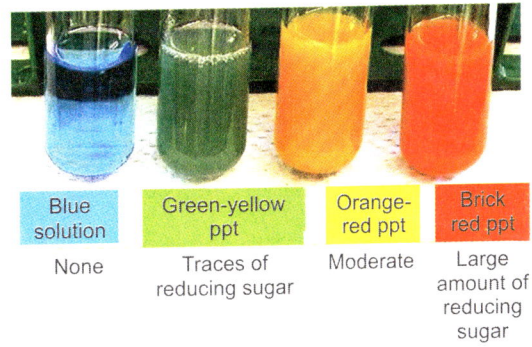

B

Fig. 9.1A and B: Benedict's qualitative test for urinary glucose

Calculation: Suppose, we have tested 20 ml of diluted urine (1:10 dilution)

So, 20 ml diluted urine contains 0.05 gm of sugar

Or, 20 ml undiluted urine (original urine) contains 0.05 gm × dilution factor = 0.05 × 10 (here)

Or, 100 ml undiluted urine contains =
$$0.05 \times 10 \times 100 \div 20 \text{ gm}$$
$$= 2.5 \text{ gm\% sugar (glucose)}$$

If there is no urinary dilution, the dilution factor is 1.

Reagent Strip Method

This test is based on a specific glucose oxidase and peroxidase method, a double sequential enzyme reaction. Reagent strips differ in the chromogen used. It may be used for semiquantitative results.

$$\text{Glucose} + O_2 \xrightarrow{\text{glucose oxidease}} \text{gluconic acid} + H_2O_2$$

$$H_2O_2 + \text{chromogen} \xrightarrow{\text{peroxidase}} \text{oxidised chromogen} + H_2O \text{ (colour change)}$$

The glucose oxidase strip test is specific for glucose. It does not react with lactose, galactose, fructose or reduce metabolites of drugs.

- **Clinistix (*o*-toluidine chromogen)**: Colour changes from pink to purple. It can detect 100 mg/dl of glucose.
- **Multistix (potassium iodide chromogen)**: Colour changes from blue to brown within 30 seconds.

Note

i. False positive result may be obtained by strongly oxidising cleaning agents in the urine container.
ii. Use of sodium fluoride as a preservative causes false negative results.
iii. High specific gravity of urine decreases colour development.
iv. All reagent strips should be protected from humidity, otherwise it will reduce the reactivity.
v. For optimal result, of this enzymatic reactions, urine should be kept at room temperature.

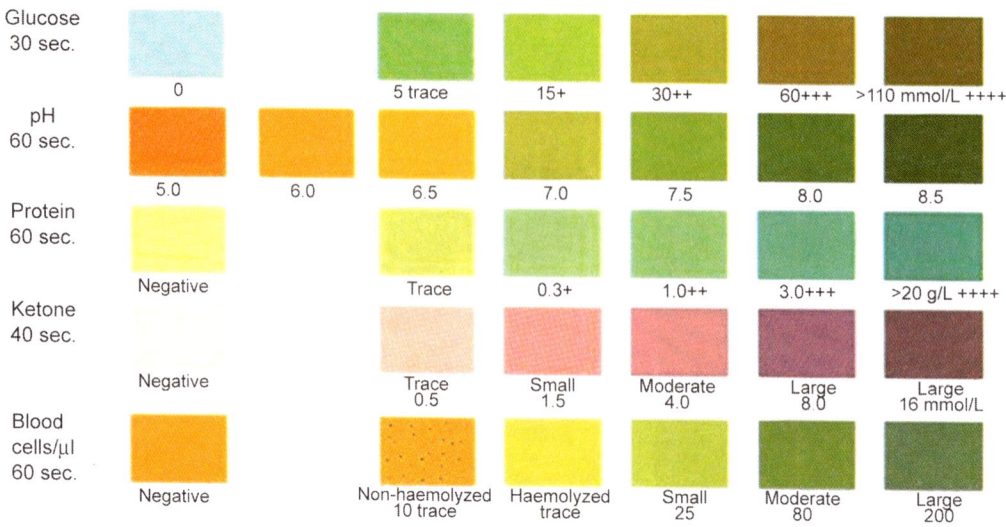

Fig. 9.2: Multistix for chemical examination of urine

- **Chemstrip (aminopropyl-carbazol chromogen)**: Colour changes from yellow to orange-brown at 60 seconds.
- **Chemstrip ^uG_c (tetramethylbenzidine chromogen)**: These strips have different sensitivities to urine glucose, range is 60 mg/dl to 5 gm/dl. Colour change at 2–3 minutes.

Sugar in Urine and its Significance

1. **Glycosuria with hyperglycaemia**
   - Diabetes mellitus
   - Other endocrine disorders: Hyperthyroidism, hyperpituitarism, acromegaly, Cushing's syndrome, phaeochromocytoma.
   - Pancreatic diseases: Haemochromatosis, cystic fibrosis (late stage), carcinoma, severe chronic pancreatitis.
   - CNS dysfunction: Intracranial injury, tumours or haemorrhage (especially in hypothalamus)
   - Drug induced: Thiazides, corticosteroids, ACTH, oral contraceptives
   - Massive metabolic derangement: Uraemia, sepsis, cardiogenic shock, severe burns, advanced liver disease.

2. **Glycosuria without hyperglycaemia**
   - Renal glycosuria: Normally, sugar does not come into urine unless it is >180 mg/dl in blood. But in case of renal glycosuria renal threshold for urinary sugar is reduced. So, sugar appears in without high blood sugar level.
   - Renal tubular dysfunction: Fanconi's syndrome, galactosaemia, cystinosis, lead poisoning, multiple myeloma.
   - Pregnancy (differentiate it from gestational diabetes)

3. **Non-glucose sugars in urine**
   - *Galactose:* Galactosaemia in newborn due to deficiency of galactose-1-phosphate uridyltransferase or galactokinase.

Table 9.3: Comparison between Benedict and reagent strip (glucose oxidase) methods for urinary sugar detection

Test result	Benedict's test	Reagent strip (glucose oxidase) method
1. True positive	• Glucose • Galactose • Lactose • Fructose • Maltose • Pentose	• Glucose
2. False positive	• Ascorbic acid • Homogentisic acid • Salicylates • X-ray contrast media • Anti-tubercular drugs • Levodopa • Stress, excitement	• Hydrogen peroxide (H_2O_2) • Hypochlorite in container • Pregnancy and lactation • Stress excitement
3. False negative		• Ascorbic acid • Homogentisic acid • Large amount of salicylates • Deteriorated reagent strips

- *Lactase:* May appear in urine in late pregnancy or during lactation.
- *Fructose:* During parenteral feedings with fructose and in association with inherited enzyme deficiencies that cause benign essential fructosuria.
- *Pentose:* Ingestion of large amounts of fruits, causing the excretion of L-xylose and L-arabinose.
- *Sucrose:* After ingestion of very large amounts of sucrose. It gives negative results with glucose oxidase or copper reduction tests. (Sucrose is not a reducing substance.) It can be separated by chromatography.

4. **Tests for protein in urine (proteinuria):** Normal urine contains up to 150 mg/day or 10 mg/dl (1–14 mg/dl) of protein depending on urine volume.

The proteins in urine are derived from plasma and urinary tract. Albumin and small molecular plasma globulins constitute about 2/3rds of the protein, and 1/3rd is the glycoprotein secreted by the thick part of the ascending loop of Henle and possibly the distal tubule. This glycoprotein is known as Tamm-Horsfall protein. It is believed that this protein forms the matrix of all casts. It forms a meshwork of fibrils which may trap cells, cell fragments or granular material. Enzymes and proteins from tubular epithelial cells, immunoglobulin A in secretions of urinary tract, other desquamated cells and leukocytes are other proteins found in very small amount in normal urine.

Plasma proteins with MW < 50,000–60,000 pass through the glomerular membrane and are normally reabsorbed by proximal renal tubular epithelial cells. Albumin which has MW of 69,000 is filtered out only in small amount. Immunoglobulin light chains, retinol binding protein, β_2-microglobulin and lysozyme are excreted in small amounts. Anderson in 1979, demonstrated more than 200 urinary proteins.

Qualitative or Semiquantitative Tests

Heat and Acetic Acid Test

Principle of the test: Urinary proteins are coagulated and denatured by heat and thus rendering the solution turbid (turbidometric method). Acetic acid (3%) is added to the urine to make it slightly acidic. It facilitates the precipitation of protein, and in addition, avoid false positive results due to precipitation of phosphates which are nomal constituents of urine. But excessive amount of acid or alkaline medium should be avoided as it may produce meta-proteins (acid or alkaline) which are not coagulated by heat.

Method: Take 10 ml urine in a clean test tube (15 ml capacity) or two-thirds portion of the test tube. Hold the test tube at the bottom with a test tube holder and start heating the upper half-inch or inch of the column of urine (keep the open end of the test tube away from you). If white cloudiness appears, it may due to protein or phosphates. Add 2–3 drops of 3% acetic acid. If the cloudiness disappears it is due to phosphates, but if the cloudiness persists, it is due to protein in urine. If cloudiness appears when heated and disappears when cooled down it is Bence-Jones protein.

Results
- Negative: No cloudiness
- Trace: Hardly visible cloudiness
- 1+: Cloudiness present but no granular flocculation
- 2+: Heavy and granular cloudiness but no flocculation
- 3+: Dense cloud but no marked flocculation
- 4+: Thick, curd-like precipitate and coagulation.

Sulphosalicylic Acid Test

Take 2 ml of centrifuged (clear) urine specimen. Add equal volume of 3–5% sulphosalicyclic acid solution. Invert to mix and

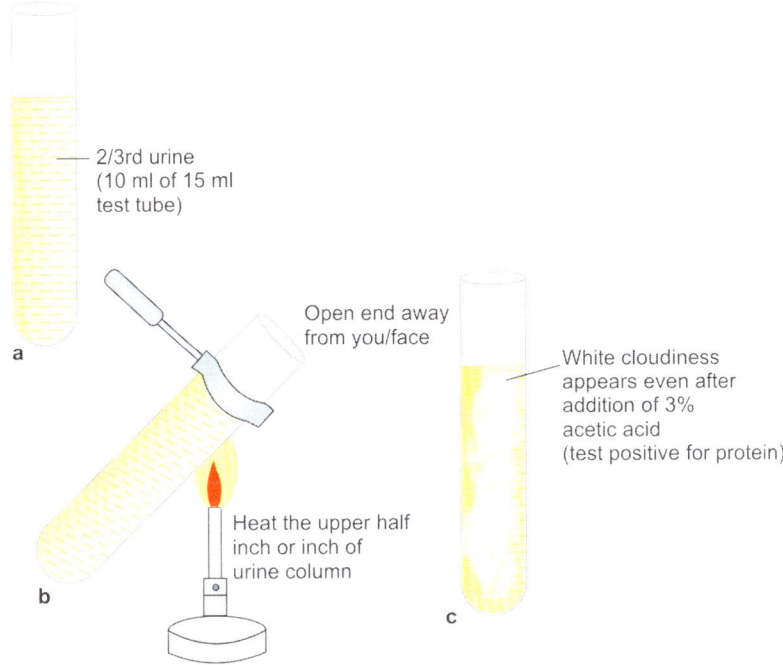

Fig. 9.3: Schematic diagram of different steps (a, b and c) of heat and acetic acid test for urinary protein detection

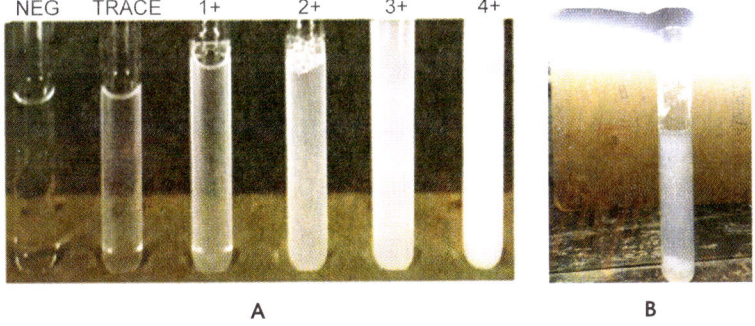

Fig. 9.4A and B: (A) Interpretation of heat test for detection of urinary protein; (B) Showing 2+ positivity

wait for 10 minutes. Note the degree of turbidity.
- Negative: No turbidity (<0.005 gm%)
- Trace: Faint turbidity (0.01 gm%)
- 1+: Distinct turbidity but no granulation (0.01–0.05 gm%)
- 2+: Turbidity with granulation but no flocculation (0.05–0.2 gm%)
- 3+: Turbidity with granulation and flocculation (0.2–0.5 gm%)
- 4+: Clumps of precipitate (>0.5 gm%)

Sulphosalicyclic acid test is more sensitive than heat test. It can detect 5–10 mg/dl of urinary protein.

Heller's Nitric Acid Test

Take 1 ml of concentrated nitric acid (fuming) in a test tube first. Then add 2 ml urine by the side of test tube with the help of a pipette and make a layer on the top of acid. A whitish ring appears at the junction of the two fluids due to formation of metaprotein

Detection

a. *Heat coagulation test*

5 ml of urine and heat the upper part of the tube—agglutination is formed in the upper part

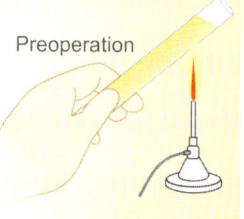

b. *Heller's test*

3 ml conc HNO_3 + 3 ml of urine on side of TT—**white ring** at the junction indicate albumin

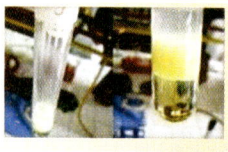

c. *Sulphosalicylic acid test*

6 drops of 20% SSA (aqueous) on 5 ml urine—if **clouds**—albumin

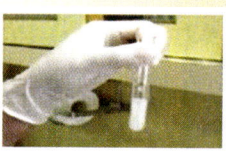

Fig. 9.5: Three methods for detection of urinary protein (albumin)

which appears as precipitates. It is due to presence of albumin in urine.

Reagent Strip Method

This test is based on protein charge and change in pH. As proteins carry a charge at physiologic pH, their presence elicits a pH change. The reagent strip is impregnated with tetrabromophenol blue buffered to an acid pH of 3 or tetrachlorophenol tetrabromosulfopthalein. This area is yellow in the strip in the absence of protein. Colour changes to a shade of green, depending on the type and concentration of protein present in 30–60 seconds.

Quantitative Estimation of Protein in Urine

Esbach's Method (by Albuminometer)

i. **Esbach's reagents**
   - Picric acid: 05 gm (which precipitates albumin)
   - Citric acid: 10 gm (which dissolves phosphates)
   - Distilled water: 500 ml

ii. **24 hours urinary sample:** Collect 24 hours urine sample in a clear container. Make the urine clear by filtering it and acidifying with 10% acetic acid. If the specific gravity is >1.025, then urine should be diluted (1:2, or 1:3, or 1:4

Table 9.4: Comparison between reagent strip test and sulphosalicylic acid test for detection of proteinuria

Parameter	Reagent strip test	Sulphosalicylic test
1. Principle	Colorimetric	Acid precipitation
2. Sensitivity	5–10 mg/dl	20 mg/dl
3. Type of test	Screening	Confirmatory
4. Indicator	Colour change	Turbidity
5. Proteins detected	Albumin only	All (albumin, myoglobin, haemoglobin, Bence Jones protein)

depending on SG), so that albumin precipitates do not float.

iii. **Esbach's albuminometer:** This is a thick-walled glass tube with 'R' mark above and 'U' mark below. At the lower part of the tube there is a few graduations with numerical markings. Also, there is a wooden stand to keep this glass tube.

Method: The albuminometer is filled with filtered and acidified urine sample (specific gravity <1.025) up to mark 'U'. Then Esbach's reagent is added up to the mark 'R'. It is then well mixed and kept in the stand in vertical position for 24 hours.

Result: The level of precipitate deposited at the bottom of the albuminometer is measured by graduation and is expressed in gm/litre. To get gm%, the result should be divided by 10.

Principle of the test: Albumin combines with picric acid in acid environment and forms the salt 'albumin picrate' which deposits at the bottom.

Tubidimetric Method

Here, colorimetric readings are taken against blanks and calculation done accordingly to get the result. As for example, sulfosalicylic acid turbidity method. It provides an accurate estimation of urinary protein.

Patterns of Different Proteinuria

1. **Glomerular pattern:** In healthy person, albumin is not lost in urine, because of the same negative charge of protein and glomerular capillary wall which causes repulsion. But in disease (glomerulone-phritis), there is loss or reduction of the fixed negative charge on the glomerular capillary wall that allows albumin to permeate into Bowman's space in large amount, more than which can be reabsorbed by proximal tubular cells. Glomerular disease often causes heavy proteinuria (>3–4 gm/day).

When serum protein is lost in urine, other proteins of similar size or charge are also lost. As for example, transferrin, prealbumin, α_1-acid glycoprotein, α_1-antitrypsin and antithrombin. Protein with larger size or molecular weight (MW) does not appear in urine till the glomeruli are not totally damaged, e.g. β-lipoprotein and α_2-macroglobulin.

2. **Tubular pattern**: Here, glomerulus is normal but there is defective tubular reabsorption of protein. These urinary proteins are usually of low MW. As for example, light chain immunoglobulin, lysozyme, α_1-microglobulin and β-globulin like β_2-microglobulin. Tubular pattern of proteinuria is seen in renal tubular diseases like cystinosis, Wilson's disease, Fanconi's syndrome, renal transplant rejection and pyelonephritis. The amount of proteinuria is lower than with glomerular diseases and usually 1–2 gm/day.

Tubular proteinuria may be missed by the reagent strip test because of absent or very low amount of albumin and presence of other protein(s). However, it may be detected by other methods.

3. **Overflow proteinuria**: It is due to excessive production of certain proteins and subsequent loss in urine as it overflows. This overflow proteinuria is seen in haemoglobinuria, myoglobinuria and loss of immunoglobulins in urine. These proteins are not associated with glomerular or tubular disease initially but may cause renal disease later on. Myoglobinuria causes acute tubular necrosis and haemoglobinuria becomes toxic when the patient is dehydrated.

Causes of Proteinuria

Heavy Proteinuria (>3–4 gm/day)

- Nephrotic syndrome: Different types of primary and secondary glomerulone-phritis.
- Malignant hypertension

- Amyloidosis (primary, secondary and with multiple myeloma)
- Toxaemia of pregnancy
- Drugs (penicillamine)
- Heavy metals (gold, mercury)
- Renal transplant rejection
- Sickle cell disease

Moderate Proteinuria (1-3 gm/day)

- Different chronic glomerulonephritis
- Nephrosclerosis
- Multiple myeloma
- Radiation nephritis
- Diabetes nephropathy (mild)

Minimal Proteinuria (<1 gm/day)

- Chronic pyelonephritis
- Nephrosclerosis
- Chronic interstitial nephritis
- Acute diffuse post-streptococcal glomerulonephritis (nephritic syndrome)
- Congenital diseases: Polycystic kidney disease, medullary cystic disease.
- Renal tubular disease
- Hypertension (not malignant)
- Lower urinary tract infection
- Haemoglobinuria with severe haemolysis
- Fever, severe emotional stress
- Exercise

Bence Jones Proteinuria

Bence Jones protein is a group of similar proteins with molecular weight about 2500 (light chain globulin). The most characteristic of this protein is its behaviour on heating. Whereas ordinary plasma albumin and globulin begin to precipitate between 60°C and 70°C, Bence Jones protein begins to precipitate between 40°C and 60°C (lower temperature) and then redissolves as the temperature reaches boiling point. Subsequent cooling reprecipitates the protein and boiling redissolves it.

Cause of Bence Jones proteinuria
- Multiple myeloma and other plasma cell dyscrasia (most common cause)
- Malignant lymphoma
- Other rare causes: Chronic myeloid leukaemia (CML), osteomalacia, osteosarcoma, cancer metastasis to bone.

Tests for Bence Jones Protein

1. **Heat test:** A white coagulum of Bence Jones (BJ) protein develops on heating at 40–60°C and redissolves on boiling. On cooling down, the precipitates reappear at 40–60°C. Further cooling to room temperature, the protein will be invisible.

   Albumin is often present along with BJ protein. It can be separated by filtering hot, through a hot filter funnel. BJ protein comes through leaving the albumin behind on the filter paper. On cooling the filtrate, the BJ protein reprecipitates (at 40–60°C) and can then be completely redissolved by heating to boiling point again.

2. **Bradshaw test:** Take 1 ml of concentrated hydrochloric acid in a test tube. Then add 2 ml of urine by the side of the test tube with the help of a pipette. BJ protein is precipitated by the acid giving a white ring at the junction of the two fluids.

Table 9.5: Grading of albuminuria

Condition	mg/24 hours urine	mg/litre urine	mg/g creatinine	µg/min	µg/mg creatinine
Normal	<30	<20	<20	<20	<30
Microalbuminuria	30–300	20–200	20–300	20–200	30–300
Overt albuminuria	>300	>200	>300	>200	>300

3. **Osgood and Haskin's test**: In a test tube, mix 0.5 ml of 50% acetic acid, 1.5 ml of saturated sodium chloride solution and 2.5 ml of urine. A precipitate at room temperature on addition of the salt solution, strongly favours the presence of BJ protein. Heat the mixture gradually. If BJ protein is present is urine, then precipitate increases at 40–60°C and redissolves on boiling. Albumin and globulin usually appear only on heating, and boiling has no effect on the amount of the precipitate.
4. **Urine electrophoresis:** Urine is concentrated and run on electrophoresis just like blood. If BJ protein is present, it will appear as dense band in the gamma globulin region (M-band).
5. **Toluenesulphonic acid (TSA) test:** Add 1 ml of TSA reagent to 2 ml of urine (reagent should flow by the side of test tube). Mix well. A precipitate appears within 5 minutes, if BJ protein is present.

Test for Ketone Bodies in Urine (Ketonuria)

Ketone bodies are the products of incomplete fat metabolism, and their presence may be indicative of acidosis. Ketone bodies are synthesized in the liver by condensation of acetyl CoA associated with impaired carbohydrate metabolism. Three types of ketone bodies are:

i. Acetone [$CH_3.CO.CH_3$]
ii. Acetoacetic acid [$CH_3.CO.CH_2.COOH$ (also known as diacetic acid)]
iii. β-hydroxybutyric acid [$CH_3.CHOH.CH_2.COOH$]

Their accumulation in blood known as ketoacidosis and presence in urine is known as ketonuria.

In ketonuria, three ketone bodies present in urine in the following percentage:
- Acetoacetic (diacetic) acid (20%)
- Acetone (20%)
- β-hydroxybutyrate (about 58%)

Acetone is formed non-reversibly from acetoacetic acid. β-hydroxybutyric acid (3-hydroxybutyrate) forms reversibly from acetoacetic acid.

$$\text{Acetoacetic acid} \xrightarrow{-CO_2} \text{acetone}$$

$$\text{Acetoacetic acid} \underset{-2H}{\overset{+2H}{\rightleftharpoons}} \beta\text{-hydroxybutyrate}$$

Causes of Ketonuria

- Uncontrolled diabetes mellitus
- Chronic starvation (due to increased tissue especially fat catabolism)
- Pregnancy toxaemia with vomiting
- In infants and children: Acute febrile diseases and toxic states accompanied by vomiting and diarrhoea.
- The use of low carbohydrates diet for weight reduction.
- Glycogen storage disease and other inherited metabolic diseases.
- Exposure to severe cold and heavy exercise.

A. Rothera's Test

Principle of the test: Acetone and acetoacetic acid produces a purple-coloured complex with sodium nitroprusside in an alkaline environment.

Test: Take 5 ml urine in a test tube. Saturate the urine with ammonium sulphate or ammonium chloride. A few drops of aqueous solution of sodium nitroprusside (or about 0.5 ml of 20% aqueous solution) or a pinch of powder or a crystal is added to it and well shaken to dissolve it. About 2–3 ml of concentrated ammonia (liquor ammonia) is poured down by the side of the test tube so that it forms a layer on the top of saturated urine.

Result: Presence of acetone and acetoacetic acid is indicated by the development of a purple-coloured ring at the junction.

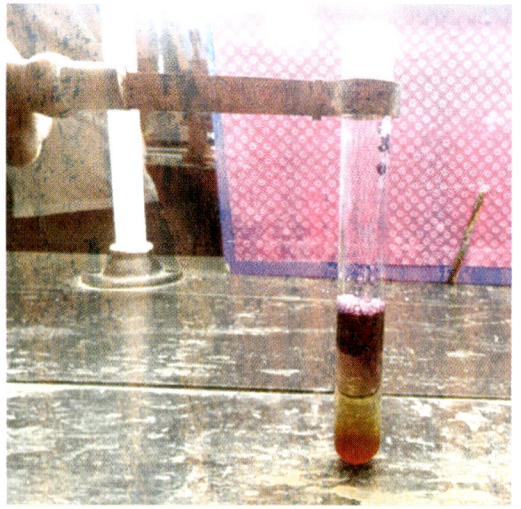

Fig. 9.6

Sensitivity: Acetone >10–25%, acetoacetic acid >1–5 mg%

> **Note**
>
> β-hydroxybutyric acid cannot be detected by routine Rothera's test. For detection of it, β-hydroxybutyrate has to be oxidised by addition of H_2O_2 to acetoacetic acid.

Take 5–6 ml of diluted urine (1:10) in a test tube. Add 2–3 drops of acetic acid to it. Mix well. Then boil it for 4–5 minutes to drive away acetone and acetoacetic acid which are present in urine. Now, add 1 ml of H_2O_2 (hydrogen peroxide). Warm gently, cool it and perform the routine Rothera's test (if β-hydroxybutyric acid is present, it has been converted to acetoacetic acid).

B. Gerhardt's Ferric Chloride Test

This is not a very sensitive test. Precipitate the phosphates in 5 ml of freshly voided urine with 10% ferric chloride solution, drop by drop. Filter it and add more ferric chloride solution to the filtrate (phosphates free). If a purple-red colour appears, it indicates presence of ≥0.05% of acetoacetic acid. Sensitivity for acetoacetate <80 mg/dl.

A similar colour may be given by salicylic acid and salicylates. If the heating is done after adding the ferric chloride, the colour already formed disappears if it is due to acetoacetate (diacetic) acid but salicylates are unaffected by boiling the urine and the colour persists.

C. Salicylaldehyde Method

Behre and Benedict (1926) developed a method in which the ketone bodies of all types are converted into acetone. This acetone then reacts with salicylaldehyde in the presence of alkali. The amount of red coloured di-acetone (hydroxybenzal) thus formed is measured colorimetrically.

D. Legal's Test

Like Rothera's test, here also sodium nitroprusside is used. Take 10 ml of urine in a test tube and add a few crystals of sodium nitroprusside. Acidify the urine with glacial acetic acid, invert to mix. Pour strong liquour ammonia and wait for 5–10 minutes. A violet-coloured ring indicates a positive test.

Reagent Strip Method

The test is based on nitroprusside (sodium nitroferricyanide) reaction for ketones. **Chemstrip** contains sodium nitroferricyanide and glycine which react with acetoacetic acid and acetone in an alkaline medium to form a violet dye. The test is read at 1 minute and it detects about 10 mg/dl of acetoacetic acid and 70 mg/dl of acetone. **Multistix** contains buffers and sodium nitroferricyanide, which react with acetoacetic acid, producing pink-marron colour within 15 seconds. The reagent can detect 5–10 mg acetoacetic acid/dl of urine. It does not react with acetone.

Blood in Urine

Haematuria: Presence of increased number of RBCs (intact) in urine is known as haematuria.

Important
Read package insert before use. Do not touch test areas. Store at temperature between 15°–30°C. Do not remove desiccants. Be sure to replace cap immediately and tightly

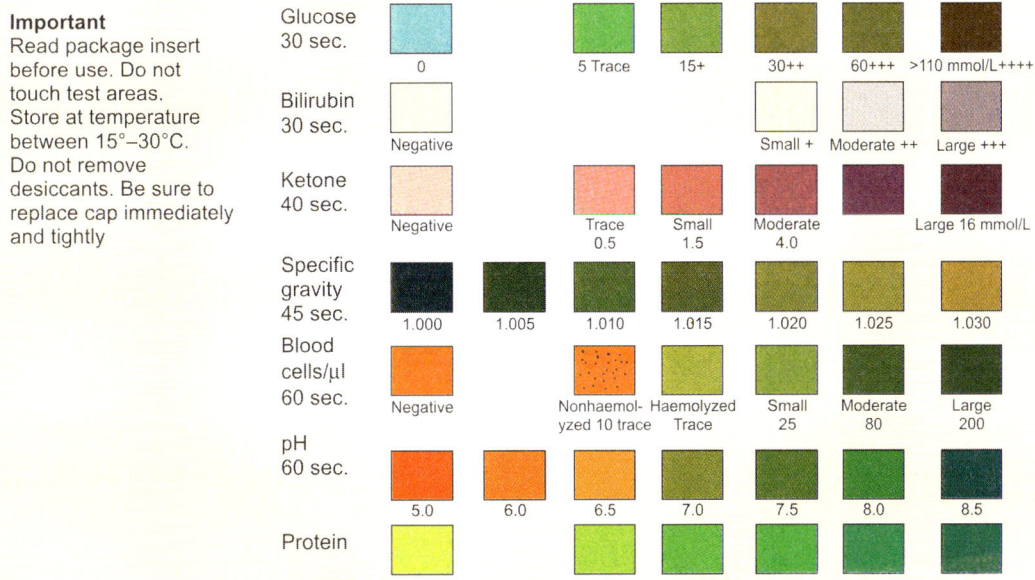

Fig. 9.7: Multisticx for urine examination

Haemoglobinuria: Presence of haemoglobin or blood pigments (Hb) in urine in absence of RBCs is called haemoglobinuria.

Causes of Haematuria

a. **Pre-renal cause:** Blood dyscrasias (haemophilia, leukaemia, purpura), subacute bacterial endocarditis, acute febrile conditions, malignant hypertension, anticoagulant therapy, drug reactions.
b. **Renal causes:** Glomerulonephritis, acute pyelonephritis, hydronephrosis, tuberculosis of kidney, stone in kidney, renal vein thrombosis, Wilms' tumour.
c. **Post-renal causes**: Haemorrhagic cystitis, carcinoma prostate, enlarged prostate, carcinoma bladder, salpingitis.

Causes of Haemoglobinuria

- Paroxysmal nocturnal hemoglobinuria (PNH)
- Autoimmune haemolytic anaemia
- Cold haemoglobinuria
- Mismatched blood transfusion
- Black water fever
- Marching haemoglobinuria
- Gas gangrene
- Snake venom poisoning

Test for Blood (Haematuria and Haemoglobinuria)

- Orthotoluidine test
- Benzidine test
- Guaiacum test

Both orthotoluidine and benzidine tests are highly sensitive tests compared to guaiacum test.

Orthotoluidine test: Pinch of orthotoluidine is dissolved in 2 ml glacial acetic acid in a test tube. Add 10–15 drops of urine and shake well. Then 4 ml of 30% H_2O_2 is added. Development of greenish-blue colour indicates presence of blood in urine.

Principle of the test: Haemoglobin and myoglobin (iron porphyrin products) release oxygen from hydrogen peroxide. This oxygen causes oxidation of orthotoluidine and develops a blue colour.

Benzidine test: Take equal volume of saturated solution of benzidine in glacial acetic acid and hydrogen peroxide (say 4 ml each) in a test tube. Take 4 ml of urine in another test tube. Add 4 ml of the mixed reagent (from the first tube) to urine. Developement of blue colour indicates presence of haemoglobin or occult blood in urine. This is very sensitive test.

Microscopic Examination of Urine

Use a clean fresh morning sample (midstream) whenever possible. Random midstream urine is satisfactory as a screening test. Urine should be examined within one hour (preferably fresh) because cells and casts begin to lyse within 1–3 hours. If delay is presumed, then urine should be refrigerated at 2–8°C. Preservatives through not preferred but can be used during transportation and more delay is suspected.

Centrifugation of urine specimen: Take freshly void urine (10–15 ml) in a conical centrifuge tube. Centrifuge it at a moderate speed, say 2000 r.p.m. for 5 minutes. Remove the supernatant by decanting into another test tube. The centrifuged deposit along with remaining fluid is resuspended in the first tube. This is taken out by a pipette and a drop is placed on a slide and covered with a coverslip (18 mm square). Remove bubbles if any.

Microscopy: Examine urinary sediment first under low power then under high power, vary the light intensity for seeing different casts.

1. Renal epithelial cells, RBCs, WBCs are identified under HP (high power) objective and counted in 10 representative HP fields.
2. Crystals are identified under LP (low power) objective.
3. Casts are identified under LP but finer details are confirmed under HP objective.
4. Others: Yeast, bacteria, parasites are identified under HP objective and number given per HP field.

In most instances, an unstained sediment is sufficient for reporting, However, if there is difficulty, then **Sternheimer and Malbin stain** may be used.

For identifying cellular structure and bacteria a drop of **methylene blue** solution can be used. Alternatively, **crystal violet safranin** stain can be used to identify cellular elements. Sometimes a peroxidase stain (myeloperoxidase or MPO) is used to differentiate renal tubular cells and neutrophils (pus cells). Neutrophil is MPO positive while tubular cells are negative.

Urinary sediments are divided into two broad classes:

1. Organised element
2. Unorganised element

Organised element: Red blood cells (erythrocytes), white blood cells (leukocytes), epithelial cells, tubular cast, broad cast and other casts, bacteria and others (yeast, parasites, spermatozoa, etc.)

Unorganised element: Crystals in normal acid urine (amorphous urates, crystalline urates, crystalline uric acid and calcium oxalate), crystals found in normal alkaline urine (amorphous phosphate, crystalline phosphate, calcium carbonate, ammonium biurate), crystals found in abnormal urine (cysteine, leucine, tyrosine and drug crystals).

Organised Elements in Urine

Red Blood Cell (Erythrocytes)

Red cells are identified by their smaller size, round shape, often with crenated margins (due to exosmosis). It should be distinguished from yeast cells. The finding of >2 RBC/HPF is abnormal. Causes of increased RBCs in urine or haematuria are:
- Renal disease: Glomerulonephritis, interstitial nephritis, hydronephrosis, trauma, polycystic kidney, malignant nephrosclerosis, tuberculosis, calculi.

- Lower urinary tract disease: Urinary tract infection or UTI (acute and chronic), stricture ureter and urethra, urinary bladder tumour and calculus.
- Extrarenal disease: Tumour of the colon, rectum and pelvis, salpingitis, acute appendicitis, chyluria, diverticulitis.

Dysmorphic erythrocytes: Fairley in 1982, observed that aberrant or dysmorphic erythrocyte morphology is specific in detecting glomerular bleeding. These distorted cells are better visualised under phase-contrast microscopy. When ≥80% of RBCs are undistorted and uniform, then bleeding is due to non-glomerular causes (i.e. from tubular cause or associated with calculi or may be due to urinary tract disease). Fassett in 1982, pointed out that normal persons usually have a mixture of distorted and undistorted RBCs in urine.

Leukocytes (Pus Cells)

They are identified by their nucleated structure with uneven margin. Leukocytes are bigger than RBC and do not lyse with addition of 2% acetic acid like RBC. But the acid however, accentuates the nucleus that appears as dark dots inside the cell. Normal urine shows 0–5 WBC/HPF, but in female their number is a little bit higher.

An increased number of WBCs (pus cells) in urine indicates renal infection which can be in the urinary bladder (cystitis) or in the kidney (pyelonephritis)

Pyuria: When more number of WBCs is found in urine (≥10 WBC/10 HPF). Pyuria can also be detected by reagent strip (leukocyte esterase dipstick test) which has a sensitivity of 90% and specificity of 80%. The reagent strip test is specially used when neutrophils swell and exhibit Brownian movement in hypotonic urine with pyuria. Because of this Brownian movement, moving granules appear as refractile and these cells are called **glitter cells**.

Renal Epithelial Cells

In normal urine, their number is 2–3/HPF in male and 8–10/HPF in females. The renal epithelial cells are 3 types:

i. **Transitional (urothelial) cells:** These cells are originate from renal pelvis, ureter, urinary bladder and prostate (in men). These cells are 2–3 times the size of a leukocyte (from 40 to 200 µm) and they are round or pear-shaped with a tail like process.

When stained with **Papanicolaou (Pap) stain**, transitional cells have dark blue nuclei with variable amount of pale blue cytoplasm. Another helpful clue is the presence of 'endo-ecto cytoplasmic' rim.

ii. **Squamous cells:** These cells originate from distal one-third of the urethra and vagina, vulva of women. These cells are large and flat with abundant cytoplasm and small round central nuclei. Margins are often folded. If stained with **crystal violet safranin**, nuclei are purple and cytoplasm pink to violet.

iii. **Small round or polygonal (parabasal) cells:** They originate from kidney tubules. Normally these cells are not present in urine and their presence indicates some renal diseases.

Casts

Casts are normally formed as colourless translucent gels from protein in the tubules of nephron (e.g. hyaline cast). Cast formation is increased when larger than normal amounts of plasma proteins enter the renal tubules. Most of these excess proteins are usually albumin although Bence Jones immunoglobulin, haemoglobin and myoglobin also take part in cast formation. The plasma protein probably react or combine with Tamm-Horsfall protein to form less translucent casts and glomerular casts unlike hyaline cast which is translucent.

In a normal person, very few are seen in the urinary sediment (mostly hyaline casts).

Increased number of casts is seen in widespread kidney disease when many nephrons are involved.

Classification of urinary casts
- Matrix casts: Hyaline cast, waxy cast
- Inclusion casts: Granular casts (proteins, cell debris), fat globules, haemosiderin granules, crystal (uncommon), melanin granules (rare)
- Pigment casts: Haemoglobin, myoglobin, bilirubin, drugs.
- Cellular casts: Erythrocytes and RBC remnants, leukocytes (neutrophil, lymphocytes, monocytes, histiocyte), renal tubular epithelial cells, mixed cells (more than one above mentioned cells).

Hyaline casts: These are clear (like glass) homogenous, transparent, cylindrical with parallel walls. Hyaline casts have a low refractive index and better seen under reduced light. They dissolve rapidly in alkaline urine or standing urine. They are translucent with brightfield microscopy but are easily visualised with phase-contrast microscopy. Increased number is seen in:
- Normal person after strenuous exercise
- Chronic renal failure
- Diabetic nephropathy
- Glomerulonephritis and pyelonephritis
- Congestive heart failure

Waxy casts: These casts are more opaque than hyaline casts because of high refractive index and have yellowish tinge. With brightfield microscopy, waxy casts are homogenously smooth in appearance. Their margins are sharp even in subdued light.
- Tubular inflammation and degeneration
- Chronic renal failure
- Acute and chronic renal allograft rejection

When waxy casts are unusually broad, these are known as **renal failure casts**.

Fatty casts: These are light yellowish bodies with a transverse split, associated with chronic renal disease or amyloid disease. They contain refractile fat droplets mixed with certain amount of granular material. Commonly found in nephrotic syndrome. Visible fat droplets are triglycerides or cholesterol esters.

Granular casts: These are hyaline casts containing large granules embedded in coagulated proteins. These granules are disintegration of epithelial cells or leukocytes which are trapped into the protein matrix.
- Glomerular and tubular disease
- Tubulointerstitial disease
- Renal allograft rejection
- Pyelonephritis, viral infections, chronic lead poisoning
- Coarse granular casts with haematuria in renal papillary necrosis
- Fine granules (calcium phosphate precipitant) in hyperparathyroidism.

RBC (red blood cell or erythrocyte) casts: Glomerular injury (mostly due to immune cause) allows erythrocytes to escape into the tubules. With concomitant proteinuria, RBC casts are formed in the distal nephron. In urine, these casts appear yellow under low power objective. A prerequisite for the identification of RBC cast is that red blood cell outlines be sharply defined in at least part of the cast. If there are many RBCs, the matrix may not be visible. RBC casts are best seen with phase-contrast microscopy. With supravital staining (crystal violet or brilliant cresyl blue or new methylene blue). Erythrocytes are colourless or lavender in a pink matrix.
- Acute glomerulonephritis (nephritic syndrome)
- Subacute endocarditis
- Renal infarction
- IgA nephropathy
- Lupus nephritis

WBC (leukocyte) casts: WBCs usually enter tubular lumen from renal interstitium. They enter through and between tubular epithelial cells. So, by and large WBC casts reflect tubulointerstitial disease. WBC casts may also be present in glomerular disease owing to the chemotactic effect of complement, interstitial nephritis, lupus nephritis and even in nephritic syndrome, but most common cause is pyelonephritis.

Renal tubular epithelial cell casts: Causes of these casts are:
- Acute tubular necrosis
- Viral disease (e.g. cytomegalovirus disease)
- Exposure to various drugs
- Heavy metal poisoning
- Ethylene glycol and salicylate intoxication
- Acute allograft rejection

Unorganised Elements in Urine

Crystals are found in urine in normal as well as in abnormal condition. Phosphates, urate and oxalates are common and found in normal urine. So, presence of these crystals has a little clinical significance. Oxaluria and phosphaturia are mostly related with dietary factors and digestive disorders respectively.

Crystals Found in Acid Urine

- *Calcium oxalate:* Refractile, octahedral, folded, envelop shaped. Occasionally dumbbell shaped or spherical appearing.
- *Amorphous urates:* Reddish yellow granules. They dissolve by heat (60°C) and sodium hydroxide. But when treated with acetic acid they do not dissolve but converted to uric acid crystals.
- *Uric acid:* Reddish brown or yellow, rhombic plates or prisms.

Crystals Found in Alkaline Urine

- *Triple phosphate (crystalline phosphate):* Composed of ammonium, magnesium, phosphate. These are colourless, refractile, six-sided prisms with oblique ends referred to as coffin lids. Occasionally leaf-like or feathery forms.
- *Amorphous phosphate:* Colourless fine granular precipitate
- *Calcium carbonate:* Small granular or colourless spherical.
- *Ammonium biurate:* Yellowish brown, apple thorn-like crystal.

Crystals Found in Abnormal Urine

- *Leucine:* Oily appearing spheres with radial and concentric striations
- *Tyrosine:* Fine yellowish silky needles in clumps
- *Cysteine:* Hexagonal, colourless, refractile plates
- *Drug crystals:* Radiographic media, ampicillin (high dose), sulphonamide may be found in urine.

Chyluria

It refers to milky-white urine resulting from ruptured lymphatics in the wall of urinary bladder or kidneys. The lymph containing fat droplets enters into urine which also contains RBCs. Sometimes, there may be clot formation due to presence of excessive fibrinogen.

Composition of chyle

- *Fat:* Average 2–3 gm/dl, finely dispersed. Special stain Sudan III and Oil red O. By adding equal volume of chloroform and ether, fat will be dissolved and milky colour disappears.
- *Protein:* Present in variable amount
- *Deposit:* WBCs, RBCs and microfilariae when caused by filarial infection.

Causes

i. Late stage filariasis
ii. Pregnancy or childbirth
iii. Abdominal tumours or lymph node enlargement
iv. Partial nephrectomy
v. Thermal ablation of a kidney lesion

Urine and Pregnancy Test

There are two types of pregnancy tests; one uses a urine sample, the other uses a sample of blood.

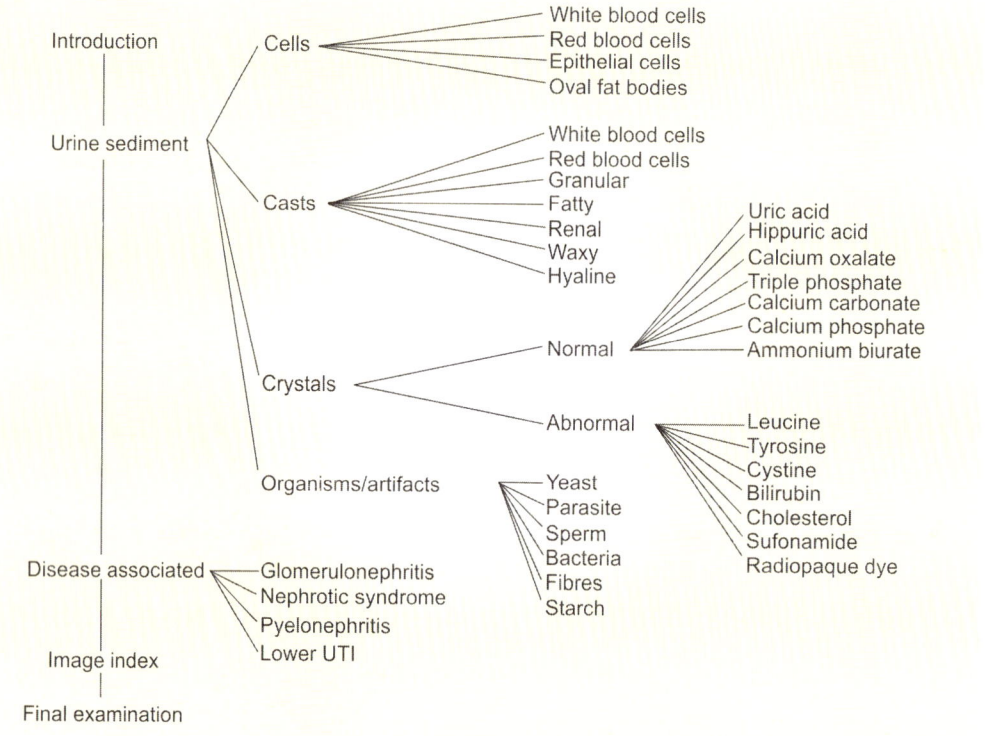

Fig. 9.8: Microscopic findings of urinary sediment

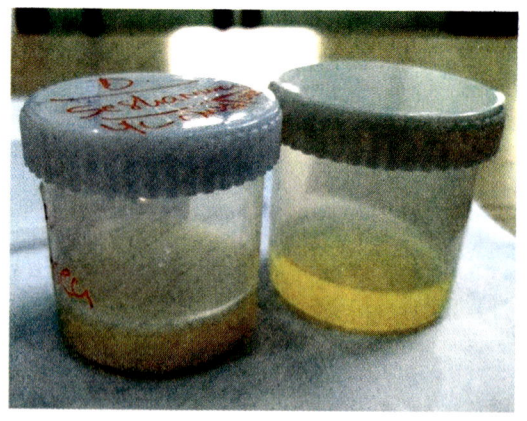

Fig. 9.9: Left container has chyluria and right container has normal urine. Note the milky-white colour of chyluria compared to pale yellow colour of normal urine

A pregnant woman's placenta produces hCG, also called pregnancy hormone. It (hCG) is a glycoprotein produced by trophoblastic cells beginning about 10 days after conception when the fertilised egg attached to the uterine wall. hCG is a dimer, the alpha subunit is nonspecific (shared with FSH, LH and TSH) but the beta subunit is unique to hCG.

During the first 8–10 weeks of pregnancy, hCG level normally increase very rapidly. This level reaches its peak at about 10th week of pregnancy and the gradually decline until delivery.

hCG urine tests are commonly sold in kits and they detect β (beta) subunits of hCG.

Test method: Take first morning urine sample as it contains more amount of β-hCG after 2 weeks of conception. For strip test, dip it into container containing urine sample up to maximum line. For cassette test, put 2 drops of urine in the specified sample well. Wait for 5 minutes and notice for colour bands (red in colour) in the **control (C)** and **test (T)** area.

Table 9.6: Urinalysis in various renal/urinary system diseases

Diseases	Macroscopic urinalysis	Microscopic urinalysis
1. Acute glomerulonephritis	• Gross haematuria • Proteinuria • Smoky urine	Erythrocytes, erythrocytes and blood casts, epithelial casts, hyaline and granular casts
2. Chronic glomerulonephritis	• Haematuria • Proteinuria	Epithelial casts, granular casts, leukocytes, erythrocytes, waxy casts
3. Acute pyelonephritis	• Turbid • Occasional proteinuria • Bad smell or odour	WBC cast, numerous neutrophils (many in clumps) epithelial casts, granular and waxy casts, bacteria
4. Chronic pyelonephritis	• Occasional proteinuria	Leukocytes, broad waxy casts, granular and epithelial casts, bacteria
5. Nephrotic syndrome	• Proteinuria (heavy) • Fat droplets	Fatty and waxy casts, cellular and granular casts, oval fat bodies
6. Cystitis	• Haematuria (gross or microscopic)	Plenty of WBCs, RBCs, transitional epithelial cells, histiocytes, bacteria
7. Acute tubular neoplasm	• Haematuria • Occasional proteinuria	Necrotic and degenerated renal epithelial cells, WBC, RBC, granular cast, epithelial casts, waxy cast, broad casts
8. Urinary tract necrosis	• Haematuria	Atypical large epithelial cells with enlarged hyperchromatic nuclei, WBC, RBC

Table 9.7: Differences between haematuria and haemoglobinuria

Haematuria	Haemoglobinuria
1. Haematuria is the presence of red blood cells in urine	1. Haeglobinuria means haemoglobin (free in plasma not in red blood cells) in abnormally high in concentration in urine
2. Urine is smoky	2. Urine is coca cola/red coloured as haemoglobin is converted to acid haematin in presence of oxygen
3. After centrifugation RBC deposits are found and seen under microscope	3. After centrifugation no RBC deposit
4. Common causes are urinary tract infections, nephrolithiasis (stones in kidney, bladder or ureter), polycystic kidney disease, benign prostatic hyperplasia, glomerular causes (glomerulonephritis)	4. Common causes are any haemolytic anaemia with primarily intravascular haemolysis in which RBCs are destroyed and released haemoglobin (free haemoglobin) found in plasma
5. Tests: Orthotoluidine test, benzidine test and dipstick test	5. Same as haematuria tests

Pathology Practicals

Table 9.8: Comparison of haematuria, haemoglobinuria, and myoglobinuria

Parameter	Haematuria	Haemoglobinuria	Myoglobinuria
Colour of urine	Normal/smoky/red/brown	Pink/brown/red	Red/brown
Colour of plasma	Normal	Pink	Normal
Urine microscopy	Many RBCs	Occasional RBCs	Occasional RBCs
Urine test based on peroxiadase activity	+	+	+
Serum creatine kinase	Normal	Normal	Marked increase
Serum haptoglobin	Normal	Low	Normal

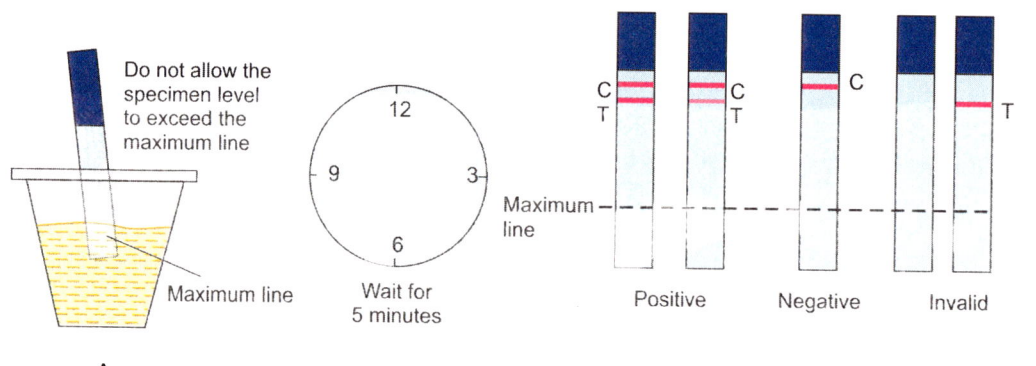

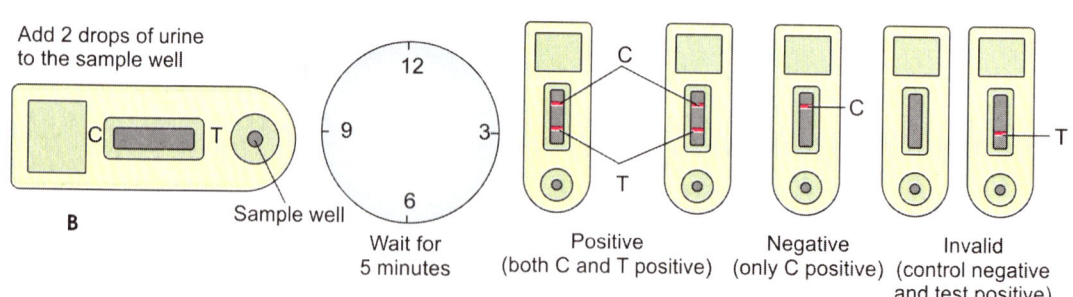

Fig. 9.10A and B: (A) Strip test; (B) Cassette test. C: Control, T: Test

Interpretation
- **Positive**: When both control and test give colour band **(red in colour)**
- **Negative**: When band in control area but no band in test area
- **Invalid**: Control negative but band in test area.

Principle of test: Antiserum anti-β-hCG and enzyme conjugate used in the control and test area. If the urine contains β-hCG, it combines with anti-β-hCG and enzyme conjugate fixed on C and T areas and gives red colour band.

VIVA VOCE

Q1. For routine examination of urine, which sample is preferred?
Ans: The morning sample is preferred as urine is concentrated and large volume of urine can be obtained. However, any fresh sample collected any time of the day is suitable but test should be done within 2 hours. If delay is anticipated, urine specimen should be refrigerated.

Q2. Which sample is preferred for culture of urine?
Ans: Midstream (clean-catch) fresh sample of urine after proper cleansing of glans penis in the male or vulva in the female.

Q3. How is 24-hour urine sample collected?
Ans: The first morning sample (say 8 AM) is discarded. All subsequent urine samples are collected in a clean and dry container (1.5 to 2 litre bottle with a cap). The last urine sample is the next day's first morning sample (say 8 AM).

Q4. What is renal glycosuria?
Ans: Normal renal threshold for glucose in humans is 180 mg/dl. This renal threshold is lowered in renal glycosuria (<180 mg/dl). So, glycosuria occurs even the blood sugar is below 180 mg/ml (normal threshold). This happens because of the defect in the tubular cells of the kidneys that decreases the reabsorption of glucose. Causes may be hereditary, cystinosis, Wilson's disease or as part of Fanconi syndrome. It may be acquired also (certain drugs, acute pyelonephritis) and sometimes in pregnancy.

Q5. What is alimentary glycosuria?
Ans: Sometimes, blood glucose level rises above renal threshold (180 mg/dl) physiologically after a meal. If may cause glycosuria. But it disappears after 2 hours of consumption of meal.

Q6. What is low and fixed specific gravity of urine?
Ans: Normal specific gravity (SG) of urine is 1.015–1.025. Low and fixed specific gravity is called when it becomes 1.008–1.010 and is fixed. Causes are:

i. Chronic glomerulonephritis (end stage renal disease), as the concentrating power of renal tubules are either low or lost due to damage to renal tubules.
ii. In ADH (anti-diuretic hormone) deficiency, the concentrating power of the tubules is lost. Hence, SG is low and fixed though the tubules are healthy.
iii. It is also seen in arteriosclerotic kidney, and cause is same, i.e. damaged tubules.

Q.7. In heat test of urinary protein detection, why is upper part of the tube is heated and not the lower part of the tube?
Ans: When upper part of the tube is heated, the protein flocculate in upper part and haziness is seen. This haziness is compared to the unheated lower part which serves as control.

In addition, by doing so, the convection current is not produced which may disturb the hazziness. On the contrary, if lower part of the tube is heated, convection current will be produced, which will go upwards and make the whole urine specimen in the tube hazy. If there is trace or a little urinary protein is present, it will be missed as there is no control.

Q8. In Benedict's (semiquantitative) test, why is fixed volume of 5 ml Benedict's reagent and 8 drops (0.5 ml) of urine is used?
Ans: As this is a semiquantitative test and is graded from traces to 4+ based on colour changes, the ratio of reagent volume and urine volume should be fixed for accurate result and quantity of the urinary protein. If ratio is changed, the test will lose its semiquantitative nature and will be qualitative purely.

Q9. How are RBCs distinguished from air bubbles under microscope?

Ans: In unstained wet specimen of urine, RBCs are of same size, yellowish and double-contoured. But air bubbles have variable size with a dark halo and absent double-contour.

Q10. What is functional proteinuria?

Ans: When there is no organic lesion present but proteinuria occurs due to renal vasoconstriction. The causes are excessive exercise, exposure to heat and cold and emotional stress.

Q11. What is postural proteinuria?

Ans: Some people excrete more protein than normal range when they are in standing position. This proteinuria disappears, if the person lies down. The probable cause is venous vasoconstriction during standing posture.

Q12. What is microalbuminuria?

Ans: Microalbuminuria is defined as urinary albumin excretion of 30–300 mg/day, or 20–200 µg/min. It is a marker of general vascular dysfunction and nowadays is considered a predictor of both kidney and heart patients (hypertension). It is used to identify early kidney damage like diabetes mellitus. More than 300 mg albumin (macroproteinuria) indicates advanced kidney disease. In India, patients with type II diabetes of less than 1 year, the prevalence of microalbuminuria was 24.7% and macroproteinuria was 6.2%. In the US, approximately 6% of men and 9.7% of women have microalbuminuria.

10
Lumbar Puncture Needle, Cerebrospinal Fluid and Other Body Fluids

Cerebrospinal fluid (CSF) is produced in the choroid plexuses (70%) and the remainder is formed around the blood vessels and along the ventricular walls. It is produced at a rate of 500 ml/day. It leaves the ventricular system through the medial and lateral foramina, flowing over the brain and spinal cord surface with the subarachnoid space.

The functions of CSF are to collect wastes, circulate nutrients, cushion and lubricate the central nervous system. Resorption of CSF occurs at the arachnoid villi. Total volume of CSF is 90–150 ml in adults and 10–60 ml in neonates.

Blood–brain barrier: When a dye (trypan blue) is injected in living animal/human, it results in staining of all tissues except brain and spinal cord. It was explained by postulation of an existence of a blood–brain barrier. Anatomically, this barrier represents the barrier in the capillary endothelium in contact with astrocyte foot processes. On the other hand, blood CSF barrier is represented by the choroid plexus epithelium and the endothelium of all cerebral capillaries in contact with CSF that accounts for different concentrations of solutes in plasma and CSF. Certain substances in the CSF are tightly regulated by specific transport system (e.g. H^+, K^+, Ca^{++}, Mg^{++}, HCO_3^-), whereas other like glucose, urea and creatinine diffuse freely. Water, chloride, carbon dioxide and oxygen also diffuse rapidly through the barrier easily.

LUMBAR PUNCTURE (LP) NEEDLE

It is a sterile long slender needle with a stilette. It is about 10 cm long and has a bore of 1–1.5 mm.

Lumbar Puncture Method

Evaluation of lumbar puncture (LP) is essential for the diagnosis of clinically suspected infectious meningitis, subarachnoid haemorrhage, leptomeningeal neoplastic disease and noninfectious meningitis.

Relative contraindication of doing LP: Local skin infection in the lumbar area, suspected spinal cord mass lesion, suspected intracranial mass lesion, any bleeding diathesis

Haematological work up: A functional platelet count is >50,000/mm³, and/or INR <1.5 are advisable to perform LP safely.

LP Technique

Proper position of the patient is important. Two different positions can be used:
i. *Lateral decubitus position:* Most common and routinely performed.
ii. *The sitting position:* Less common, preferable in obese patients.

Table 10.1: Reference values of CSF in adults

Parameter	Conventional units	SI units
i. **Protein**	15–45 mg/dl	0.15–0.45/L
• Prealbumin	2–7%	
• Albumin	56–76%	
• α_1-Globulin	2–7%	
• α_2-Globulin	4–12%	
• β-Globulin	8–18%	
• γ-Globulin	3–12%	
ii. **Electrolytes**		
• Osmolality	280–300 mOsm	280–300 mmol/L
• Sodium	135–150 mEq/L	135–150 mmol/L
• Potassium	2.6–3.0 mEq/L	2.6–3.0 mmol/L
• Chloride	115–130 mEq/L (720–760 mg%)	115–130 mmol/L
iii. **pH**		
• Lumbar fluid	7.28–7.32	
• Cisternal fluid	7.32–7.34	
iv. **Other constituents**		
• Glucose	40–80 mg/dl	2.4–5.6 mmol/L
• Ammonia	10–35 µg/dl	6–20 µmol/L
• Creatinine	0.6–1.2 mg/dl	45–92 µmol/L
v. **pO$_2$**	40–44 mm Hg	
vi. **pCO$_2$**		
• Lumbar fluid	44–50 mm Hg	
• Cisternal fluid	40–46 mm Hg	

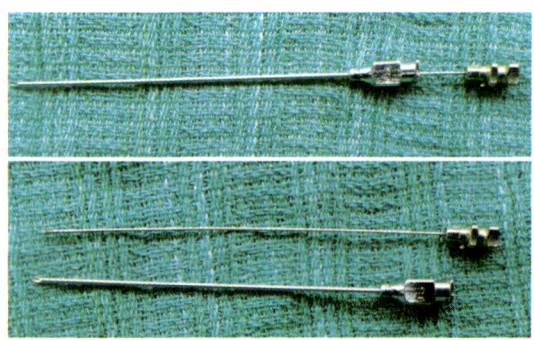

Fig. 10.1: Lumbar puncture (LP) needle

In both the positions, the patient should be instructed to flex the spine as much as possible. In the lateral decubitus position, the patient is instructed to assume the foetal position with the knee fixed towards the abdomen. In the sitting position, the patient should be blend over a table with his/her head resting on folded arm.

The entry site for a LP is below the level of the conus medullaris, which extends to L1–L2 in most adults. Thus, L3–L4 or L4–S1 interspace can be utilized for entry site. The posterior superior iliac crest should be identified and the spine palpated at this level. It represents the L3–L4 interspace, with the other interspace referred from this landmark. The midpoint of the interspace between the spinous processes represents the entry point for the thoracocentesis needle.

Overlying skin is properly cleansed with antiseptics. The skin and fascia of lumbar space selected for puncture are infiltrated with 1–2% lignocaine. Wait for 3–5 minutes.

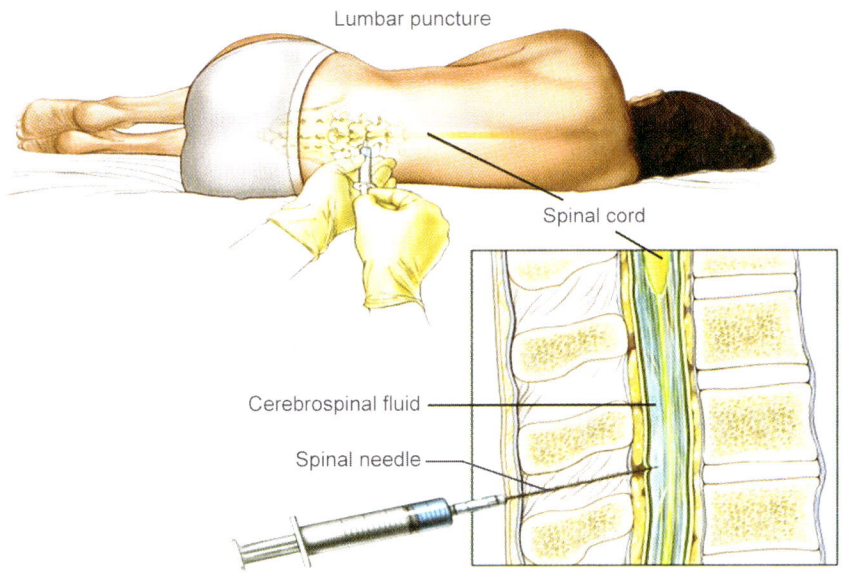

Fig. 10.2: Lumbar puncture technique

Properly sterilized LP needle with stilette within it is pushed forward and slightly upward in midline between L3 and L4 vertebrae till a peculiar "give-way" sensation the needle is felt. The stilette is then removed. Pressure of CSF may be measured by fitting the nanometer to the needle or by counting drops (normally 60 drops/minute).

The CSF is then collected (total 10–15 ml) in 3 sterile tubes/vials. One tube is used for cytological, second for biochemical and the third for microbiological examinations.

Once, the required amount of CSF is collected, the stilette should be replaced and the LP needle is quickly withdrawn.

Postprocedure: To minimize the chance of a post-LP headache, the patient should be instructed to lie prone for at least 3 hours. If a headache develops then bed rest, hydration, and oral analgesics are often helpful.

NORMAL VALUES OF CSF

- Appearance: Clear and colourless
- Normal opening adult pressure: 90–180 ml of water in an adult in the lateral decubitus position
- Cell count: Adults: WBC → 0–5 cells/mm^3, RBC → $0/mm^3$
  Newborns: WBC → $0-30/mm^3$, RBC → $0/mm^3$

Table 10.2: Differential cell count

Cell type	Adults (%)	Neonates (%)
• Lymphocytes	62 ± 34	20 ± 18
• Mononuclear cells and monocytes	36 ± 20	72 ± 22
• Neutrophils	2 ± 5	3 ± 5
• Histiocytes	Rare	Rare
• Eosinophils	Rare	Rare
• Ependymal cells	Rare	Rare

Macroscopic Examination

i. **Turbidity** or cloudiness begins to appear with WBC count >200 cell/mm^3 and RBC count >400 cells/mm^3.

ii. **Clot formation** in CSF may be seen in patients with traumatic taps, complete spinal block (Froin's syndrome), suppurative or tuberculous meningitis.

iii. **Xanthochromia:** The CSF is centrifuged, and the supernatant fluid is compared with a tube of distilled water. Xanthochromic CSF is pink, orange or yellow due to RBC lysis and haemoglobin break down. Pale pink, orange xanthochromia is noted after subarachnoid haemorrhage. Yellow xanthochromia is derived from bilirubin. It develops 12 hours after a subarachnoid bleeding, reaches peak at 2–4 days and persists for 2–4 weeks.

    CSF xanthochromia may also be due to bilirubin in jaundice patients, artifactual red cell lysis caused by detergent contamination of the needle or tube, carotinoids (orange) in dietary hypercarotenemia, and rifampicin therapy (red-orange).

iv. **Protein coagulum:** Normal CSF does not show protein coagulum. Fibrin clot may form on standing when protein content is very high (>1000 mg%). A fine **cobweb or spider web coagulum** is seen in tuberculous meningitis when CSF is allowed to stand overnight. This cobweb coagulum may contain tubercle bacilli which may be seen after staining with ZN stain.

CSF Pressure

It is directly related with the pressure in jugular veins and vertebral veins. So, it is decreased in circulatory collapse and is increased in:

- Congestive cardiac failure (CCF)
- Superior mediastinal syndrome
- Breath holding, physical straining, pressure against abdomen.

CSF pressure is also increased if there is raised intracranial tension, such as:

- Meningitis, encephalitis, meningoencephalitis
- Cerebral tumour, cerebral abscess
- Cerebral oedema
- Cerebral hemorrhage

Indications for Collection of CSF

A. **Diagnostic indications**
  - Meningitis, encephalitis, meningoencephalitis
  - Subarachnoid haemorrhage (SAH)
  - Central nervous system (CNS), syphilis
  - Spinal cord tumour
  - Multiple sclerosis
  - Intracranial haemorrhage due to injury
  - Intracranial space occupying lesion
  - Differential diagnosis of cerebral infarction versus intracerebral haemorrhage: Almost in 80% of cases, the latter show blood or xanthochromia.

B. **Therapeutic indications**
  - Relief of intracranial pressure
  - Removal of exudate or blood from subarachnoid space
  - Introduction of anti-meningococcus or anti-tetanus serum
  - Introduction of spinal anaesthesia, radiographic contrast media or drugs.

Contraindications of Doing LP

- Spinal cord tumour
- Brain tumour at cerebropontine angle
- Septicaemias
- Brain abscess (chance of spreading)
- Recent intracranial haemorrhage
- Patient is having convulsions (epilepsy)
- Cardiovascular disease (advanced)

Complications of LP

- Postpuncture persistent headache
- Death due to asphyxiation especially in infants
- Paresis followed by paralysis in cases of spinal cord tumour
- Implantation of skin and subsequent development of implantation dermoid if stylette is not used.
- Development of cerebellar coning followed by sudden death if there is increased intracranial pressure/tension.

Differential Cell Count

A differential performed in a Neubauer's counting chamber is unsatisfactory as low cell numbers have poor precision and identifying the cell type beyond granulocytes and mononuclear cells in a wet preparation. To improve precision and accuracy, different methods have been adopted:

i. **Cytocentrifuge**: It is recommend method for all body fluids including CSF. From 30 to 50 cells can be concentrated from 0.5 ml of normal CSF. This is rapid, and allows Romanowsky staining of air-dried cytospins.

ii. **Filtration method**: It provides excellent cell recovery slightly better preservation than cytocentrifuge but more time-consuming and costly. Romanowsky stain cannot be used. But the advantages are the ability to concentrate large volumes of CSF for cytological examination or culture while retaining the fluid filtrate for additional studies.

iii. **Sedimentation method**: It provides high quality smears, but the yield is not as good as filtration method. These methods are more cumbersome than cytocentrifugation.

Disease Detected by Laboratory Examination of CSF

1. **High sensitivity, high specificity**
   Bacterial, tuberculous and fungal meningitis
2. **High sensitivity, moderate specificity**
   - Subarachnoid haemorrhage
   - Viral meningitis
   - Multiple sclerosis
   - Paraspinal abscess
   - Central nervous system syphilis
3. **Moderate sensitivity, high specificity**
   Meningeal malignancy
4. **Moderate sensitivity, moderate specificity**
   - Viral encephalitis
   - Subdural haematoma
   - Intracranial haemorrhage

BODY CAVITY FLUID

The pleural, peritoneal and pericardial serous cavities usually referred to as body cavities and are lined by single layer of mesothelial cells. These mesothelial cells are made up of flattened or cuboidal epithelium, which is supported by a rich network of capillaries, lymphatics and loose connective tissue. The visceral and parietal surfaces are separated by a potential space which usually contains 10–50 ml fluid (pleural fluid 10–20 ml, peritoneal fluid 10–50 ml and pericardial fluid 10–50 ml). This fluid is pale yellow, clear serous fluid which acts as lubricant.

Normally, serous fluid has a glucose concentration similar to those of blood, a pH 7.0 and protein concentration of <2 gm%. The cellular contents are a few mesothelial cells and occasional lymphocytes.

Accumulation of serous fluid is called effusion, e.g. pleural effusion, peritoneal effusion and pericardial effusion. It can be transudate or exudate.

Laboratory Investigations

Specimen: Specimen (body cavity fluid) should be collected aseptically. The fluid should be collected in 3 sterile containers (test tubes/vials)—one for cytological examination, one for biochemical and other for microbiological examinations.

1. *Physical examination:* This includes macroscopic examination, determination of specific gravity and others.
2. *Microscopic examination:* Examination for total cell count and differential cell count (stained smear). Look for any neoplastic/malignant cell.
3. *Chemical examination:* Usually done for protein and occasionally for glucose, chloride and LDH, mucin or clotting test also reflects the behaviour of certain proteins.
4. *Laboratory culture*: To identify the particular infective organism.

Mucin clot test: Addition of 2–3% acetic acid to fluid.

Table 10.3: CSF findings in some common disorders

	Normal	Subarachnoid haemorrhage	Pyogenic/ bacterial meningitis	Viral meningitis	Tuberculous meningitis	Fungal meningitis
CSF pressure	50–180 mm H$_2$O	↑	↑↑↑	N/↑	↑↑	↑
Colour	Crystal clear or colourless	Blood stained Xanthochromic	Turbid cloudy or opalescent	Clear	Clear/slightly turbid	Slightly turbid/clear
Coagulum of protein	Absent	Absent	Big protein clots within few minutes	Absent	Fine, thread-like cobweb or spider coagulum	Present as thread-like
Protein content	15–45 mg/dl	↑	↑↑↑ (100–600 mg%)	↑ (60–80 mg%)	↑ (80–140 mg%)	↑ (60–160 mg%)
Glucose	40–80 mg%	Normal	Decreased 10–20 mg%	Normal/increased	Decreased (20–50 mg%)	Decreased (20–50 mg%)
Chloride	720–760 mg%	Normal/slightly increased	Decreased	Decreased	Marked decreased	Marked decreased
Total cell count	1–4/mm^3	Increased RBC	1000–10,000 or more/mm^3	5–300/mm^3	100–600/mm^3	40–400/mm^3
Cell type	Lymphocytes	RBC	Mostly neutrophils (>90%)	Lymphocytes	Mostly lymphocytes (>90%)	Neutrophils and/or lymphocytes; eosinophils in coccidioides
Gram stain	Nil	–	Gram-positive or gram-negative cocci or bacilli found	–	–	–
ZN stain	Nil	–	–	–	Acid-fast bacilli	–
PAS/GMS or fungal stain	Nil	–	–	–	–	Positive, filaments or spores of fungus

Table 10.4: Differences between transudate and exudate

Parameters	Transudate	Exudate
• Colour and appearance	Pale yellow, clear	Cloudy or haemorrhagic opaque
• Cause	Increased hydrostatic pressure or diminished colloidal oncotic pressure of blood	Increase capillary permeability due to various agents
• Specific gravity	<1.015	>1.015 (usually ≥1.018)
• Protein	<1 gm%	>2 gm%
• Glucose	Normal (15–30 mg%)	Low
• Fibrin	Poor	Rich, may form fibrin clot
• LDH (lactate dehydrogenase)	Normal	Increased
• Fluid/serum protein ratio	<0.5	>0.5
• Fluid/serum LDH ratio	<0.6	>0.6
• Cell count	Few	Many
• Cell type	Few mesothelial cells, occasional lymphocytes	Many inflammatory cells as per cause
• Bacteriological study	Negative	Usually positive if inflammatory causes, negative if neoplastic cause

Synovial Fluid

Synovium refers to the tissue lining synovial tendon sheaths, bursae and diarthrodial joints except for the articular surface. Synovium is composed of 1–3 cell layers which form a discontinuous surface overlying fatty, fibrous or periosteal joint space.

Synovial fluid is an imperfect ultrafiltrate of plasma combined with hyaluronic acid produced by the synovial cells. Small ions and molecules like glucose and urea cross easily into the joint space and their concentration is similar to plasma. But large molecules are absent or are present in only trace amounts. Synovial fluid acts as a lubricant and adhesive and provides nutrients for the avascular articular cartilage.

Normal Synovial Fluid

Volume in a joint: 0.1–2.0 ml

Colour and appearance: Transparent, straw colured

Chemical composition
- Protein: 1–3 gm/dl (albumin 55–70%, α_1-globulin 6–8%, α_2-globulin 5–7%, β-globulin 8–10%, γ-globulin 10–14%)
- Hyaluronate: 0.3–0.4 gm/dl
- Glucose: 70–110 mg/dl
- Uric acid: 2–8 mg/dl
- Lactate: 10–20 mg/dl

Cytology: Usually 1–2/mm^3 (lymphocytes or histiocytes; a few synovial cells). Maximum range up to 20/mm^3.

Investigations of Synovial Fluid

1. **Inflammatory fluid:** Turbid, and yellow. Cell count 3000–5000/mm^3. Protein content is elevated, viscosity diminished and glucose level normal or low. This may be due to gouty arthritis, other

Table 10.5: Causes of pleural, peritoneal and pericardial effusion

Fluid type	Pleural	Peritoneal	Pericardial
1. Transudate	• CCF (congestive heart failure) • Nephrotic syndrome (hypoproteinaemia) • Hepatic cirrhosis	• CCF • Nephrotic syndrome • Hepatic cirrhosis	—
2. Exudate	**Neoplasms** • Bronchogenic carcinoma • Metastatic cancer • Lymphoma • Malignant mesothelioma **Infections** • Tubreculosis • Pyogenic pneumonia • Viral pneumonia • Mycoplasmal pneumonia **Others** • Trauma • Pulmonary infarct • SLE • Rheumatic disease	**Neoplasms** • Hepatocellular carcinoma • Metastatic cancer • Lymphoma • Malignant mesothelioma **Infections** • Tuberculosis • Bacterial peritonitis • Appendicitis (secondary bacterial peritonitis) **Others** • Trauma • Bile peritonitis • Pancreatitis	**Neoplasms** • Metastatic cancer • Lymphoma **Infections** • Tuberculosis • Bacterial pericarditis • Fungal pericarditis • Viral or mycoplasmal pericarditis **Others** • Trauma • Myocardial infarction • SLE • Rheumatic disease

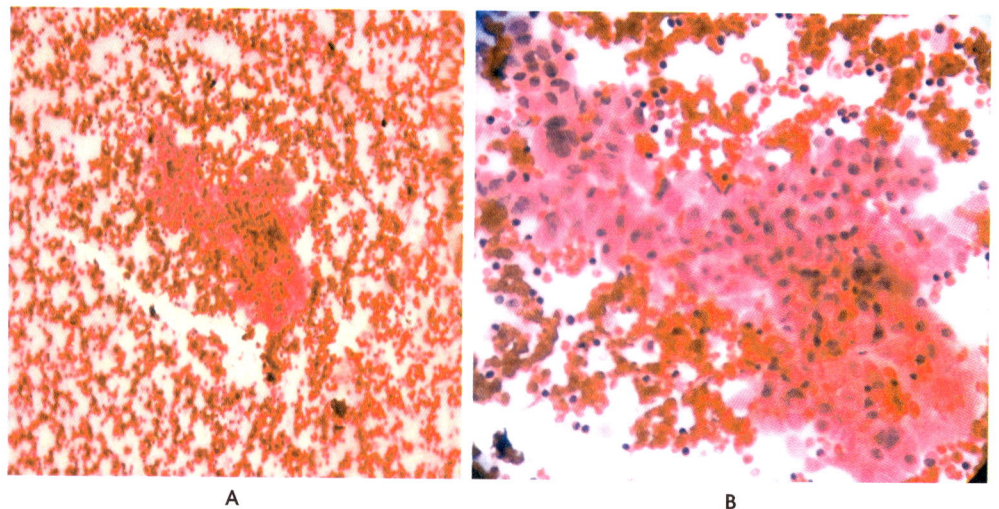

Fig. 10.3A and B: Granuloma in pleural fluid. (A) Low power view; (B) High power view. Granuloma is formed by clusters of epithelioid histiocytes (macrophages)

inflammatory arthritis and occasionally septic arthritis.

A fair number of plasma cells is found in rheumatoid arthritis (>500/mm³). In septic arthritis, the neutrophil count is high and go up to 50,000/mm³. The enzyme lactate dehydrogenase (LDH) is elevated in rheumatoid arthritis, gouty arthritis and infectious (septic) arthritis.

2. **Non-inflammatory fluid:** It is clear, viscous and amber-coloured. WBC count is <200/mm³ (mostly mononuclear cells). Protein is low and glucose normal (transudate). Seen in trauma and osteoarthritis.

Mucin Clot Test (Ropes Test)

Addition of acetic acid to synovial fluid precipitates hyaluronate into a mucin clot, which may be graded as good, fair and poor. Mucin clot reflects the polymerization of synovial fluid hyaluronate.

Mucin

Mucin is a mucopolysaccharide or glycoprotein which is the chief constituent of mucus.

Principle of test: It measures how well-polymerized the hyaluronic acid is.

Test method: A few drops of synovial fluid are added to 10 ml of 5% acetic acid in a beaker and swirled for 1–2 minutes. The result is interpreted as:
- **Good mucin clot:** A solid clot in a clear solution
- **Fair mucin clot:** A soft clot in a slightly turbid solution
- **Poor mucin clot:** A friable (crumby) clot in a turbid solution
- **Very poor mucin clot:** No clot, turbid fluid

Inflammation in the joint space damage the hyaluronic polymers, shortening them.

Good mucin clot: Ostearthritis, trauma, haemophilic arthritis.

Fair mucin clot: Lupus and rheumatoid arthritis

Poor and very poor mucin clot: Septic and crystalline (gout) arthritis, gonorrhoea.

Polarised Microscopy

Crystals and cellularity are analysed by polarized microscope. Needle-shaped crystals of monosodium urate (usually intracellular) are seen in gouty effusions. Rhomboid shaped crystals are seen in pseudogout and chondrocalcinosis.

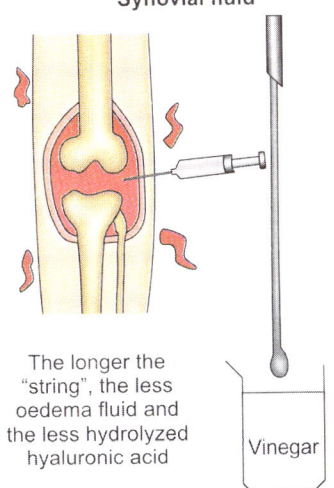
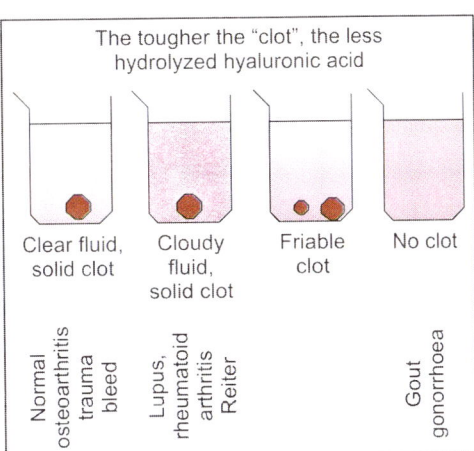

Fig. 10.4: Mucin clot test (Ropes test)

Table 10.6: Synovial fluid in normal and in disease conditions

Finding	Normal	Disease category			
		Group I (noninflammatory)	Group II (inflammatory)	Group III (infections)	Group IV (haemorrhagic)
• Appearance	Clear, straw coloured	Yellow, transparent	Yellow, cloudy, turbid or bloody	Yellow and purulent	Xanthochromic or red-brown
• WBC count	0–150/ml	<3000/ml	3000–75,000/ml	50,000–200,000/ml	50–10,000/ml
• Neutrophil percentage (%)	<25%	<30%	>50%	>90%	<50%
• RBC (if any)	No	No	No	Yes	Yes
• Glucose content	0–10 mg/dl	0–10 mg/dl	0–40 mg/dl	20–100 mg/dl	0–20 mg/dl

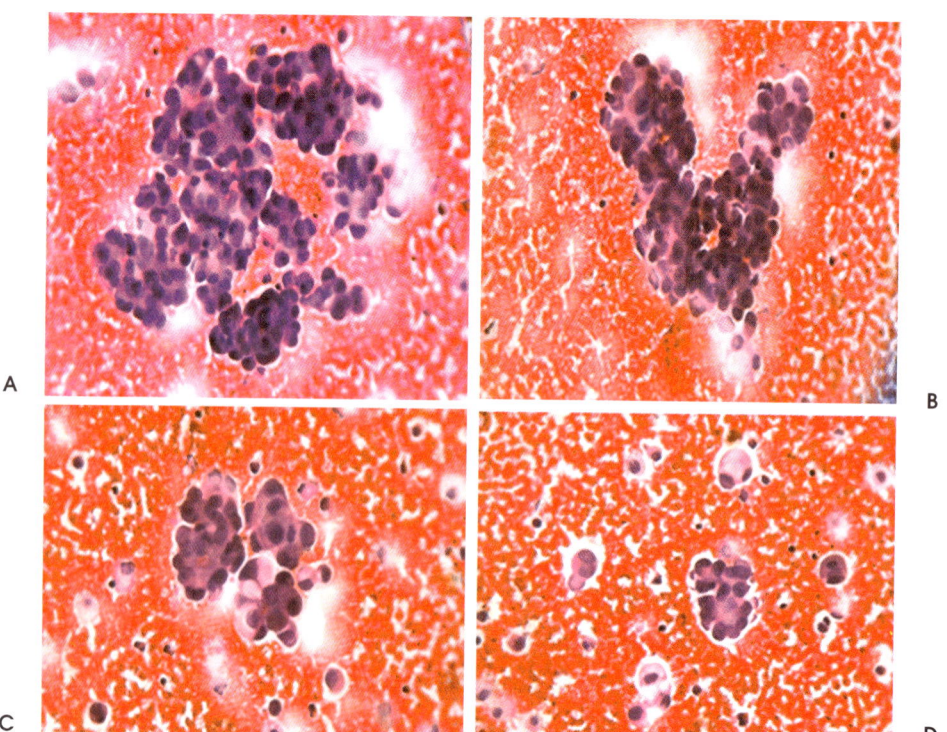

Fig. 10.5A to D: Adenocarcinoma cells in fluid cytology (peritoneal fluid). (A) Low power view showing sheets and papillary pattern of malignant cells (MGG × 100); (B) Low power view showing sheets and papillary pattern of malignant cells (Pap × 100); (C) High power view showing mucin vacuoles among tumour cells (Pap × 400); (D) High power view showing adenoid/pseudoglandular pattern of tumour cells. Few signet ring cells are also seen in the background (Pap × 400)

Table 10.7: Distinguishing feature among reactive mesothelial cells, mesothelioma and adenocarcinoma cells (exfoliated)

Feature	Reactive mesothelium	Mesothelioma (malignant)	Adenocarcinoma
1. Cellularity	Variable	High (offen)	Variable
2. Edges of group of cells	Berry like group (<10 cells) with scalloped contour, 'window' present	Berry like groups with scalloped contour, 'window' present.	Large clumps (>10 cells), smooth contoured cohesive group with "hard" edges
3. Cell sheets	May be seen but single cell is also seen	Rare	Not found
4. Acinar structures	Not found	May be found	Common
5. Papillary structures	Rare	May be found	May be found
6. Multinucleated cells	Occasional	Frequent	May be found
7. N:C ratio	Low, a little cell to cell variation	Low, a little cell to cell variation	High, cell to cell variation
8. Nuclei	Round with smooth contour	Enlarged nuclei with smooth contours	Anisonucleosis, often with irregular contours
9. Nucleoli	May be prominent	Often macronucleoli	Often prominent
10. Cytoplasm	Abundant and dense with peripheral fuzziness	Abundant and dense with peripheral fuzziness	Variable amount, not dense, sharp borders
11. Cytoplasmic vacuolation	May be found	May be found	Often present
12. Cytoplasmic mucin (vacuoles)	Absent	Absent	Often present
13. Cytoplasmic glycogen (vacuoles)	Often found	Often abundant	May be found
14. Cytoplasmic lipid (vacuoles)	Frequent small perinuclear vacuoles	Frequent, small perinuclear vacuoles	Seen in cases of clear cell carcinoma of kidney
15. Electron microscopy (scanning EM or SEM)	Majority show vesicles or blebs covering the surfaces. A few cells are covered by regular microvilli (MV) and show openings of pinocytic vacuoles	Numerous, long, slender microvilli	Short, plump, microvilli

Light's Criteria for Pleural Fluid

There are three parameters:

1. Pleural fluid protein/serum protein ratio >0.5.
2. Pleural fluid LDH/serum LDH ratio >0.6.
3. Pleural fluid LDH greater than two-thirds of the upper limits of normal of the serum LDH.

If at least one of the above three criteria is present, the fluid is virtually always an exudate.

If none is present, the fluid is always a transudate.

VIVA VOCE

Q. 1. What are the different uses of lumbar puncture needle?
Ans:
i. Most important use is to draw CSF (cerebrospinal fluid)
ii. It may also be used for aspiration from pleural cavity, peritoneal cavity or from joint spaces.

Q. 2. Why is L_3–L_4 or L_4–L_5 vertebra chosen for lumbar puncture?
Ans: Spinal cord in humans extends up to L_1 vertebra level. So, if aspiration is done between L_3–L_4 or L_4–L_5 level, there will be no damage to spinal cord and CSF is collected safely. But in small children, conus medullaris extends lower than in adults, so puncture is done L_4–L_5 or lower.

Q. 3. When CSF pressure is high, why lumbar puncture is contraindicated?
Ans: It may cause herniation of cerebellum and coning of medulla which may be fatal.

To prevent this, precaution is taken if it is to be done. After introduction of lumbar puncture needle, stylet is partially and slowly withdrawn so that CSF comes drop by drop and not in a jet as CSF pressure is high.

Q. 4. How would you differentiate between haemorrhage due to pathological cause and traumatic tap?
Ans:

Parameters	Pathological	Traumatic tap
i. Presence of blood in subsequent collection from 3rd–4th tube onwards	Present in all tubes	Absent
ii. Xanthochromia (yellowish colour) of the supernatant CSF	Present	Absent
iii. Latex agglutination test for cross-linked fibrin derivative D-dimer specific for fibrin degradation	Present	Absent
iv. Haemosiderin laden macrophages and/or erythrophagocytosis under microscope	Present	Absent

Q. 5. What is the significance of coagulum in CSF?
Ans: Fibrin clots may be formed on standing when protein content in CSF is very high (>1000 mg/dl, normal 15–45 mg/dl).

In tuberculous meningitis, fine cobweb (thread-like) coagulum is often seen in CSF when it is allowed to stand overnight (prolonged time). This cobweb coagulum may take up tubercle bacilli which may be detected by ZN stain.

Q. 6. What is the normal volume of different body cavity fluids and how does it appear?
Ans: Peritoneal cavity contains 10–50 ml, pericardial cavity contains 10–50 ml and pleural cavity contains 10–20 ml of serous fluid. It appears as a pale yellow, clear serum fluid and serves as friction lubricant.

Q. 7. What is fibrinous exudate?

Ans: Exudates have higher protein content (>2 mg/dl). When fibrinogen enters body fluid the sample clot after collection and is called fibrinous exudate.

To prevent this, EDTA may be added to the collecting vial/tube.

Q. 8. What is the significance of ADA (adenosine deaminase) estimation?

Ans: ADA enzyme is related to purine metabolism and associated with immunodeficiency. Elevate ADA level is seen in tuberculous effusions irrespective of HIV status. There are two isoenzymes of ADA one in ADA-I and another is ADA-II. The ADA-II isoenzyme form is released from activated lymphocytes in tuberculosis. Level >36 U/L in fluid and >54 U/L in serum suggest tuberculosis.

Q. 9. What is the significance of high level of hyaluronic acid in serous fluid?

Ans: This is found in effusions caused by malignant mesothelioma (diffuse) and in metastatic deposits of Wilms' tumour over serous surfaces.

Higher level of hyaluronic acid in serous fluid increase the viscosity giving a honey-like consistency.

Q. 10 What is globulin test in CSF?

Ans: There are two types of tests done to detect globulins in CSF.

a. **Pandy's test:** In a small test tube, place 1–2 ml of saturated solution of phenol. To it add, 1 drop of CSF. Cloudiness against a black background indicates presence of globulin. It is reported as O (nil), 1+, 2+, 3+ or 4+.

b. **Ross Jones test:** Pour 0.5 ml of clear CSF over 1 ml of saturated solution of ammonium sulphate in a test tube. A thin white ring is formed at the juncture of two fluids. If it disappears on mixing, then it is reported as 1+. Heavy cloudiness persists even after mixing is reported as 4+.

Part III

Histopathology and Cytopathology

11. Histological Techniques
12. H and E (Haematoxylin and Eosin) and Other Special Stains
13. HP Slides (Light Microscopy)
14. Cytology: Exfoliative and FNAC

11
Histological Techniques

Histological techniques are a series of processes by which the tissues are prepared for microscopic examination. It starts with fixation and continues with dehydration, clearing, embedding, cutting and staining.

When the tissues are removed from the body (e.g. surgical excision) or blood supply is cut off; tissues begin to decompose. This is due to lack of oxygen and other essential metabolites and also from the accumulation of carbon dioxide and other toxic metabolites in the cell and due to activation of different autolytic enzymes. Some tissues are decomposed rapidly, whereas others are slow to decompose. The rapidity is proportional to the natural metabolic activity of the tissue. This is the basic of rapid decomposition in liver, pancreas, convoluted tubules in kidney.

To minimize the decomposition and to preserve as nearly as possible the natural activity of the cells; the tissues are put in a suitable fixative (usually 10–20 times of volume of surgical specimens). Fixation is defined as a complex series of chemical and physical events which prevents or at least minimizes tissue decomposition and it differs for the different groups of chemical substances found in the tissues. There are other reasons of fixation. In most of the cells, there is an outer complex membrane containing the fluid protoplasm. The protoplasm is a mixed, true and colloidal solution of carbohydrates, proteins, lipids, salt, organic acid and enzymes. Many of these substances would have been lost if tissues had not been fixed.

The aims of fixation are

- Prevention of tissue autolysis and bacterial attack.
- To coagulate various tissue proteins/elements and make them insoluble.
- To maintain the shape and volume of the tissues during subsequent procedures (e.g. clearing, embedding, etc.).
- To prevent loss of tissue substances or rearrangement of tissues ingredients.
- To facilitate the staining reaction by acting as a mordant.
- To keep tissues as close to their natural state and to minimize change of natural colour and appearance.

Types of Fixatives

Fixatives may be of two types—primary and secondary.

Primary fixatives: Only one fixative or mixture of fixatives is used for specified period. Examples: 10% formalin, glutaraldehyde, Bouin's fluid, Carnoy's fixative, Zenker's fluid, etc.

Secondary fixatives: The use of two fixatives in succession. In other word, use of secondary fixative after the tissue is already fixed with previous fixative (primary fixative). As for example, after primary fixation in buffered formalin, tissues are kept in secondary fixative of mercuric chloride formaldehyde solution. Advantages of this sublimate post-fixation are that tissues are more easily cut and flatten better, also they give better staining quality. Likewise tissues fixed with glutaraldehyde may be post-fixed with osmium tetroxide which makes the membranes relatively permeable and better stained. This secondary fixation is also known as **post-fixation or post-chromatin**.

Classification of Fixatives

- **Aldehyde (protein cross-linking agents):** Formaldehyde, glutaraldehyde
- **Protein denaturing agent:** Acetic acid, methyl alcohol, ethyl alcohol
- **Oxidizing agents:** Osmium tetroxide, potassium dichromate, potassium permanganate
- **Physical agents:** Microwave, heat
- **Other cross-linking agents:** Carbodimides
- **Miscellaneous:** Picric acid, mercuric chloride

Routine Formalin Fixatives

This is a fixative which is most commonly used in histological laboratories. The reaction between fixative and tissue proteins is usually mild with a short reaction time. Cross-links between proteins are formed and the reaction starts with basic amino acid lysine. Lysine amino acid which is on the exterior aspect of the protein molecule can only react.

Aldehyde fixation may denature proteins to some extent apart from their primary role in forming crosslinks. As most of the proteins are not denatured, tissues fixed with aldehyde may be used for IHC (immunohistochemistry).

The commercially available solution contains 30–40% formaldehyde gas by weight and is called **formalin**. So, a 10% formalin fixative gives 4% formaldehyde gas for tissue fixation. Most laboratories prefer 10% buffered or 10% formal saline as fixative.

Formal saline (10%)
- Water (preferably distilled): 900 ml
- Sodium chloride: 9 gm
- Formalin (40% formaldehyde): 100 ml

10% formalin (4% formaldehyde)
- Formalin (40% formaldehyde): 100 ml
- Distilled water or tap water: 900 ml

Neutral buffered formalin (10%)
- Water (preferably distilled): 900 ml
- Farmalin: 100 ml
- Sodium dihydrogen phosphate monohydrate ($Na_2 H_2 PO_4 . H_2O$): 4 gm
- Disodium hydrogen phosphate anhydrous ($Na_2 HPO_4$.): 6.5 gm

Protein Denaturing Agents as Fixative

Alcohol: This is used as 80–100% solution. It frequently shrinks and hardens the tissue. Does not preserve chromatin well but good for demonstration of glycogen, plasma cells, amyloid, iron and uric acid. Carnoy's fluid is generally used for specific purposes. Alcohol denatures and precipitates proteins probably by disrupting hydrogen bonds. Ethyl alcohol is used as a fixative for enzymes.

Acetic acid: It is used as 1–5% aqueous solution. It is good for nuclear fixation and has rapid penetration (so, fixation time is less). Disadvantage of this fixative is that it forms pigments if used with formalin. Also, it causes haemolysis of RBCs.

Carnoy's fixative
- Absolute alcohol: 60 ml
- Chloroform: 30 ml
- Glacial acetic acid: 10 ml

Table 11.1: Advantages and disadvantages of formalin fixative

Advantages	Disadvantages
• It is cheap, relatively stable (when buffered) and easy to prepare • Tissue penetration is good • Does not make tissues very hard or brittle • Allows most routine stainings • Frozen section is possible with formalin fixed tissues • Natural colour may be restored • Most commonly used fixative and is the best fixative for the nervous system (brain)	• It may cause dermatitis and asthma in allergic individuals • It is slow to act (less tissue penetration) • There may be formation of dark brown artefact granules especially in tissues containing much blood (e.g. spleen, liver) • Reagent grade formalin (contains 10% methanol in addition to formaldehyde) is unsuitable for electron microscopy as methanol denatures protein. However, pure formalin is suitable • Gradual loss of basophilic staining of nucleus and cytoplasm. So, prolonged fixation is not advisable • Loss of myelin reactivity when Weigert iron haematoxylin stain is used

Zenker's fluid
- Distilled water: 950 ml
- Potassium dichromate: 25 gm
- Mercuric chloride: 50 gm
- Glacial acetic acid: 50 gm
- Fixation time: 4–24 hours followed by prolonged wash.

Bouin's fluid
- Saturated aqueous picric acid solution: 75 ml
- Formalin (40% formaldehyde): 25 ml
- Glacial acetic acid: 5 ml

TISSUE PROCESSING, MICROTOMY AND PARAFFIN SECTIONS

Tissue Processing

Tissue contains intracellular as well as extracellular water which should be removed as paraffin wax (commonly used as embedding medium) is not miscible with water. Also, most fixatives are water based (like formalin). So, there must be some processes which remove this water and allow paraffin wax impregnation. The whole process is called tissue processing.

Table 11.2: Advantages and disadvantages of alcohol fixative

Advantages	Disadvantages
• Methyl alcohol (80–100%) is excellent fixative for smears • Ethyl alcohol is used as a fixative for enzymes • Carnoy's fixative is used for urgent biopsy (paraffin processing within 5 hours) • Good fixative to demonstrate glycogen, alkaline phosphatase, etc.	• Should be used at 0° C or cooler, otherwise cause marked shrinkage • Distorts morphology and hardens the tissue • Contraindicated for lipid study • Although glycogen can be demonstrated it cause polarization (steaming of protoplasm to one pole of the cell) of glycogen granules

Table 11.3: Choice of fixative for different cellular components or surgical specimens

Surgical specimens/tissue components	Choice of fixative
• Routine specimen/general surgical specimen	• 10% buffered formalin
• Glycogen	• Bouin's fluid (picric acid fixative) or alcohol fixatives (absolute alcohol)
• Fat/lipid	• Osmic acid
• Golgi bodies	• Osmic acid
• Enzymes	• Ethyl alcohol
• Smears (blood or cytologic smears)	• Methyl alcohol
• Urgent biopsies	• Carnoy's (alcohol) fixative
• Electron microscopy	• 3% glutaraldehyde, osmium tetroxide
• Nuclei	• Mercury fixative (Zenker), acetic acid
• Cytoplasm	• Potassium dichromate
• Gastrointestinal hormones	• Carbodimide
• Metachromasia	• Mercury fixative (Zenker's fluid)
• Testis	• Bouin's fluid, buffered formalin
• Nucleic acid (DNA and RNA)	• Carnoy's fluid
• Mucoprotein	• Glutaraldehyde
• Neuroendocrine granules	• Ethanol, methanol, acetone
• Cholesterol and its esters	• Bouin's fluid, Zenker's fluid
• Glycoprotein	• Chromates
• Gouty crystals (monosodium urate)	• Absolute alcohol
• Intermediate filaments	• Carnoy's fluid, Methacar n
• Trephine/bone marrow biopsy	• Zenker's formalin (previously called B_5)

The steps in tissue processing are:
- **Dehydration:** Common agents are ethyl alcohol/ethanol/acetone, methyl alcohol, isopropyl alcohol and dioxane.
- **Clearing**: Common agents are xylene (xylol), toluene (toluol), chloroform, citrus fruits oil, paraffin and Histoclear.
- **Impregnation:** Common agents are paraffin wax, other waxes (like ester wax, polyester wax), resins (acrylic, epoxy), agar, gelatin, and celloidin.
- **Embedding**: Final stage with paraffin blocks.

Dehydration

This step removes water and fixative from the tissue and replaces then with dehydrating fluid. Naturally dehydrating fluid should mix with and has water affinity so that it can easily penetrate the tissue cells. The best reagent is ethanol or ethyl alcohol.

1. **Ethyl alcohol (ethanol):** It is a clear colourless flammable liquid. It is used as graded alcohol beginning with 70%, then to higher grades, e.g. 85% or 95%. But for delicate tissues like embryo, animal tissues or brain it should be more gradual (begins with 50%). As it is hydrophilic, it is miscible with water and many other organic solvents.

2. **Acetone:** This is also a clear and volatile, colourless, flammable fluid which is miscible with water, ethanol and many organic solvents. Through it has rapid action, it has poor tissue penetration and prolonged use may cause tissue brittleness. It is cheaper than ethanol but more amount (at least 10 times the volume of tissue) is needed.

3. **Methanol:** It is highly toxic but can substitute ethanol, rarely used nowadays.
4. **Isopropyl alcohol:** Becoming very popular as it is cheaper and no excise duty is required as in alcohol. It is miscible with water, ethanol and most organic solvents It is recommended for microwave over processing method.
5. **Dioxane (diethyl dioxide):** It has the advantage of being miscible with water, alcohol, xylene, balsam and paraffin wax. The dioxane can be reused after removing the water from dehydrating fluid with calcium chloride or quick lime ($CaOH_2$). But it is toxic and in not recommended for routine use.

Clearing

This step replaces the dehydrating fluid and embedding medium (paraffin wax). So, this stage acts as a bridge between dehydration and subsequent embedding. When the dehydrating fluid is totally replaced by these agents, the tissue looks translucent, hence the name clearing agent came.

1. **Xylene (xylol)**: This is an excellent clearing agent but immersion must not be prolonged (>3 hours) as it makes tissue hard and brittle. It is cheap and can be used with celloidion section. This is not suitable for lymph nodes and brain, as it makes them very brittle.
2. **Toluene (toluol):** It has almost similar properties to xylene but has the advantage of not making the tissues hard and brittle.
3. **Chloroform:** It is slower in action than xylene. It causes a little brittleness and is recommended for nervous tissue, eye, granulation tissue, lymph nodes and larger tissue block (up to 1 cm) can be processed. It is non-inflammable but highly toxic. Unlike other clearing agents it does not make tissues translucent.
4. **Citrus fruit oils:** It is extracted from orange and lemon rinds. It is nontoxic and miscible with water. But it has the disadvantage of dissolving out small mineral deposits in tissues (copper, calcium).
5. **Paraffin wax:** Recently introduced as a clearing agent because of its cheapness. Time of immersion is similar to chloroform.
6. **Histoclear:** It has been recently introduced. This nontoxic agent is derivative of food-grade material and has much promise.

Impregnation

This step involves replacement and clearing agent with the embedding medium. This impregnating medium fills all natural cavities, interstices and spaces of the tissue. It makes the tissues sufficiently firm to allow thin section cutting but without alteration of the spatial relationship of the tissues and cellular components and also not to distort the tissues. Subsequently, making of blocks is done with embedding medium. Usual duration is 1–3 hours. Paraffin is the most commonly used impregnating medium used in the routine histological laboratory.

Embedding

Tissues which have been impregnated in paraffin wax is put in freshly melted paraffin wax is put in freshly melted paraffin wax and allowed to solidify. This can be done by using metal containers like tissue Tek, Leukhart's L or paper boats, etc. The tissues should be carefully oriented so that the surface to be cut is placed downwards. Commonly two methods are used in histology namely paraffin wax, resins and celloidion method.

- **Paraffin wax:** It is probably the most popular embedding medium as it is cheap, easily handled and section cutting is easier. Melting point ranging between 40–70° C. Wax with higher melting point has higher hardness. Wax with a melting point of 54–58° C is preferred for routing use. Sometimes, substance like bee wax, rubber ceresin, dental wax, diethylene glycol are added as additive to increase the hardness of paraffin wax hence, more thin sections can be cut.

- **Resins:** This is particularly used for thin sections for high resolution for electron microscopy and for undecalcified bone.
- **Celloidion:** Celloidion or its variant **low viscosity nitrocellulose (LVN)** was popular large tissue and for nervous tissue (like eye). Sections are cut by base sledge or a sliding microtome.
- **Agar:** It does not have sufficient support for sectioning friable tissue pieces after fixation. After solidification in molten agar, tissues are embedded in paraffin wax.
- **Gelatin:** Its main use is in frozen sectioning.
- **Paraplast:** It is a mixture of purified paraffin wax and synthetic plastic polymers whose melting point is 56–57°C. Sections can be cut without cooling the block face by ice. Ribbon like sections are more easy to cut and does not tend to crack. Large blocks and bone blocks may be cut easily as it is more resilient than paraffin wax.
- **Carbowax:** Alcohols with more carbon atoms (≥12) are solid at room temperature and may be used in tissue embedding. Alcohol with 12–18 carbon atoms are suitable for this purpose. Carbowax (polyethylene glycol) is good for this purpose. Carbowax is soluble in and miscible with water, hence embedding may be done directly from the formalin fixation bypassing the first dehydration and second clearing steps of normal tissue processing. Normally, four changes of carbowax (70%, 90% and two changes of 100%) are used at 56° C for 30 minutes, 45 minutes and 1 hour respectively with agitation.

The specimens are then put in fresh carbowax at 50° C for blocking and the blocks are immediately cooled in the refrigerator.

Table 11.4: Manual processing (2 days)

Container No.	Fluid	Time (hours)
1.	70% alcohol	1 hr (9.00 AM–10.00 AM)
2.	95% alcohol	1 hr (10.00 AM–11.00 AM)
3.	95% alcohol	2 hr (11.00 AM–1.00 PM)
4.	100% alcohol	1.5 hr (1.00 PM–2.30 PM)
5.	100% alcohol	1.5 hr (2.30 PM–4.00 PM)
6.	100% alcohol	1.5 hr (4.00 PM–5.30 PM)
7.	100% alcohol	**Over night**
8.	Xylene	1 hr (9.00 PM–10.00 PM)
9.	Xylene	1.5 hr (10.00 PM–11.30 PM)
10.	Paraffin wax	1.5 hr (11.30 PM–1.00 AM)
11.	Paraffin wax	1.5 hr (1.00 AM–2.30 AM)
12.	Paraffin wax	2.5 hr (2.30 AM–5.00 AM)
		Total = 16.5 hours

As carbowax is very hygroscopic, blocks and sustained sections must not come in contact with water or ice and are stored in dry, airtight containers.

Automated Tissue Processing

Many histopathological laboratories nowadays use automatic tissue processors to process tissues. These machines have reduced the processing time compared to manual time (at least 24 hours). Other advantage is superior quality of tissue processing due to constant agitation.

There are two types of automated tissue processor:
- Open (hydraulic)
- Closed (vacuum)

Open (hydraulic) type: Usually there are 11 to 12 stations.
- 1 jar: Formalin (optional)
- 6 jars: Graded alcohol
- 3 jars: Xylene
- 2 jars: Molted paraffin wax

Closed (vacuum) type: Different processing fluids are moved in and out of a single station sequentially. Enclosed tissue processor is advantageous over open type, as in case of any electric fault, this machine sounds an alarm and automatically stop.

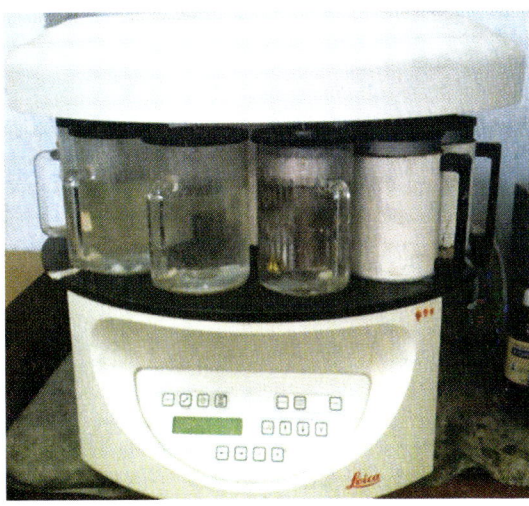

Fig. 11.1: Automatic tissue processor (closed or vacuum type) with different jars (stations) containing processing fluid

Table 11.5: Overnight schedule (automation technique)

Container No.	Fluid	Time (hours)
1.	10% formalin	0
2.	70% alcohol	½ hr
3.	95% alcohol	½ hr
4.	100% alcohol	½ hr
5.	100% alcohol	1 hr
6.	100% alcohol	1 hr
7.	100% alcohol	1 hr
8.	100% alcohol/xylene	½ hr
9.	Xylene	1 hr
10.	Xylene	2 hr
11.	Paraffin wax (molted)	2 ½ hours
12.	Paraffin wax (molted)	4 hours
		Total time = 14½ hours

Most laboratories use an overnight schedule of approximately 14–18 hours. In case of weekend and holidays, when delay is required, then the tissues are kept in first container with 10% formalin.

Microtomy

Microtomy is the process by which tissues are sectioned by microtomes and these sections are attach to a surface for visualization by microscopes. A microtome (from Greek *micros*, meaning "small" and *temmein*, meaning 'to cut') is a tool used to cut extremely thin slices of material, known in histology as **sections**.

Microtomes are basic instruments for microtomy and are designed for accurate cutting of sections (thin slices). Generally there are several types of microtome:
- Rotary microtome
- Rocking microtome
- Sliding microtome
- Freezing microtome
- Ultrathin microtome
- Rotary rocking microtome
- Base sledge microtome
- Vibrotome

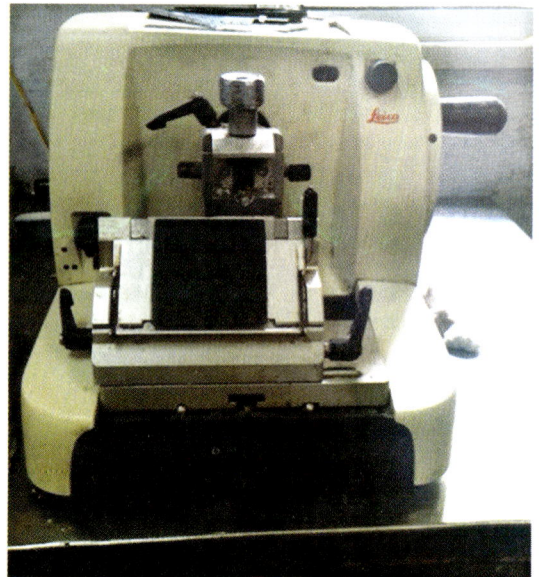

Fig. 11.2: Rotary microtome (manual type)

Rotary microtome: This microtome was invented by Minot in 1885-1886. Probably this is the most popular microtome for routine paraffin wax embedded tissues. Serial sections can be cut conveniently. A large number of paraffin blocks can be cut. Electrically driven rotary microtomes are costlier compared to manual microtomes and are used when the control is necessary to produce ribbons for serial sections. Electrically driven or manual rotary microtomes are used in cryostats for frozen sections.

Disadvantages
i. Only a small length of knife is available for cutting, so large blocks cannot be cut (cutting facet base sledge microtome).
ii. Celloidion embedded blocks cannot be cut (cutting facet sliding microtome).
iii. Relatively costlier than other microtomes.

Rocking microtome: It was used in the past and Cambridge rocking microtome was most commonly used. It is cheap and was also used in cryostats first. But hard tissue cannot be cut and size of block should be small.

Base sledge microtome: This microtome is favoured when large blocks and very hard tissues should be sectioned. In neuropathology, this microtome is preferred as large blocks of brain are made. It is also good for resin embedded undecalcified bone. But consistent thin sections are difficult to cut unlike in rotary microtome.

Sliding microtome: This machine is dangerous as knife is taken along with runners to the block and knife guards cannot be attached. It was used in the past for celloidion embedded blocks cutting.

Rotary rocking microtome: This microtome has the advantage of making flat surface to the tissue block. It is usually used in cryostat though paraffin embedded blocks can also be cut.

Vibratome: Here a vibrating knife is used which oscillates variably according to the voltage supplied through a transformer when passed through a tissue during section cutting, its main use in some enzyme demonstration in unfixed, unfrozen sections.

Microtome Knives

Four types of microtome knives in use are:
- Wedge shaped
- Plano concave
- Biconcave
- Tool edge

Wedge-shaped knife: This is the most common microtome knife used nowadays for section cutting. The sides of the wedge knives are inclined at an angle of approximately 15° **(wedge angle)**. Surfaces of these knives are highly polished so that sections will move on surface and will not adhere to surface. This minimizes chances of folding, distortion and facilitates ribbon formation.

Plano concave: This knife is used in sliding microtome for sectioning celloidion embedded material.

Biconcave: This is not recommended for normal routine work as rigidity is sacrificed because of its shape. But a very keen edge can be produced.

Tool edge: This kind of knife is rigid and is recommended for use in hardest of tissues and embedding media. So, it is preferred for resin embedded undecalcified bone. This type is used in Jung K microtome.

Knife Materials

Knives used for microtomy are made from good quality tool steel or high carbon, tempered from the tip inwards for one-third of the width of knife. Hardness preferred for these knives is about 700 on **Vickers hardness**. Knives with higher hardness are difficult to sharpen and knife edges become brittle.

Disposable blade (made of steel) is the most common type used for routine paraffin embedded sectioning. Other types are glass knives, Tungsten carbide tipped knives, diamond knives, stellite tipped knives.

Paraffin Section Cutting

The numbered paraffin block is secured in place in the microtome object clamp. The object holders are adjusted so that top of the paraffin block just touches the knife edge. After placing the knife in position, both the **clearance angle** and **angle of slope** should be adjusted. A clearance angle of 3–4° and angle of slope of 40° are found to be satisfactory.

After trimming the paraffin block (10–15 µm thickness), melting ice is placed on suitable area of the block for few minutes. This is to give the tissue and paraffin wax a similar consistency so that sections can be cut with ease. For routine purpose, sections are cut at 4–5 µm thickness. Some tissues are cut at 3 µm (e.g. kidney, bone marrow, trephine and lymph node biopsies) and other thicker at 5–6 µm (e.g. bone and brain).

The sections are taken out and placed in floating out bath. Usually water bath is used and temperature of water should be 10° C below the melting point of paraffin wax.

After that, the whole length of section (ribbon which contains 6–8 sections) is placed on a slide coated with adhesive. As adhesive Mayer's egg albumin—glycerol, poly-L-lysine or **3-aminopropyltriethoxy-silane (APES)** is used.

Note

Clearance angle: This is the angle between the front face of the paraffin block and the lower facet of knife which is facing the paraffin block.

Blocking out Moulds

For making paraffin blocks, tissues after processing (impregnation) are placed within liquid paraffin and to solidify to prepare paraffin blocks. These paraffin blocks are prepared in several containers.

- **Leuckhart's embedding irons**: These consist of two L-shaped pieces of heavy brass or similar metal. Advantages are adjustability to give wide variety of block sizes, even blocks with parallel sides.
- **Tissue-Tek system**: This system has stainless steel base moulds in which the tissue block is embedded. A plastic mould is then placed on top and filled with wax.
- **Peel-A-Way**: These are disposable thin plastic embedding molds. When paraffin wax has solidified, the plastic walls are simply peeled off, hence the name.
- **Plastic moulds**: Convenient for use.

Mounting Media and the Sections

After cut paraffin sections are placed on slides with adhesives, the sections are stained. These stained sections are covered with mounting media and covered with coverslips. *Mounting is the placing of mounting media on the stained tissue section and covering it with coverslips.*

The main function of mounting media is to make stained sections visible under microscope. Therefore, it should have refractory index (RI). close to the glass (RI 1.5) as light passes through glass slides and coverslips. Other functions are: To fill the tissue and tissue cavities, to prevent damage to the section, easy handling, storage and to release entrapped air bubbles. Common

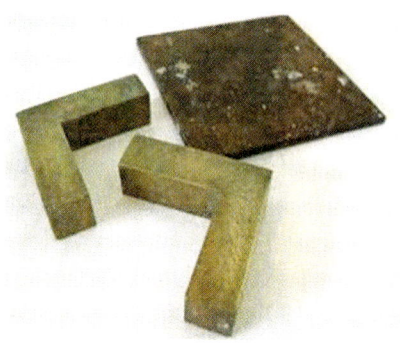
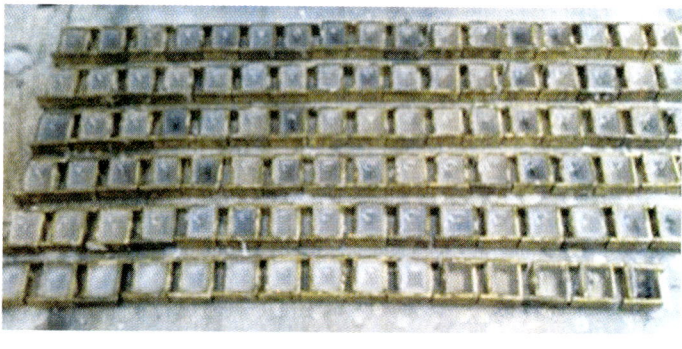

Fig. 11.3A and B: (A) Leuckhart's embedding iron without paraffin (embedding medium); (B) Leuckhart's embedding iron after proper arrangements with paraffin (embedding medium)

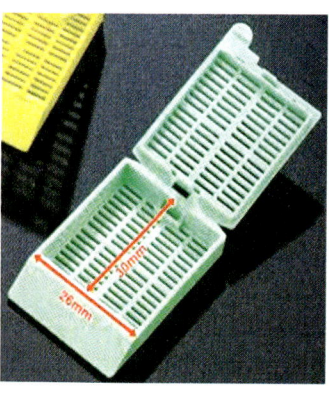
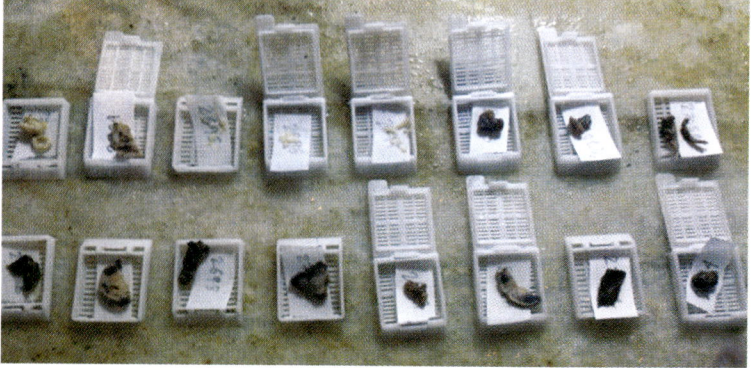

Fig. 11.4A and B: (A) Plastic mould with open lid; (B) Plastic moulds containing surgical specimens after grossing

mounting media are Canada balsam (RI 1.5) and **DPX or distrene dibutylpthalate xylol** (RI 1.52). Others are glycerine jelly, Apathy's medium, Farrant's medium, etc.

Decalcification

The presence of calcium salts and other minerals in bone and other calcified tissues prevents the preparation of good histologic sections by routine methods. Incomplete removal of these minerals results in ragged and torn sections and in damage to the cutting edge of the microtome knife.

Decalcification is a routine procedure which makes bone and calcified tissue compatible with the embedding media for cutting a microslide (section) and the subsequent staining. The most ubiquitous media is paraffin wax. Decalcification adjusts the hard substance of bones to the softness of paraffin. Some media, like resins do not require decalcification at all. Bones are the main object of decalcification but other surgical specimens like calcified tumors, atheromatous plaques, calcified heart valves also require decalcification.

Classification of Decalcifying Agents

1. **Acid solutions**

   A. Strong or inorganic acids: Nitric acid (HNO_3), hydrochloric acid (HCl), formalin—nitric acid, Perenyi's fluid

   B. Weak or organic acid: Aqueous formic acid, formic acid—formalin, buffered formic acid, others like acetic acid and picric acid as components in Bouin's, Carnoy's fixative or Zenker's fixative.

2. **Chelating agents**: Ethylenediaminetetra-acetic acid (EDTA), formalin EDTA.

3. **Ion exchange resins**

4. **Electrophoretic method or electrolytic ionization**

5. **Microwave technique.**

Time Requirement for Decalcification

- Aqueous nitric acid (5–10% solutions): 24–48 hours
- von Ebner's fluid (HCl): 36–37 hours
- Formalin (formol) nitric acid: 24–48 hours
- Formic acid (5–10%): 1–10 days depending upon the thickness of the tissue and degree of calcification.
- EDTA: For small bone/spicules <1 week, for dense cortical bone 6–8 weeks
- Electrophoretic method: 6–8 hours

VIVA VOCE

Q1. Why the tissues are fixed in fixative(s)?
Ans:
i. Prevention of tissue autolysis and bacterial attack (putrefaction).
ii. To preserve the cell elements, most importantly nuclei and cytoplasm. Fixative coagulates, various tissue proteins/elements and make them insoluble.
iii. To maintain the shape and volume of the tissues during subsequent procedures (e.g. clearing, embedding, etc.)
iv. To facilitate the staining reaction by acting as mordant.
v. To keep tissues as close to their natural state and to minimize change of natural colour and appearance.

Q2. Why 10% formalin or neutral buffered formalin is most commonly used as fixative?
Ans:
i. It is relatively cheaper and easy to prepare.
ii. The reaction between fixative and tissue proteins are usually mild with a short reaction time.
iii. It penetrates well and cause a little cell shrinkage. It maintains normal colour of large specimen.
iv. It permits many staining methods in histologic sections.

Q3. What is secondary fixation (post-fixation/post-chromatin)?

Ans: It is use of two fixatives in succession. The first one is the primary fixatives and the second one is the secondary fixative. The primary fixative is usually 10% formalin and secondary fixatives are often those contain mercuric chloride, such as formal sublimate or Helly's solution.

The second fixative reflexes the tissue so that some of its characteristics can be obtained. It must be remembered that secondary fixation does not give same results as would have been obtained if the secondary fixative had been applied to fresh, unfixed tissue.

Advantage of this sublimate post-fixation (secondary fixation) is that tissues are more easily cut and flatten better. Also, they give better staining quality.

Q4. What is the role of clearing agent in tissue processing?

Ans: Clearing agent (xylene or toluene) is a solvent of wax, helps to replace alcohol in dehydrated tissue and thus it facilitate paraffin wax penetration into tissue. Clearing agent must be miscible with alcohol. It usually makes the tissue transparent, hence the name. But some clearing agents do not make tissue transparent, so the better terminology would be 'de-alcoholisation agent'.

Q5. What is decalcification?

Ans: The presence of calcium salts and other minerals in bone and other tissue prevents the preparation of good histologic sections by routine methods. Incomplete removal of these minerals results in ragged and torn sections and in damage to the cutting edge of the microtome knife.

Decalcifying agents remove those minerals and adjust the hard substance of bone to the softness of paraffin wax. Apart from bones, other surgical specimens like calcified tumours, atheromatous plaques, calcified heart valves also require decalcification.

Common decalcifying agents are strong acids (nitric acid, hydrochloric acid), weak acids (aqueous formic acid, acetic acid, picric acid) and EDTA (ethylenediaminetetraacetic acid).

Q6. What is microtome?

Ans: A microtome (from the Greek *mikos*, meaning "small" and *temmein*, meaning "to cut") is a tool used to cut extremely thin sections (4–5 micron thickness routinely). Uses are:

- Traditional histology techniques, sections are stained and viewed under microscopes.
- Frozen sections procedures: Uses freezing microtome or microtome cryostat.
- Electron microscope: Usually transmission electron microscope (TEM)
- Botanical microtomy: Sledge microtomy is used.
- Spectroscopy (especially infrared spectroscopy or FTIR)
- Fluorescent microscopy
- Recently laser microtome: It uses femtosecond laser instead of mechanical knife.

Q7. Why rotary microtome is most commonly used?

Ans: Although most rotary microtomes are manual, some are automatic or semi-automatic, where the advancement of the block and speed of cutting are controlled by a foot pedal or a digitally keypad at one's fingertips. Main advantages are:

i. Ideal for cutting serial section and making ribbons
ii. Heavier knife is use, so less vibration
iii. Cutting angle to knife is adjustable
iv. Ability to cope with harder tissue
v. Can be used in cryostat for frozen sections
vi. Heavier, so more stable

Q8. What are the disadvantages of rotary microtome?

Ans:
i. Only a small length of knife is available for cutting, so large blocks cannot be cut.
ii. Celloidion embedded blocks cannot be cut.
iii. It is relatively costlier.

Q9. What is frozen section?

Ans: The basic principle in frozen section is to freeze the tissue (–5° to –25°C commonly –23°C), so that the water within the tissue transforms into ice. The tissue becomes firm. The ice acts as embedding medium (like paraffin wax in routine tissue processing) and sections are cut by a special microtome known as cryostat.

The frozen section was pioneered by the Dr Louis B. Wilson in 1905.

Q10. What are advantages of frozen sections?

Ans:
i. They are indispensable for rapid diagnosis during operations (to know the tumour type, margin involvement, etc.), i.e. 'on-table' diagnosis of malignancy.
ii. For certain staining procedures these are essential, e.g. fat staining by Oil red O, some methods in CNS and silver impregnation methods.
iii. Ideal to demonstrate enzymes in tissues.
iv. Also used in immunofluorescent method and in immunocytochemical method.

Q11. What are the disadvantages of frozen section?

Ans:
i. Only individual section is obtained. No serial section or ribbon possible.
ii. Staining of unfixed tissues is not as satisfactory as paraffin embedded permanent sections.
iii. Structural details are somewhat distorted during section cutting as no embedding medium (like paraffin) is used.
iv. Sometimes freezing artefacts are produced due to improper techniques. These include presence of ice crystals in tissues, separation of mucosal and other epithelial surfaces, nuclear vacuolization and ballooning.

H and E (Haematoxylin and Eosin) and Other Special Stains

A good routine histologic stain must be able to stain nuclei and cytoplasm but also connective tissue. A properly stained histologic section by haematoxylin and eosin differentiates and distinguishes the nuclei, the cytoplasm and connective tissue. The nuclei appear blue, whereas the cytoplasm and connective tissue fibres will have shades of pink. As it can stain and differentiate well all these structures, so it is the most popular routine stain.

Haematoxylin is used in conjunction with eosin as routine stain. Usually 0.5–1% aqueous solution of eosin is used as a counterstain, though some prefer phloxine (0.5–1%) as a counter stain. Phloxine gives a brighter and vivid red stain but eosin is more informative as it differentiates better. Some other counterstains are orange G, Bordeaux red and Biebrich scarlet.

Haematin (oxidation product of haematoxylin) is inadequate as a nuclear stain without the presence of a mordant. So, Haematoxylin solutions are classified according to which mordant is used.

- **Alum haematoxylin:** Ehrlich's hematoxylin, Harris's hematoxylin, Mayer's hematoxylin, Cole's hematoxylin, Gill's haematoxylin and Carazzi's haematoxylin.
- **Iron haematoxylin:** Weigert's haematoxylin, Verhoeff's hematoxylin, Loyez's hematoxylin, heidenhain hematoxylin.
- **Tungsten hematoxylin:** Phosphotungstic acid Haematoxylin (PTAH)
- **Lead hematoxylin**
- **Molybdenum Haematoxylin**
- **Haematoxylin without mordant**

PRINCIPLE OF ALUM HAEMATOXYLIN STAINING

The mordant used in alum Haematoxylin is aluminum either potash alum (aluminium potash sulfate) or ammonium alum (aluminium ammonium sulfate).

Initially, the nuclei become red after staining, which turn blue or blue black when stained sections are washed in weak alkali. Practically, tap water can be used for washing as it is alkaline enough to produce desired colour change. Sometimes, alkaline solutions like Scott's tap water, saturated lithium carbonate or 0.5% ammonia in distilled water is used for this colour change. *This process of changing colour from red to blue is called 'blueing'.*

Progressive staining: Here, the sections are stained for a predetermined time, so that the nuclei become well stained but the background is relatively under stained.

Regressive staining: In this procedure, the sections are first over stained, and then excess stain is selectively removed in acid alcohol. Advantage of this staining procedure is that the degree of staining is controlled (some tissue elements retain more stain/dye compared with others. Hence, the nuclei take good staining, whereas the cytoplasm and background are perfectly clear.

Harris Alum Haematoxylin

Composition of alum haematoxylin
- Hematoxylin: 2.5 gm
- Absolute alcohol: 50 ml
- Ammonia or potassium alum: 50 gm
- Distilled water: 500 ml
- Mercuric oxide: 1.5 gm or sodium iodate: 0.5 gm
- Glacial acetic acid: 20 ml

Preparation: The Haematoxylin is dissolved in the absolute alcohol and it is then added to previously prepared alum solution (alum in distilled water). The two solutions are mixed well. The mixture is now heated to boiling point and mercuric oxide or sodium iodide is added. Then the mixture is rapidly cooled by plunging the flask in cold water or into a sink containing ice pieces. The solution is ready for staining.

Addition of glacial acetic acid is optional but is preferred, because this gives more precise and selective nuclear staining. Filter before use when previously made solutions are used.

Advantages: It is a good nuclear stain and is used for general purpose. As the nuclear staining is very clear, it is also used in exfoliative cytology. In routine histologic sections, Harris's Haematoxylin is used regressively but in exfoliative cytology it is used progressively.

Disadvantages: Nuclear stain fades after a few months which is also seen in other chemically ripened alum Haematoxylin (of natural ripening of Ehrlich's alum hematoxylin). In stored solution, there is formation of a precipitate after few months and the solution is not good for staining. At this stage, the stain can be used by filtering the precipitate and increasing the staining time. But best thing is to use freshly prepared stain.

Standing time
- Progressive in exfoliative cytology: 4–30 seconds
- Regressive method: 5–15 minutes.

Staining Method Using Alum Haematoxylin and Eosin

- Dewax histologic sections.
- Hydrate through graded alcohol first, then to water.
- Stain the nuclei with preferred alum Haematoxylin (Harris hematoxylin) for required time.
- Wash the stained sections for 5 minutes in tap water till the blueing of the nuclei.
- Differentiate the sections, in 1% acid alcohol (1% HCl in 70% ethyl alcohol) for 5–10 seconds.
- Wash again in tap water until the sections are 'blue' for 5 minutes or less.
- Stain in 1% eosin (eosin Y is preferred) for 10 minutes.
- Wash in tap water for 1–5 minutes.
- Dehydrate through graded alcohol (70%, 95% and then 100%).
- Clearing in xylene, then mount it DPX or Canada balsam.

Result of Alum Haematoxylin and Eosin Stain

- Nuclei → Blue/black
- Cytoplasm → Varying shades of pink
- Fibrin → Deep pink
- Red blood cells → Orange/red
- Muscle fiber → Deep pink/red
- Fungal hyphae → Faintly blue
- Calcium deposits → Deep blue-black

Iron Haematoxylin

Here iron salts are used both as oxidizing agent and as mordant in the haematoxylin solutions. Ferric chloride and ferric ammonium sulphate are commonly used as iron salts.

In comparison to alum haematoxylin, iron haematoxylin can demonstrate wide range of tissue structures but staining technique is time-consuming and also it needs microscope evaluation during differentiation stage.

Weigert's Iron Haematoxylin

Composition of staining solution

i. Haematoxylin solutions
- Haematoxylin: 1 gm
- Absolute alcohol: 100 ml

ii. Iron solution
- 30% aqueous ferric chloride solution (anhydrous): 4 ml
- Hydrochloric acid (concentrated): 1 ml
- Distilled water: 95 ml

Preparation: First the solution (i) or haematoxylin solution must be allowed to ripen. For natural ripening, it takes 4–5 weeks time. It may also be prepared from a stock solution of 5% Haematoxylin in absolute alcohol (previously ripened solution). Now, mix equal part of solution (i) and solution (ii) immediately before use. When mixing is done in a test tube, it is advisable to pour solution (i) in the tube first, and then add solution (ii) as it contains concentration of HCl. The staining solution/mixture ideally should be violet-black in colour. If the colour becomes brown, then the mixture should be discarded.

Advantage: Main use is as a nuclear stain in techniques, where acid is used subsequently (e.g. picric acid in van Gieson stain). It resists removal of counterstain containing differentiating agent like picric acid. It stains nuclei black unlike blue/blue-black in alum hematoxylin. The stained nuclei will not be decolourized by light. So, it is a more permanent stain than alum haematoxylin.

Disadvantage: More time consuming and needs microscopic control for accuracy. It has been replaced by more convenient Celestine blue-alum hematoxylin. Still it is in use for CNS tissues.

Staining time: 20–30 minutes.

Heidenhain Haematoxylin

Composition of staining solution
- Iron alum solutions
  - Ferric ammonium sulfate (violet crystals): 5 gm
  - Distilled water: 100 ml
- Haematoxylin solutions
  - Hematoxylin: 0.5 gm
  - Absolute alcohol: 10 ml
  - Distilled water: 90 ml
- This solution must be kept ready for 4–5 weeks for natural ripening, or 5% stock solution (ripened) alcoholic hematoxylin: 10 ml
- Distilled water: 90 ml
- This solution is ready for immediate use.

Staining methods

1. Dewax histologic sections (either putting into xylol for 1–2 minutes or by heating).
2. Hydrate through graded alcohol to water.
3. Mordant in 5% iron alum/iron alum solution for 1 hour.
4. Rinse in distilled water (10–20 seconds).
5. Stain in Heidenhain haematoxylin solution for 1 hour.
6. Wash in running tap water until the sections are blue (usually takes 10 minutes in tap water of pH 8). Lithium carbonate may be added to water if it is not sufficiently alkaline.
7. Differentiate in 5% iron alum until the desired structure is clearly demonstrated under microscope.
8. Wash in running tap water for 8–10 minutes.
9. Dehydrate in graded alcohol (70%, 95% and then 100%).

10. Clear and mount in DPX or Canada balsam.

Advantage: It can be used to demonstrate many structures as per degree of differentiation. mitochondria, muscle striations, myelin, nuclear membrane, chromatin, chromosomes, nucleoli, centrioles, yolk and ground cytoplasm can be demonstrated which become jet black or grey black. Good for photography. The stain is permanent, if the alum is properly removed. It is applicable after use of any fixative.

Disadvantage: It is used only regressively and experience is required for good staining quality. For beginners use half-strength iron alum is advisable until they again experience.

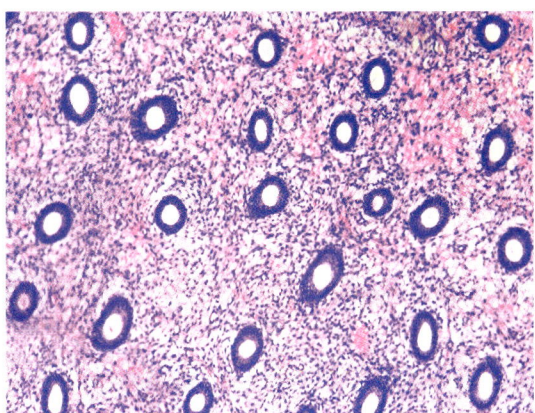

Fig. 12.1: Haematoxylin and eosin stain showing proliferative endometrium (H and E, 100X)

PERIODIC ACID–SCHIFF (PAS) STAIN

Periodic acid is a very strong oxidizing agent and under the controlled condition of the staining reaction, it reacts with the aldehyde group of the carbohydrates. This periodic acid cleaves the carbon-carbon bond in amino or alkyl amino derivatives or 1.2 glycols to form aldehydes. These aldehydes will react with fuchsin-sulfurous acid and this product combines the basic pararosaniline to give a positive result (magenta-coloured compound). This compound is chemically alkyl sulfate.

Any substance that fulfils the following criteria will give a positive result during PAS reaction (Hotchkiss, 1948).
- The substance must not diffuse away during fixation.
- It must produce an oxidation product which is not diffusible.
- The substance must have the 1.2 glycol grouping or the equivalent amino or alkyl amino derivative or the oxidation product CHOH-CO.
- Sufficient concentration of the substance must be present in the tissue to give a positive reaction (magenta color).

PAS (Periodic Acid–Schiff) Reagents

- Periodic acid solution (0.5%)
  Periodic acid: 1 gm
  Distilled water: 200 ml
- Schiff's reagent: Dissolve 1 gm basic fuchsin in 200 ml of boiling distilled water. When dissolved; cool it to 50–60°C. Add 2 gm of potassium metabisulfite and mix it. Bring the mixture to room temperature and then add 2 ml of hydrochloric acid and mix it. Also add 2 gm of activated charcoal and this chemical solution is kept at room temperature in a dark place overnight. Next morning, filter it (Whatman paper No. 1). The ideal solution after filtration should be pale yellow or clear. Store this solution at 4°C in dark container.

Staining Method

1. Deparaffinize histologic sections and bring the section to water. If Zenker's fluid is used as a fixative, remove mercury precipitate in iodine. Wash in water and decolourize in hypo solution.
2. Rinse in distilled water.
3. Oxidize in 0.5% periodic acid for 5–10 minutes.
4. Wash in running tap water for 5 minutes and rinse in distilled water.
5. Treat with Schiff reagent for 10–30 minutes

6. Wash in running tap water for 5–10 minutes.
7. Counterstain (optional) with Harris's haematoxylin for 1–3 minutes to stain the nuclei. Differentiate in 1% acid alcohol (3–5 dips). Blueing the sections in running tap water.
8. Wash in water.
9. Rinse in absolute alcohol.
10. Clear in xylene and mount in DPX or Canada balsam.

Results
- Glycogen and other PAS positive substances: Magenta/bright red.
- Nuclei: Blue
- Other tissue constituents: Yellow

PAS Positive Substances
- Glycogen, most basement membrane, amyloid, fibrin of thrombi, colloid of thyroid.
- Mucins: Intestinal glands, gastric glands, endocervical glands, salivary glands, bronchial glands, conjunctiva, prostatic gland secretion, corpora amylacea.
- Adrenal lipofuscin, many fungi, actinomycosis (clubs only), hyaline casts of kidney, cartilage matrix, ocular lens capsule, starch, zymogen granules of pancreas, beta cells of pituitary.
- Russel bodies of plasma cells, megakaryocyte granules.

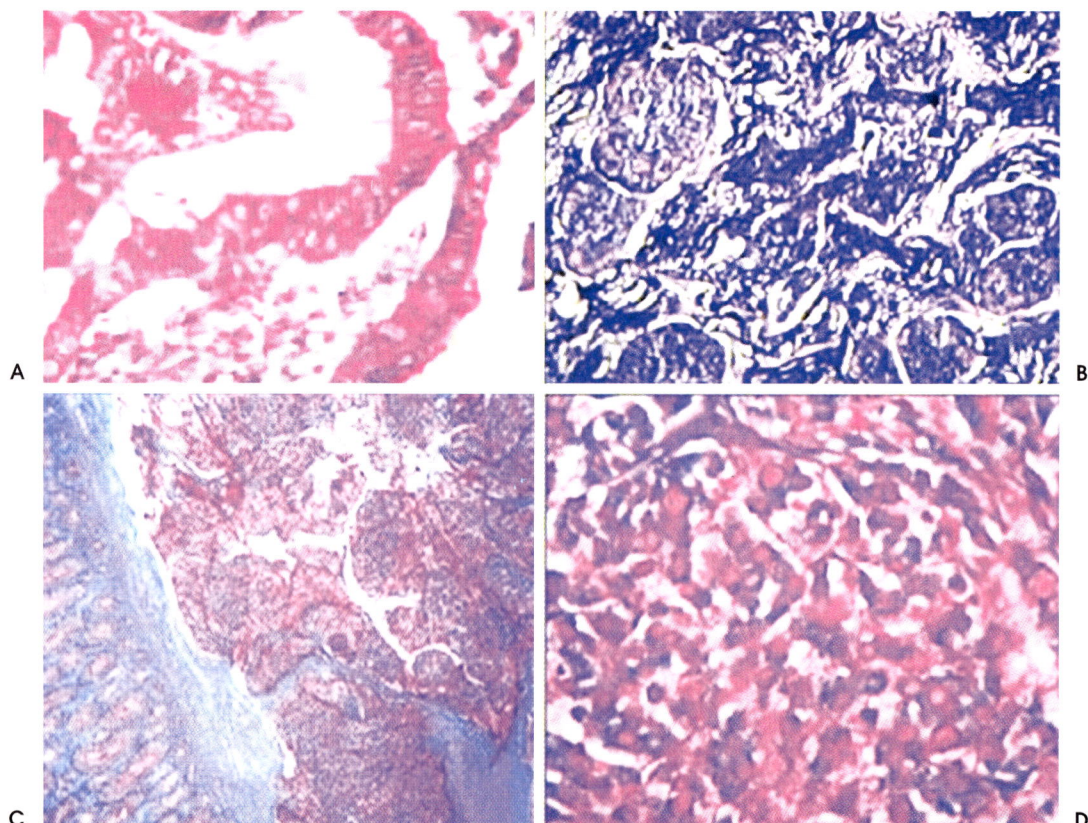

Fig. 12.2A to D: (A) Adenocarcinoma of colon showing malignant cells with neutral mucins (PAS, 400X); (B) Mucinous carcinoma showing pools of acidic mucin (alcian blue, 400X); (C) Mucinous carcinoma showing acidic and neutral mucins (combined alcian blue and PAS, 100X); (D) Signet ring cell carcinoma showing neutral mucin (combined alcian blue and PAS, 400X)

SUDAN BLACK B STAIN

Sudan black B is known as the most sensitive lipid stain. It was introduced by Lison and Dagnelie in 1935. Unlike the other Sudan dyes it can stain both phospholipid and neutral fat (compound lipids). It also can stain myelin and mitochondria.

The ability of formalin and calcium to make these lipids insoluble in acetone and other reagents used in paraffin processing, make them unsuitable for Sudan III or osmium tetroxide staining. But Sudan black B stain can be used. Ideal sections for Sudan IV staining are unfixed cryostat sections, short fixed frozen sections and cryostat sections, post-fixed in formol-calcium. Use of solvents like ethanol or acetone is not recommended for this dye, as these solvents remove a significant portion of the lipid. So, small fat droplets are dissolved out and are not detected by stain. Propylene, propylene glycol, isopropyl alcohol or ethylene glycol are better as a solvent. But 70% ethanol is still used for general purpose.

Standing Methods

1. Rinse cryostat sections in 70% ethanol.
2. Stain the slides in saturated Sudan black B in 70% ethanol for 30–120 minutes. Sections of routine formol saline-fixed tissue should be stained for 30–180 minutes at 60°C.
3. Rinse in 70% ethanol to remove excess surface dye.
4. Wash in tap water and differentiate in 70% alcohol (or in 85% propylene glycol solution for 2–3 minutes).
5. Wash in distilled water.
6. Counterstain in Mayer's carmalum for 2–3 minutes. (Mayer's carmalum: Dissolve 2 gm of carmine in 100 ml of 0.5% ammonium alum by boiling for 1 hour. Add a few crystals of thymol to prevent fungal growth, filter before use.)
7. Wash well in water.
8. Mount in glycerine jelly.

Results

- Compound lipids (phospholipids, cerebrosides): Blue black
- Nuclei: Red

OIL RED O STAIN

For this staining technique, cryostat sections, short-fixed frozen sections, unfixed in formol calcium is chosen.

Staining Solution

A saturated solution of Oil red O (0.25–0.5%) in isopropyl alcohol is kept in stock. Working solution is made by adding 6 ml of stock solution with 4 ml of distilled water. Allow the mixture to stand for 5–10 minutes and then filter it.

Staining methods

1. Cut frozen sections (relatively thick section of 8–10 µm).
2. Wash well in distilled water.
3. Rinse in 70% ethanol.
4. Stain in Oil red O staining solution for 10–35 minutes.
5. Differentiate in 70% alcohol to remove excess stain.
6. Counterstain nuclei lightly in Harris Haematoxylin for 1–2 minutes.
7. Blueing in tap water (alternatively, ammonia water may be used).
8. Mount in glycerine jelly.

Results

- Lipids: Orange to red
- Nuclei: Blue

VERHOEFF'S VAN GIESON STAIN FOR ELASTIC FIBRES

Composition of Staining Solution

- Verhoeff's staining solution
  – Stock 5% alcoholic haematoxylin: 20 ml
  – 10% ferric chloride: 8 ml
  – Verhoeff's iodine (10 dine 2 gm, potassium iodide 4 gm, water 100 ml): 8 ml

- Reagents are added as given above, then mix well; solution should be freshly prepared before use.
- van Gieson's staining solution
  - Saturated aqueous solution of picric acid: 100 ml
  - 1% acid fuchsin: 10 ml
  - Freshly prepared solution is better

Staining Methods

1. Bring histologic sections to water.
2. Stain in Verhoeff's staining solution for 15–30 minutes until sections are jet-black.
3. Differentiate in 2% ferric chloride until elastic fibres are clearly visible (rinse in water and examine under low power microscope).
4. Wash in water.
5. Place in 95% alcohol to remove iodine staining.
6. Wash in water for 5–10 minutes.
7. Counterstain in van Gieson's staining solution for 3 minutes. Blot it.
8. Dehydrate in graded alcohol.
9. Clear in xylene and mount in DPX.

Results

- Elastic fibres and nuclei: Black to blue black
- RBC, cytoplasm, background and muscle: Yellow
- Collagen: Red

Note

Do not wash the sections after van Gieson's staining (step 7). Put them directly in graded alcohol for dehydration. Otherwise, it will impair staining quality (if washed in water).

GOMORI'S SILVER IMPREGNATION STAIN FOR RETICULIN

Gomori's Silver Solution Preparation

In a test tube or flask, add 4 parts of 10% aqueous silver nitrate and 1 part of 10% potassium hydroxide. The potassium hydroxide will cause silver to deposit. Mark the volume of the fluid with a pencil/marker. Remove the supernatant fluid and wash the deposit several times with distilled water to make up to its original volume (previously marked by pencil/marker). Now, add strong ammonia drop by drop until the deposit is just dissolved. Again add 10% silver nitrate solution, to produce a light precipitate. Make the volume of this solution twice with addition of distilled water. Store in dark bottle. Filter before use. Preferably, solution should be freshly prepared but it can used for 24–35 hours.

Staining Methods

1. Bring the deparaffinized sections to water.
2. Oxidize with 1% potassium permanganate for 1–2 minutes.
3. Rinse in tap water.
4. Decolourize with 3% potassium metabisulfite for 1 minute.
5. Rinse in tap water.
6. Sensitize in 2% iron alum for 1 minute.
7. Wash in tap water for 2–3 minutes, then rise in distilled water 2–3 changes.
8. Impregnate in silver solution for 3 minutes.
9. Rinse quickly in distilled water.
10. Reduce in 10% formalin in tap water for 3 minutes.
11. Wash in running tap water for 3–4 minutes, then rinse in distilled water.
12. Tone in 1:500 gold chloride (yellow) for 5–15 minutes.
13. Rinse in distilled water
14. Place in 3% potassium metabisulfite for 1 minute to reduce toning.
15. Fix in 3% sodium thiosulfate for 1 minute.
16. Rinse in distilled water
17. Wash in water.
18. Dehydrate through graded alcohol.
19. Clear in xylene and mount in DPX.

Results

- Reticulin fibres: Black
- Collagen fibres: Purple
- Nuclei and cytoplasm: Grayish/shades of gray.

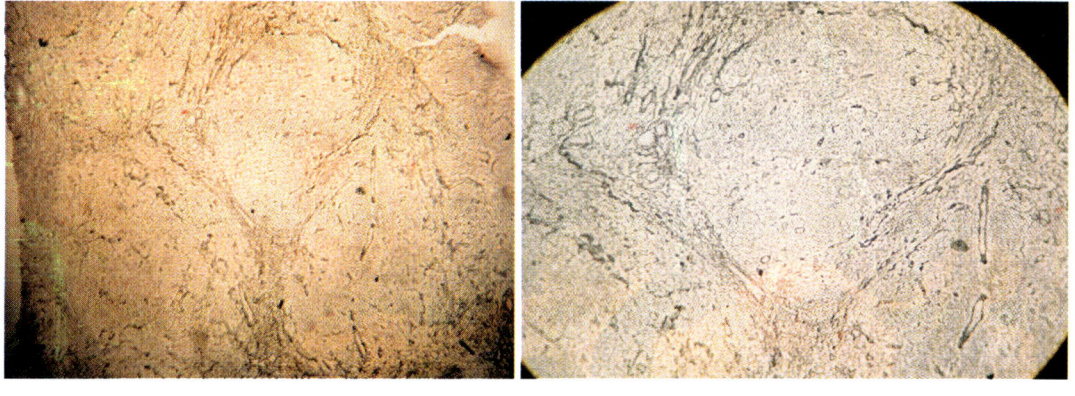

Fig. 12.3A and B: (A) Microphotograph showing reticulin fibres in cirrhotic nodules of liver (reticulin stain, low power view, 100X); (B) Microphotograph showing reticulin fibres in a cirrhotic nodule (reticulin stain, high power view, 400X).

Table 12.1: Common stains used for different connective tissues and its colour

Tissue Type	Masson trichrome	Reticulin silver	Methenamine silver	van Gieson	PTAH	H and E	PAS
Collagen	Blue green	Pale gray	Unstained	Red	Orange red	Deep pink	Pale pink
Reticulin fibres	Blue green	Black	Unstained	Yellow	Orange brown	Unstained	Pink
Elastic fibres	Pale red	Unstained	Unstained	Yellow	Orange brown	Pink	Unstained
Fibrin	Red	Unstained/grey	Unstained	Variable yellow	Variable blue	Pink	Pink or unstained
Muscle	Red	Pale grey	Pale grey	Yellow	Blue	Deep pink	Pale pink
Cartilage	Variable	Variable	Variable	Variable	Variable	Purple	Pink
Basement membrane	Blue green	Pale grey	Black	Yellow	Orange	Pink	Magenta

PTAH: phosphotungstic acid haematoxylin; H and E: Haematoxylin and eosin; PAS: periodic acid–Schiff.

VIVA VOCE

Q. 1. What is the basic principle of H and E stain?
Ans: This stain has two components; haematoxylin and eosin. Staining of nuclei is done by oxidized haematoxylin (haematin) through mordant bonds and make nuclei blue in colour. Nuclear staining is followed by counterstaining with the xanthene dye, the eosin, which colours the cytoplasm in varying shades of pink.

Q. 2. What are the results (colour) after H and E staining?
Ans: Nuclei: Blue/black

Cytoplasm: Varying shades of pink

Fibrin: Deep pink

Red blood cells: Orange/red

Muscle fibre: Deep pink/red

Q. 3. What is the principle of PAS staining?
Ans: Substances which contain vicinal glycol group or their amino or alkyl amino derivatives are oxidized by periodic acid to form dialdehydes. It combines with Schiff's reagent to form an insoluble magenta-coloured compound.

Q. 4. Which tissue components are stained by PAS staining?
Ans: It stains glycogen, neutral mucin and carbohydrate portions of glycoproteins and glycolipids.

Positive stains (magenta colour) are seen in glycogen, basement membrane, starch, neutral mucin, colloid, fungi, amoeba, cellulose, collagen (weak positive) and amyloid (weak positive).

Q. 5. What is the principle of reticulin staining?
Ans: Reticulin fibres mainly consist of type III collagen in a glycoprotein complex. It can be stained by several techniques but Gordon-Sweet's silver impregnantion method is most sensitive and most widely used stain. In this technique, hydroxyl group of adjacent hexose sugars are oxidized to aldehydes by potassium permanganate. These newly formed aldehydes then reduce silver diamine to metallic silver. This reaction can be further modified by use of silver chloride as a toner.

Q. 6. What are the results (colour) after reticulin staining?
Ans: Reticulin fibres: Black

Collagen fibres: Purple

Nuclei and cytoplasm: Grayish/shades of gray.

Q. 7. How reticulin fibres are differentiated from collagen fibres?
Ans: Reticulin fibres are fine and delicate fibres which are found along with a stronger and coarser collagen fibre, i.e. type III collagen fibre. Reticulin fibres form a delicate supporting framework for highly cellular organs like lymph nodes, liver and endocrine glands.

Reticulin fibres are gram-negative, coloured black by silver stain and isotropic (not birefringent), whereas collagen fibres are slight gram-positive, stained purple, or brown to mauve by silver stain and is anisotropic (birefringent).

Q. 8. What are elastic fibres? How are they stained?
Ans: Elastic fibres consist of elastin and glycoprotein. They are found throughout the body but most common locations are skin, respiratory system (lung, pleura), urinary bladder, ligaments, circulatory system (blood vessels).

In the Verhoeff staining technique, elastic fibres are stained black due to formation of metallic (iron)—dye (haematin) is called lake. Weigert's resorcin fuchsin also stains elastic fibres blue to black. In aldehyde fuchsin, elastin fibres are stained purple and it becomes dark brown in orcein stain.

Q. 9. When is Masson's trichrome staining used?

Ans: This is a three-step staining technique (hence the name trichrome). It stains three different categories of cell components: Nucleus, muscle and collagen.

In the first step, nucleus is stained by Weigert's iron-Haematoxylin stain followed by the second step of staining of cytoplasm and muscles with a red cytoplasmic staining of cytoplasm and muscles with a red cytoplasmic stain differentiated in phosphomolybdic acid. Lastly, staining of fibres with aniline blue or light green.

- Nuclei: Bluish black or black
- Muscle, cytoplasm, keratin: Red
- Collagen, cartilage, mucus: Blue (if aniline dye is used) or green (if light green is used)

Q. 10. What is a mordant?

Ans: The mordants form a link between the tissue and the stain. The combination of the dye and the mordant forms a compound which is capable of attracting itself to the tissue firmly. This compound is sometimes called 'lake'. The mordants are salts, usually sulpfates of aluminium, iron or chromium. Generally, double sulphates or alums are used.

13
HP Slides (Light Microscopy)

Tuberculosis of Lung
- Section shows structure of lung parenchyma.

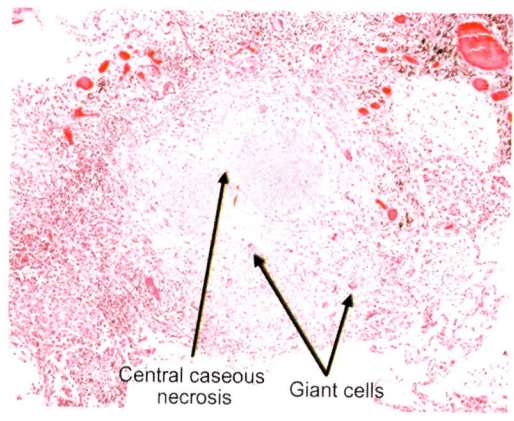

Central caseous necrosis   Giant cells

- Central granular caseation (caseation necrosis) is surrounded by epithelioid histiocytes (modified macrophages) and Langhans giant cells. Foreign body giant cells are also found.
- The tubercles are surrounded by lymphocytes and fibroblasts.

Emphysema of Lung
- There is marked enlargement of airspaces.
- Alveolar walls show thinning and destruction. Adjacent alveoli become confluent, creating large airspaces.

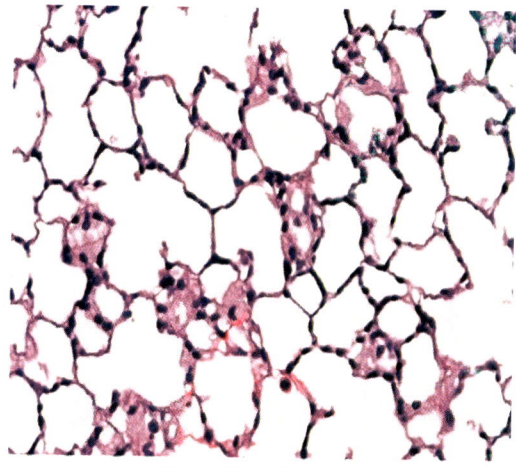

Normal lung (control)

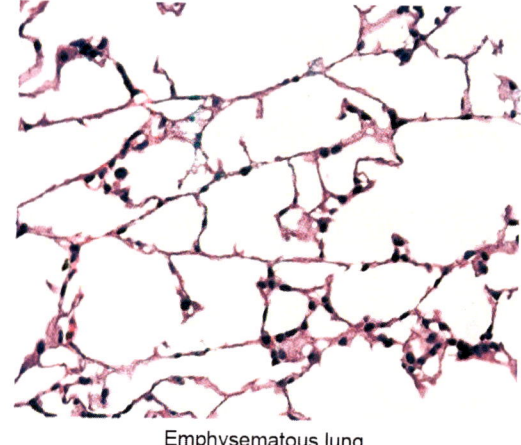

Emphysematous lung (due to cigarette smoking)

- There is loss of elastic tissue in the surrounding alveolar septae.
- Alveolar capillaries are reduced in number.

Pleomorphic Salivary Adenoma
- There is considerable variation or great heterogeneity in the histologic features within the tumour.
- It is characterized by pleomorphic or 'mixed' appearance in which both epithelial and stromal components are seen in varying proportions.
- Epithelial component: It forms various patterns like ducts, acini, tubules, sheets and strands of cells of ductal or myoepithelial cells. The ductal cells are cuboidal or columnar, whereas myoepithelial cells (basal cells) are polygonal or spindle shaped (which is PAS-positive). Focal areas showing squamous metaplasia.
- Stromal component: It is present as loose connective tissue, and as myxoid or chondromyxoid matrix which simulates cartilage (pseudocartilage). This connective tissue mucins appear as basophilic material.

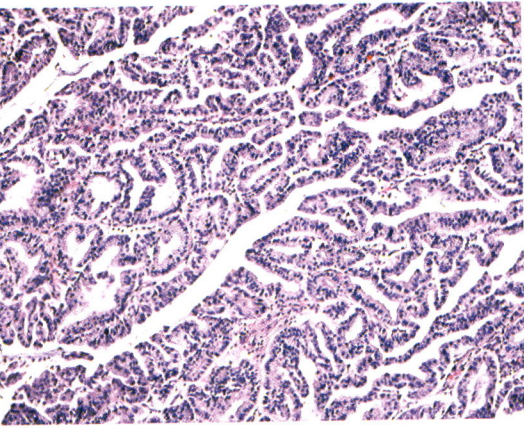

- The malignant cells have large vesicular nuclei with prominent nucleoli.
- The malignant glands are lined by tall columnar cells containing mucin resembling colonic adenocarcinoma.
- There is chronic inflammatory cell infiltration into stroma.

TB Intestine (Ileocaecal)
- There is mucosal and submucosal ulcerations.
- There is moderate to severe infiltration of chronic inflammatory cells.
- Against this background, many epithelioid granulomas are seen in all the layers of intestine, i.e mucosa, submucosa, muscularis layer and serosa.
- Both caseating and non-caseating granulomas are seen.

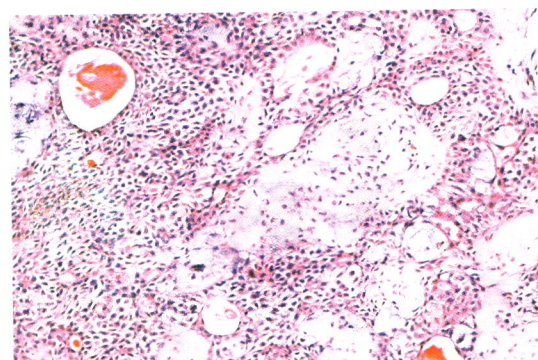

Adenocarcinoma of Stomach (Intestinal Type)
- Malignant epithelial cells arranged in tubular glands and in papillary pattern.
- Malignant epithelial cells are also arranged in sheets.

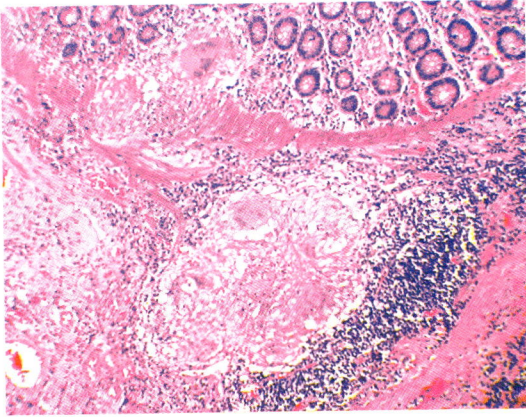

- Multinucleated giant cells of both Langhans and foreign body type are found.
- Most of the mucosal glands are unremarkable while some glands show pyloric metaplasia.

Acute Appendicitis

- There is an acute inflammatory infiltrate (neutrophilic infiltration) which extends from mucosa through the full thickness of the appendiceal wall.
- Neutrophilic infiltration is present in the muscularis layer.
- Acute inflammatory exudate is seen in the lumen.
- Focal superficial (mucosal) ulceration is noted.
- Subserosal vessels are dilated.
- Serosal layer is granular and erythematous (organized).

Clear Cell Carcinoma of Kidney

- Tumour cells with clear cytoplasm arranged in solid sheets, in trabecular (cord-like) pattern and in tubular pattern.
- Slightly irregular nuclei and nucleoli are seen in high power (40X) only. Nuclear diameter 15 µm and chromatin is open (Fuhrman nuclear grade 2).
- Mitoses are not seen.
- The tumour has delicate branching vasculature.
- The cytoplasm is abundant and clear or granular due to presence of glycogen and lipids.

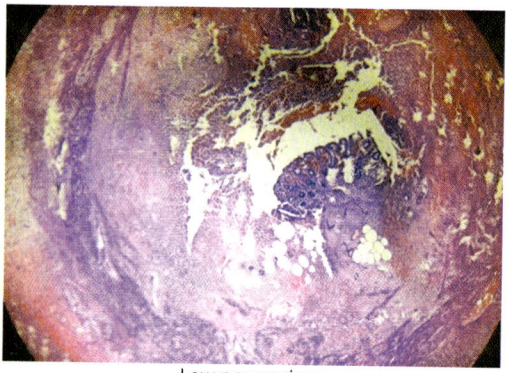

Low power view

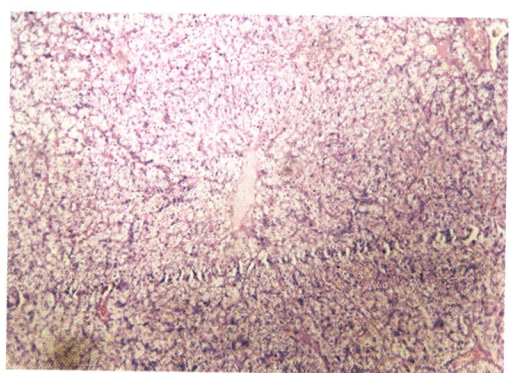

Low power view

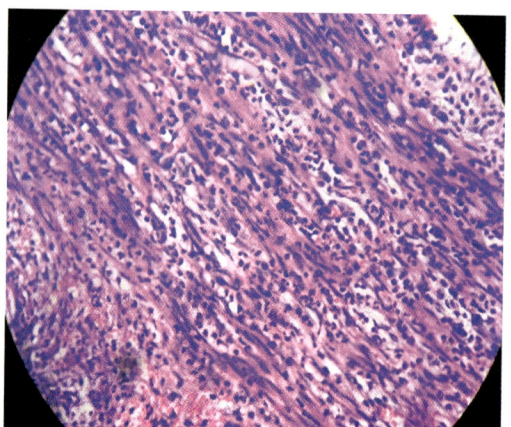

High power view

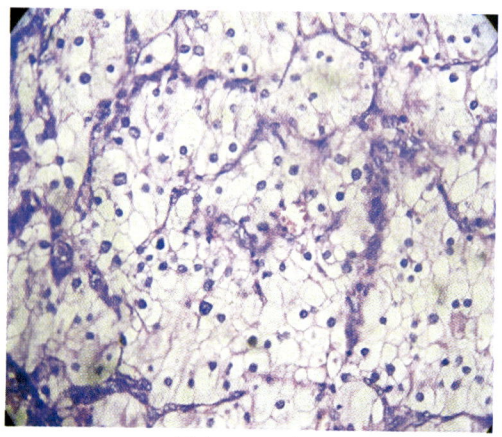

High power view

Osteogenic Sarcoma

- Tumour is composed of pleomorphic polyhedral or spindle-shaped neoplastic cells.
- The tumour cells have hyperchromatic nuclei and frequent mitoses.
- These neoplastic cells form islands of reactive new women bone (pinkish lace-like osteoid and calcified bone spicules).
- Other matrices, including cartilage or fibrous tissue, are present in varying amount.
- Bizarre tumour giant cells are present.

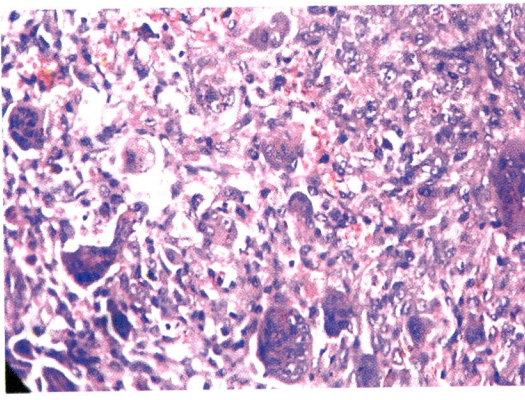

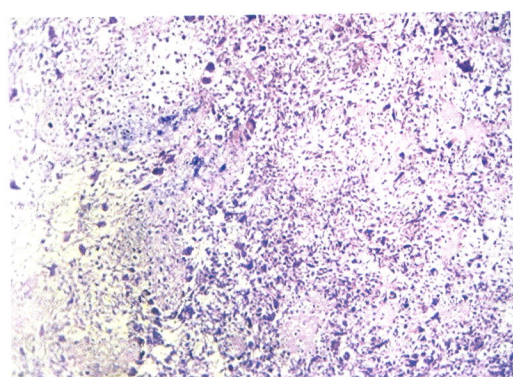

Low power view

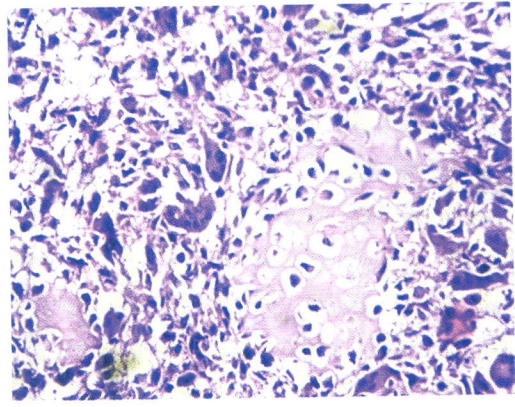

High power view

Giant Cell Tumour (of Bone)

It is a biphasic tumour composed of mononuclear uniform tumour cells (stromal cells) and giant cells.

- **Tumour cells**: They are uniform cells with indistinct cell membrane growing in a syncytium as stromal cells. The tumour cells are usually oval or round in shape.
- **Giant cells**: Numerous multinucleated osteoclast-like giant cells containing >100 nuclei are uniformly scattered among mononuclear tumour (stromal) cells. The nuclei of stromal cells resemble those of the mononuclear stromal cells. Mitoses are infrequent.

Proliferative Endometrium

- Early proliferative endometrium (days 4–7): Thin surface epithelium. Glands are small, round and straight (tubular glands) having columnar living with basal nuclei. Stroma is compact and composed of spindle-shaped cells that have scant

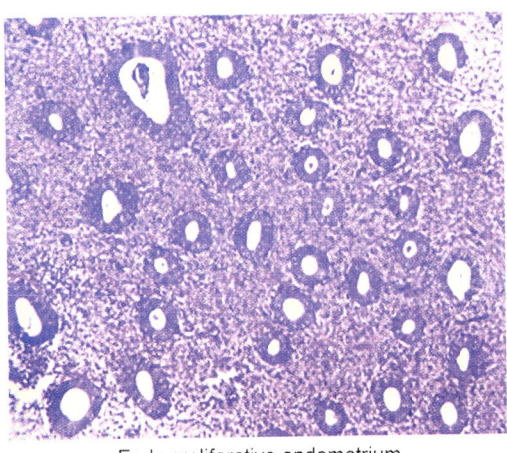

Early proliferative endometrium

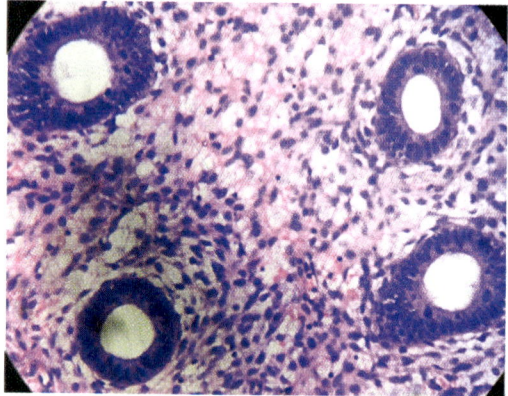

Mid-proliferative endometrium

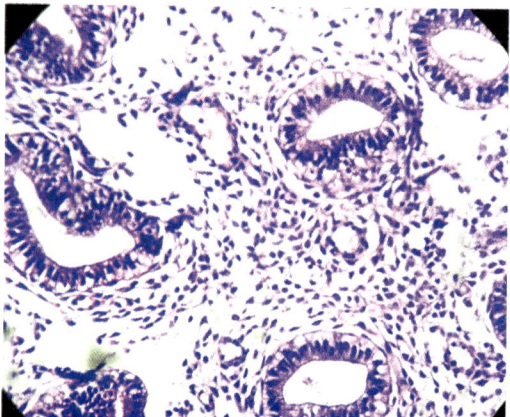

Early secretory endometrium

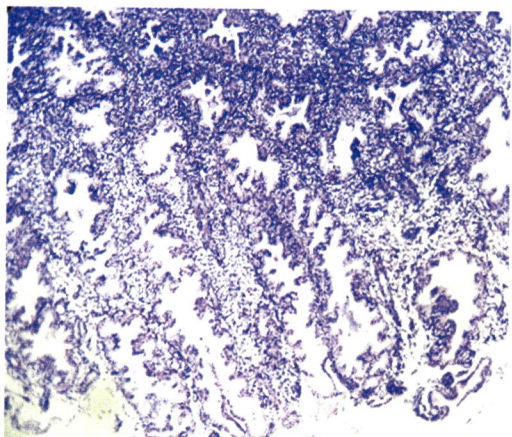

Mid-secretory endometrium

cytoplasm. Mitoses are seen both within glands and stroma. No oedema is seen within stroma. Stroma contains small, regularly distributed blood vessels.

- Mid-proliferative endometrium (8–10 days): Columnar surface epithelium. The endometrial glands are longer and curving. Variable stroma, oedema and numerous mitotic figures are seen within stroma.
- Late proliferative endometrium (11–14 days): Undulant surface epithelium. The glands are tortuous and crowded with prominent mitotic activity and pseudostratification. Subnuclear vacuoles are seen in less than 50% of glands. Stromal oedema is variable but present.

Secretory Endometrium

- Early secretory endometrium (16–19 days): Subnuclear vacuoles (secretory vacuoles beneath the nuclei) are seen >50% of glands. The glands are usually longer and tortuous. Stroma is edematous.
- Mid-secretory endometrium (20–22 days): The glands are fully coiled (**corkscrew appearance**) and lined by cells with round often vesicular nuclei. Basal vacuoles (subnuclear vacuoles) progressively push past the nuclei and become **supranuclear vacuoles**. Glandular secretion is prominent. Stromal oedema is prominent. Pseudodecidual changes seen only around spiral arterioles.
- Late secretory endometrium (23–28 days): The glands are tortuous, producing a serrated or **"saw-tooth" appearance** due to secretory exhaustion. Pseudodecidual changes in the stroma is marked as is stromal edema. Spiral arterioles become prominent as is stromal edema. Spiral arterioles become prominent as a result of thickness of their walls and cuff of predecidual stromal cells around them. There is increase in the number of **stromal granulocytes** (bean-shaped, dense nuclei, inconspicuous cytoplasm). Scattered neutrophils and occasional lymphocytes are seen in the stroma which do not imply inflammation.

Note

Stromal granulocytes once thought to derive from the endometrial stroma, now believed to originate from endometrial granular lymphocytes (NK cells).

Leiomyoma

- It is composed of smooth muscle cells which are arranged in whorls and fascicles.
- The individual smooth muscle cells are uniform in size and shape and have the characteristic oval nucleus and long, slender bipolar cytoplasmic processes.
- Mitotic figures are sparse (rare).
- Hyaline degeneration is present.

Mucinous Cystadenoma

- It is lined by a single layer of tall columnar nonciliated epithelium similar to intestinal type or endocervical (müllerian) type.
- These lining columnar cells have basally placed nuclei and large apical mucinous vacuoles.
- Nuclear stratification or nuclear atypia not present.
- Stromal invasion by tumour cells is absent and basement membrane is intact.

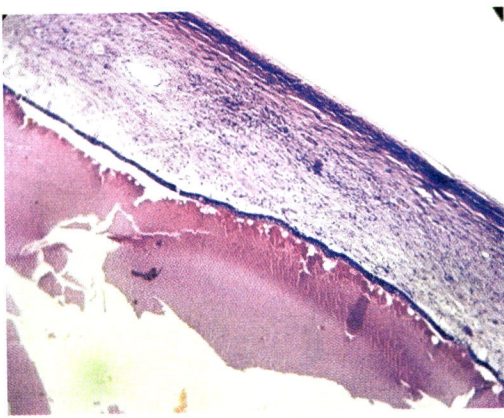

Low power view

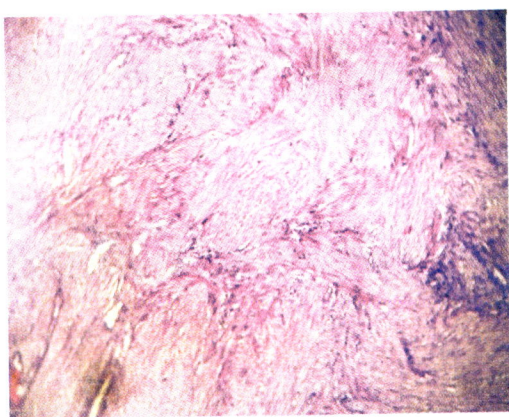

Low power

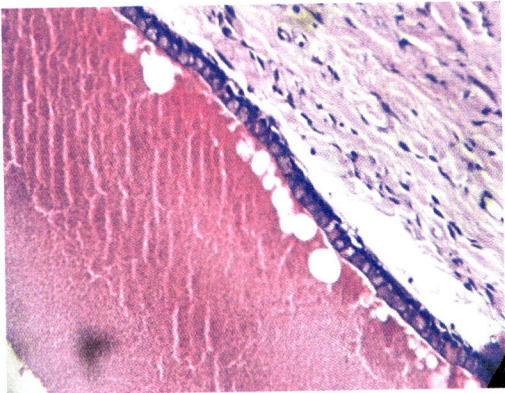

High power view

Portal Cirrhosis (Laennec's Cirrhosis or Hobnail Cirrhosis Related to Alcohol)

- Diffuse disruption in architecture of entire liver (loss of normal central vein–portal tract relationship).

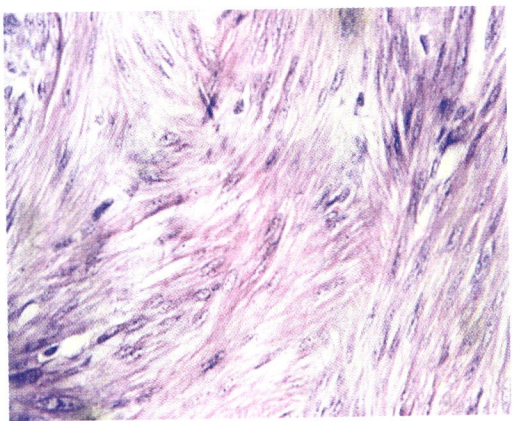

High power

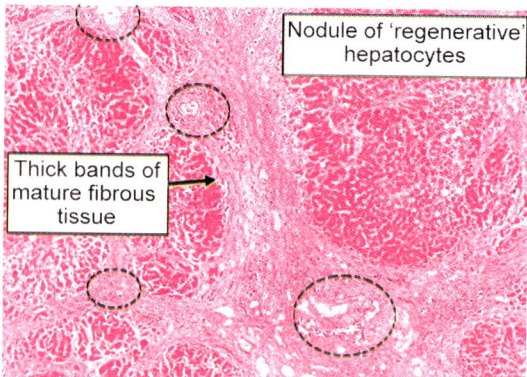

- Round-shaped parenchymal nodules of regenerating hepatocytes, i.e. regenerating nodules are seen. These nodules are small (micronodule).
- These regenerating nodules are separated by fibrous septa that bridge between portal tracts (dotted circles).
- This fibrosis occurs due to synthesis of collagen by perisinusoidal hepatic stellate cells (Ito cells).
- Within this fibrous tissue (collagenous tissue) scattered lymphocytes and proliferating bile ducts seen.

Fatty Liver

- Presence of numerous fat (lipid) vacuoles in the cytoplasm of hepatocytes around the nucleus.
- Some of these vacuoles are small and present around the nucleus (microvesicular)
- Most of these vacuoles are large, creating cleared spaces that displace the nucleus to the periphery of the cell (macrovesicular).

Note

i. Fat can be stained and demonstrated in fresh unfixed tissue by frozen section by fat stains like Sudan III, IV, Sudan black and Oil red O. (Remember in routine paraffin embedding technique fats are dissolved by organic solvents/alcohols used.)

ii. Alternatively, osmic acid can be used which acts both as fixed and fat stain.

iii. In fatty liver, **triglycerides** are deposited.

Chronic Cholecystitis

- There is chronic inflammatory cell infiltration into mucosa and other layers of gall bladder wall.
- The predominant chronic inflammatory cell is lymphocyte though plasma cells and macrophages (histiocytes) are also present.
- Focal erosion and ulceration are seen in the mucosal layer.
- Variable degree of fibrosis is noted in the subserosal and subepithelial layers.

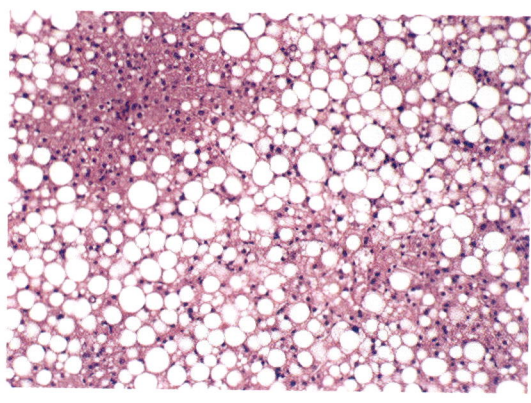

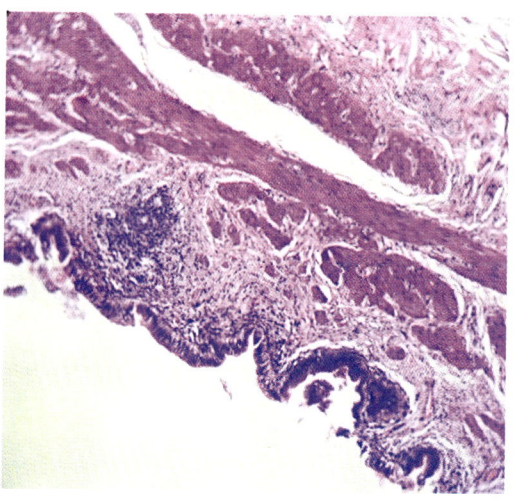

Low power view

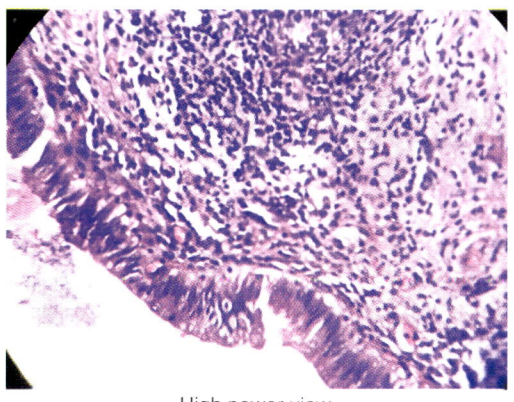
High power view

Fibroadenoma of Breast

- The tumour has a fibrous capsule (see low power view, right side).
- The tumour is biphasic which is composed of fibrous tissue element as stroma and epithelial component (ducts).
- Fibrous tissue comprises most of the tumour.

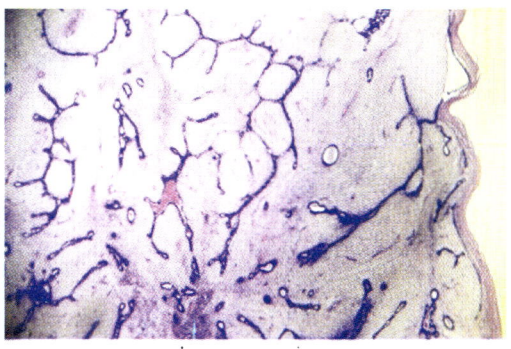
Low power view

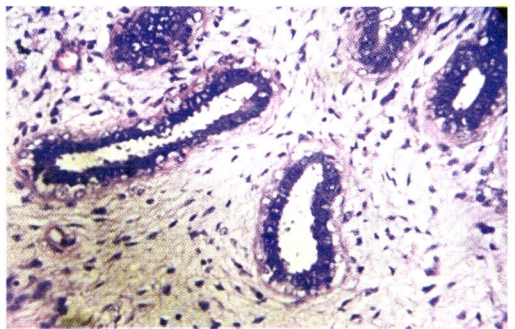
High power view

- Delicate loose fibrous stroma encloses the epithelial component consisting of gland-like or duct-like spaces lined by cuboidal or columnar cells.
- Myxoid changes are seen in the stroma.
- Two patterns are observed based on arrangements between fibrous tissue and ducts (epithelial element).
  - *Intracanalicular pattern:* In this pattern, the stroma compresses the ducts so that they are reduced to slit-like clefts lined by ductal epithelium or may appear as cards of epithelium or may appear as cards of epithelial elements surrounding masses of fibrous stroma.
  - *Pericanalicular pattern:* In this pattern, fibrous stroma encircles around patent or dilated ducts and the ducts are not compressed.
- Nuclear atypia or mitosis is not seen.

Duct Carcinoma of Breast (Moderately Differentiated)

- Malignant epithelial cells arranged in tubular glands, in cards, in sheets and in trabecular pattern.
- Malignant epithelial cells infiltrate the surrounding stroma.
- Tubule (malignant gland) formation is seen in 70% of the tumour area.
- Nuclear pleomorphism is moderate.
- Mitotic figures are increased.
- Focal necrosis and microcalcification are noted.

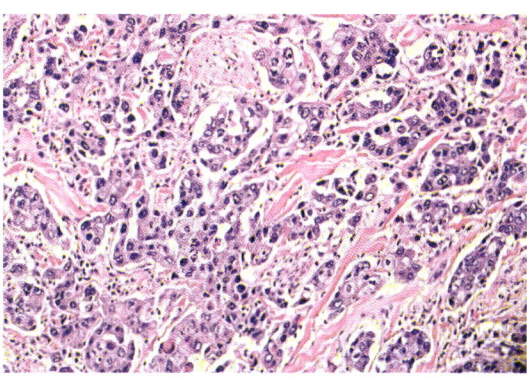

Seminoma of Testis (Classic Type)

- Sheets of uniform tumour cells divided into poorly demarcated lobules by delicate septa of fibrous tissue containing a moderate amount of lymphocytes.
- The tumour cell is large and round to polyhedral in shape.
- Tumour cell has distinct cell membrane or well defined cytoplasmic border.
- Tumour cell has abundant clear cytoplasm.
- Tumour cell has large, central nucleus with one or two prominent nucleoli.

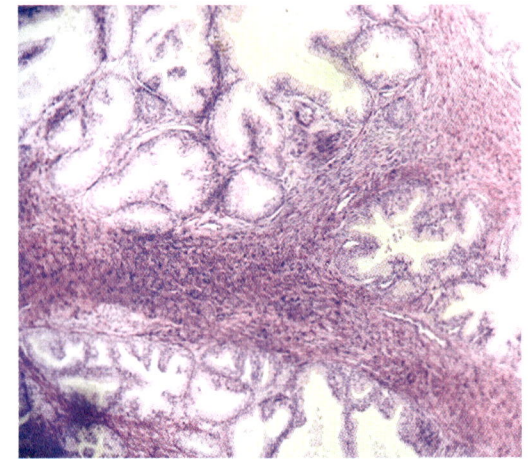

Low power view

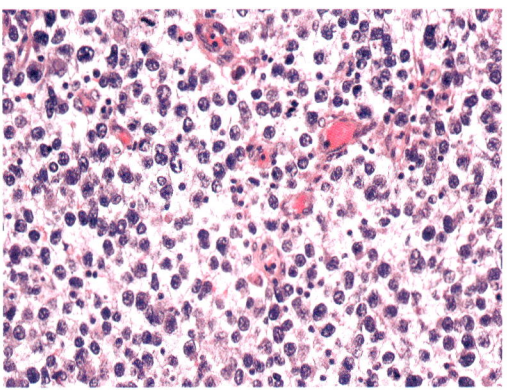

High power

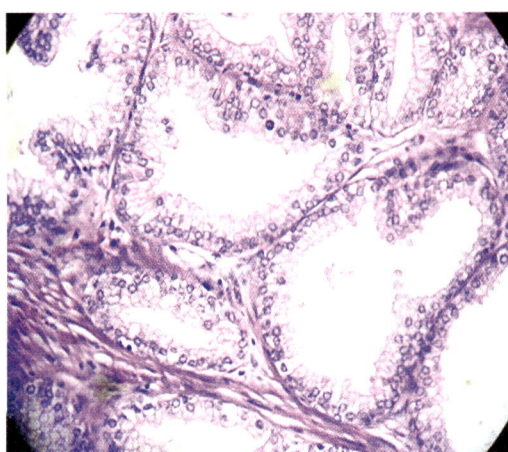

High power view

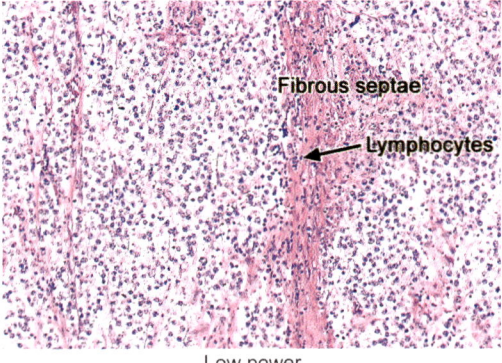

Low power

Benign Hyperplasia of Prostate (BHP) or Nodular Hyperplasia of Prostate

- There is hyperplasia of all three tissue elements in varying degree—glandular, fibrous and muscular tissue (smooth muscles).
- Glandular hyperplasia predominates and is recognized by exaggerated intra-acinar papillary infoldings with delicate fibrovascular cores.
- The glands are of benign type and the lining epithelium is two-layered: The inner tall columnar mucus-secreting with poorly-defined borders and the outer cuboidal or flattened epithelium with basal nuclei.
- Some of the glands contain eosinophilic material within lumen (corpora amylacea).
- Lymphocytotic infiltration and foci of lymphoid aggregates present.

Metastatic Deposit in Lymph Node (Metastatic Adenocarcinoma)

- There is effacement of normal lymph node architecture.
- Lymphoid tissue of normal lymph node is replaced by turmour cells.
- The tumour cells are arranged in diffuse sheets, in cords, in trabecular pattern and in glandular pattern.
- Tumour cells are also observed in sub-capsular sinuses.
- The tumour cells have high nucleocytoplasmic ratio (N:C ratio) anisonucleosis, and prominent nucleoli.

Tuberculosis of Lymph Node

- There is effacement of normal lymph node architecture.
- Many epithelioid granulomas are noted surrounded by lymphocytes and fibroblasts.
- Multinucleated giant cells of both Langhans and foreign body type are seen.
- Some of the granulomas contain eosinophilic, granular material (caseation necrosis) in the central area.

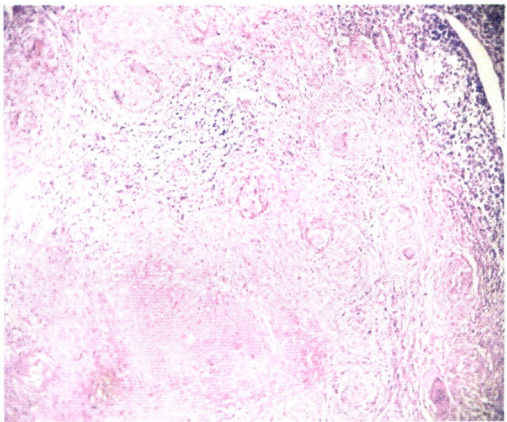

Low power view

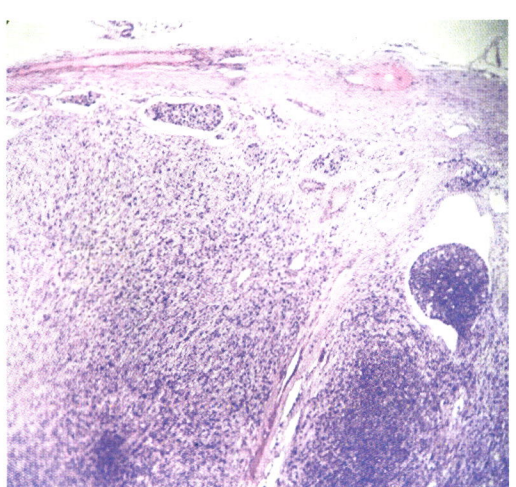

Low power view

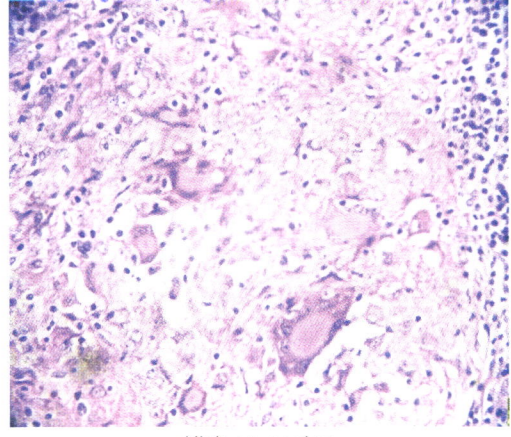

High power view

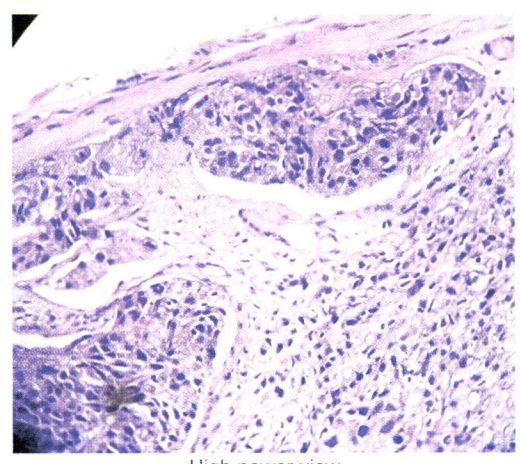

High power view

Colloid Goitre (Nodular Goitre)

- Numerous colloid filled follicles forming ill-defined nodules.

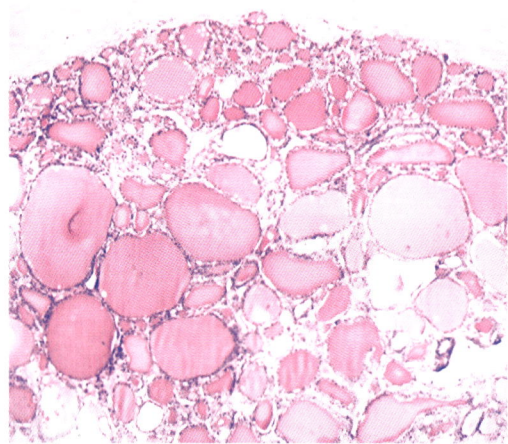

Low power view

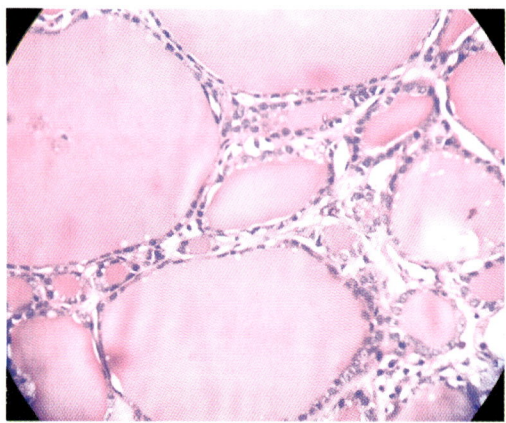

High power view

- The follicles are variably-sized (large distended to small) and are lined by flat to high epithelium.
- Few follicles show micropapillary formation.
- Colloid inside the follicles is abundant thin, pale and eosinophilic.
- Fibrous tissue deposition and scarring are noted surrounding the follicles and forming nodular appearance.
- Thin capsule is noted which separates it from surrounding compressed thyroid parenchyma.
- Foci of microcalcification are seen.

Papilloma/Squamous Papilloma of Skin (Skin Tag, Acrochondron, Fibroepithelial Polyp)

- Papillomatosis, hyperkeratosis and acanthosis of epidermis.
- It has a central fibrovascular core covered by benign squamous epithelium.
- Stroma is edematous and hypocellular.

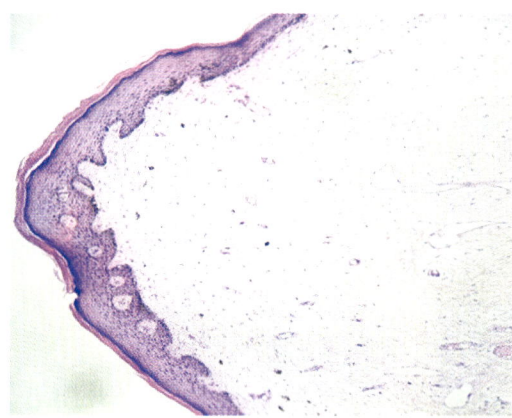

Low power view

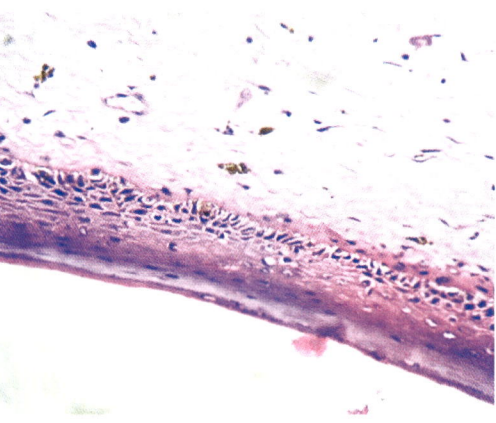

High power view

Melanoma/Malignant Melanoma of Skin

- The tumour has marked junctional activity at the dermoepidermal junction with pagetoid spread.
- From junctional layer tumour cells grow downwards into the dermis.
- Individual melanoma cells are considerably larger than normal melanocytes.

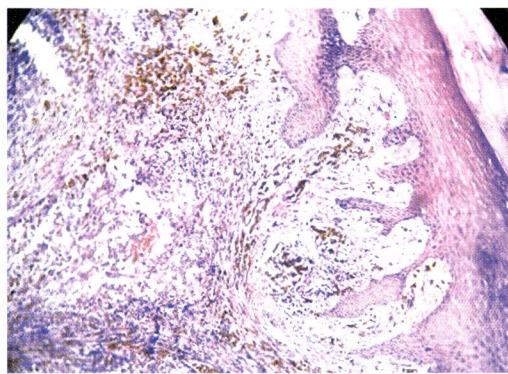
Low power view

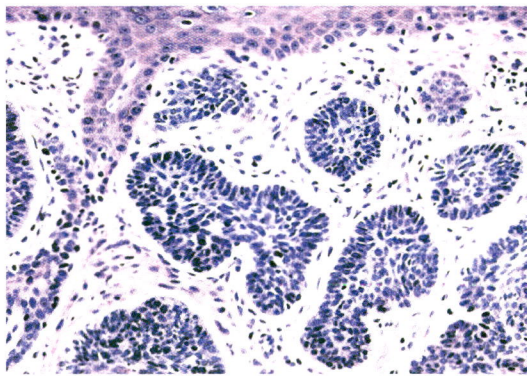

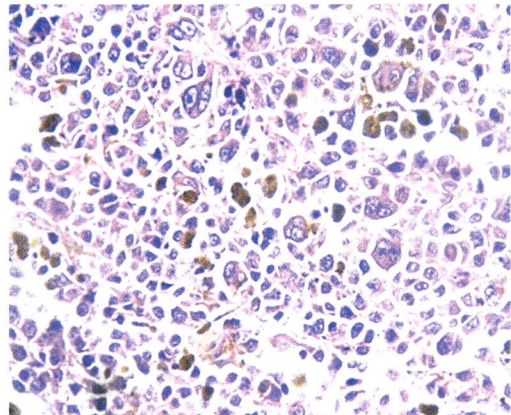
High power view

- Melanoma cells contain large nuclei with irregular nuclear contours.
- Chromatin is characteristically clumped at the periphery of the nuclear membrane.
- Nucleoli are red (eosinophilic) and prominent.
- Melanin pigments are seen both within tumour cells and in-between tumour cells.
- These brown-coloured melanin pigments in melanoma cells are fine granules unlike the benign nevi in which coarse irregular clumps of melanin are seen.
- Chronic inflammatory cell infiltrates (lymphocytes) are seen.

Basal Cell Carcinoma (Rodent Ulcer)

- There is proliferation of basaloid cells (resembling basal layer of epidermis).
- The tumour cells (basaloid cells) are arranged in lobules and clusters which are separated by stroma.
- The tumour cells have hyperchromatic nuclei and conspicuous small nucleoli.
- The cells at periphery of tumour cell clusters/islands tend to be arranged radially with their long axes in parallel alignment (**peripheral palisading**).
- The tumour cell islands are separated from dermal fibrous tissue (**cleft-like retraction artefact**).
- A few mitoses are found (sparse mitoses).
- The tumour cells have connection with the basal layer of epidermis.

Lipoma

- Lobules of mature adipose tissue (fatty tissue) cells separated by delicate fibrous septa.

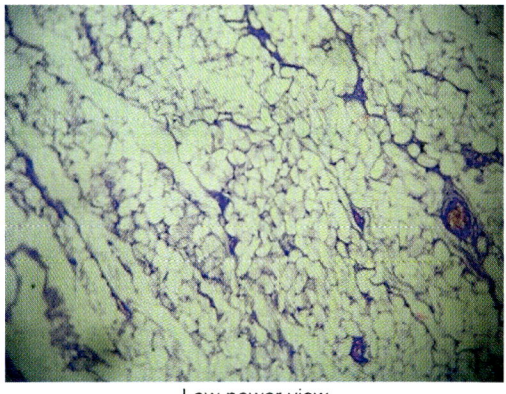
Low power view

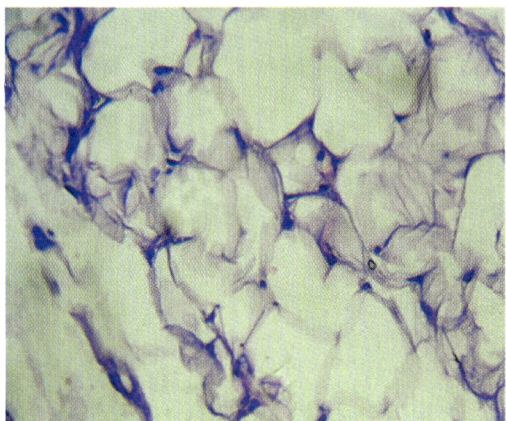

High power view

- The fat cells (adipocytes) have abundant clear lipid (fat) vacuoles and small nuclei pushed to periphery.
- Pleomorphism and nuclear atypia are absent.

Capillary Haemangioma

- Well defined lesion but lacking capsule.
- It is made up of aggregates of closely packed, thin-walled capillaries.
- These capillaries are lined by scant connective tissue stroma.

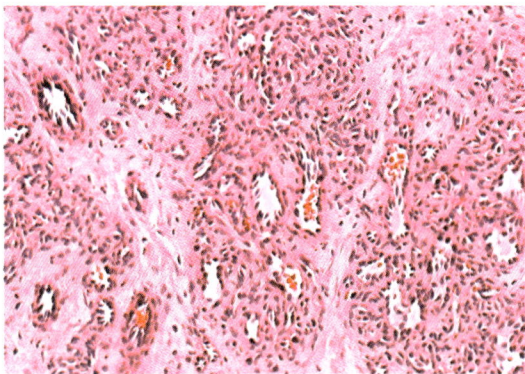

- Some of the capillaries are partially or completely thrombosed and organized.

Cavernous Haemangioma

- It is sharply defined but not encapsulated.
- It is composed of large, cavernous blood-filled vascular spaces, filled partially or completely with blood.
- The vascular spaces (dilated blood vessels) are lined by flattened endothelial cells.
- They are separated by scanty connective tissue stroma.

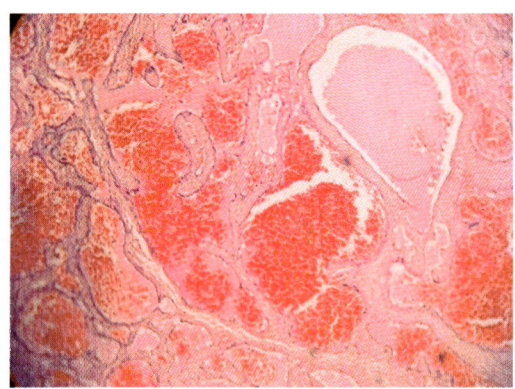

Low power view

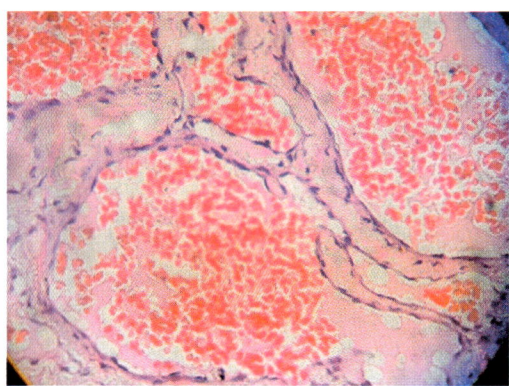

High power view

14

Cytology: Exfoliative and FNAC

Cytology is the branch of laboratory (diagnostic) medicine which deals with the study of individual cell and/or tissue fragments (microfragments) spreaded on glass slides and stained with stain(s).

Cytology came from Greek words; *kytos* means a hollow and *logia* means study of the cells. Robert Hooke (1635–1703) is considered sometimes father of cytology. But George Papanicolaou (1883–1962) was a Greek pioneer in cytopathology and inventor of Papanicolaou stain for 'Pap smear' in 1940.

Cytopathology: It is the study of cellular disease and the use of cellular changes for the diagnosis of disease.

EXFOLIATIVE CYTOLOGY

Definition

Exfoliative cytology is the microscopic examination of shed, desquamated cells from body surfaces or cells collected by rubbing, scrapping or brushing a lesional tissue surface or by tapping fluid.

The importance of exfoliative cytology in cancer diagnosis started as early as in 1950s. Exfoliative cytology means, cytological examination of stained smears of the cells, which have exfoliated, fallen or appeared in the body fluid from superficial surfaces of mother tissue.

Collection of Exfoliated Cells

1. **By collection of body fluids**
   - Mouth washings or gurgle: For oral cavity lesions
   - Gastric juice collection by Ryle's tube and syringe: For stomach lesions
   - Peritoneal fluid collection by tapping ascitic fluid or by paracentesis: For lesions of liver, ovaries and peritoneum itself.
   - Pleural fluid collection from pleural effusion: For lesions in the lung and pleura.
   - Urine collection in a clean tube: For urinary tract lesions.
   - Collection of sputum or bronchial washing: For lesions in the lungs or the bronchus
   - Joint effusions: For lesions in the joint cavity
   - Cerebrospinal fluid obtained by lumbar puncture: For lesions in the brain or the spinal cord.

2. **Scrape method:** Scraping is done by means of a wooden or spatula from the superficial surface of the tissue. Used for buccal, vaginal and cervical mucosa.

3. **Brushing:** Endoscopic brushing from lung, stomach, etc.

Exfoliated cells degenerate and distort rapidly. Hence, smears should be prepared and fixed in fixative immediately. For thick cellular discharges/fluids no centrifugation is required. But if it is watery, thin and hypocellular fluid, then it needs centrifugation. Centrifugation is done at 2000 r.p.m. for 5–15 minutes (depending on the size and concentration of suspending cells). Half of the smears are air-dried and other half of the smears are fixed.

Imprint Cytology

Procedure: On a clean glass slide, freshly cut surface of unfixed surgical specimen is gently pressed. Then these slides are fixed in 95% alcohol for a brief period and stained with Pap or H and E stain. Air-dried smears can be stained with MGG or LG stain.

Uses
1. In diagnosis of benign and malignant tumours
2. In determining parathyroid tissue, sentinel lymph nodes and adenomatous goitre
3. In certain CNS tumours like meningiomas and gliomas
4. Useful in determining the surgical resection margins.

Advantages
1. Useful as an intraoperative diagnosis and resection margin and lymph node status.
2. Immediate result.
3. Costly infrastructure or trained technician not required.
4. Tissue and cell architecture preserved.

Disadvantages
1. The depth of infiltration cannot be analysed.
2. Tumours with dense fibrous stroma cannot be interpreted.

Scrape or Brush Cytology

Another cytology technique is to gently scrape or brush some cells from the organ or tissue being tested. It may be from lesions or tumours from living persons or it may be from surgically resected unfixed specimens.

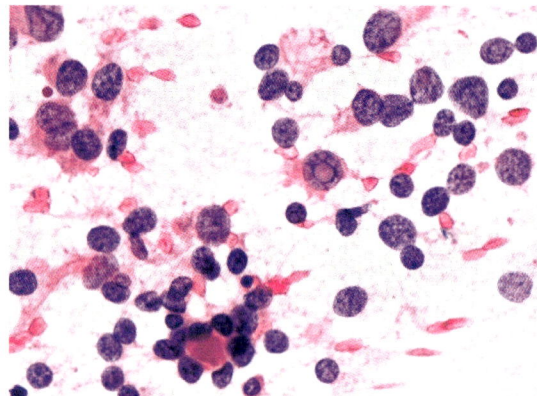

Fig. 14.1: Imprint cytology of papillary carcinoma of thyroid showing microfollicles, single cells, powdery chromatin of nuclei and intranuclear inclusions (Pap, 400X)

The best known cytology test which samples this way is the Pap test. A small spatula and/or brush is used to remove cells from the cervix for Pap test. Other areas which can be brushed or scraped include oesophagus, bronchi, mouth, bladder in living persons and ovarian tumours/other tumours as surgical specimens.

Procedure: Scrape can be done by gentle scraping over the tumour surface by scalpel blade/glass slide. For living persons, brush cytology is done by special endoscopic/bronchoscopic/cytoscopic instruments.

Barr Body (Sex Chromosome) Determination

The sex chromosome or Barr body (found in 1949 by Murray Barr and his co-workers) is the small basophilic body presents in the nuclei of epithelial cells (somatic cells) of females. The Barr body is located in the inner surface of nuclear membrane.

As per Lyon hypothesis, one of the two X chromosomes becomes inactivated in early embryonic life (blastocyst stage) and remains as **Barr body**.

There are two methods for Barr body determination:
1. Buccal smear method
2. Neutrophil method

Cytology: Exfoliative and FNAC

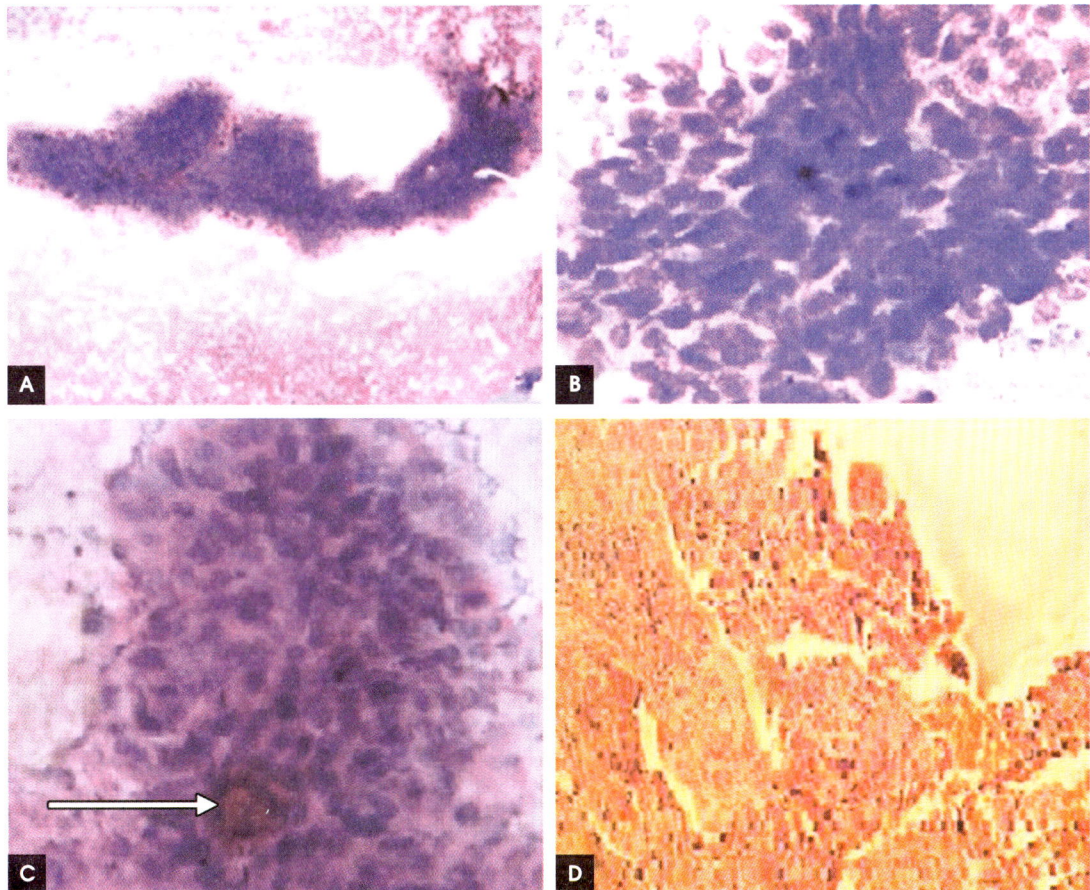

Fig. 14.2A to D: Scraping of conjunctival sqamous cell carcinoma. (A) Low power view (MGG stain); (b) High power view; (C) High power view showing a keratin pearl, marked by arrow (Pap stain); (d) Subsequent histopathological confirmation

Buccal Smear Method

Procedure: After brushing teeth, patient is asked to rinse mouth several times. The inner surface of cheek is scraped gently by edge of a tongue depressor or by Ayre's spatula. Smears are prepared on a clean glass slide and immediately fixed with alcohol. A control smear should be prepared from normal female and fixed with alcohol (95%).

Staining reagent: Orcein 0.1 gm

Glacial acetic acid solution (50% and warm): – 10 ml

Solution is cooled and mixture is prepared by shaking the bottle under running tap water. Then mixture is filtered several times to remove precipitate and debris.

Fixation of smears: Smears are fixed in at last 2 hours in acetic acid and alcohol mixture (1 ml acetic acid + 9 ml of ethyl alcohol/methanol).

Staining: Fixed smears are covered with Orcein stain for 10–20 minutes. Mount the smears with coverslips for oil immersion examination.

Microscopic examination: Only the chromatin components of nuclei are stained. Other parts of squamous epithelial cells are not stained. At least 200–300 epithelial cells of both patient and control are examined (well stained cells with chromosomes are selected for examination).

Result: Barr body (sex chromosome or X chromatin) is seen as a darkly staining small mass in contact with the nuclear membrane in the interphase nuclei of buccal cells. In normal females (XX), one Barr body is seen in 20–80% of the cells. The number of sex chromatin equals the number of X chromosome minus 1.

Interpretation: In XXX females, two Barr bodies are found. In Klinefelter syndrome (47, XXY), one Barr body is seen. In Turner syndrome (45, XO) no Barr body is seen.

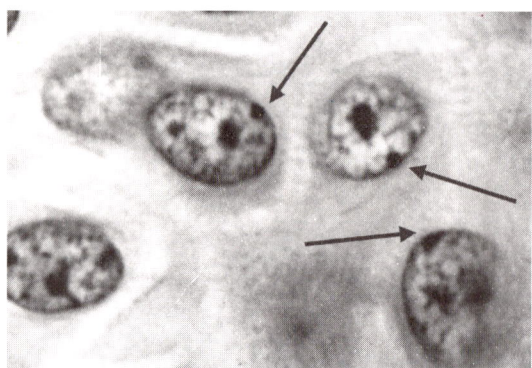

Fig. 14.3: Barr bodies (marked by arrows) in squamous epithelial cells of buccal smear (oil immersion, 1000X)

Neutrophil (Leukocyte) Method

In neutrophils, one X chromosome is visualized as a drumstick in normal females (46, XX) but not in males (46, XY). In Turner syndrome (45, XO) no drumstick is present while in Klinefelter syndrome (47, XXY), one drumstick is seen.

Procedure
1. Make few good peripheral blood smears.
2. Fix the blood smears in methanol and stain them in Giemsa stain well.
3. "Drumstick" is visualised as 1.5 micron round to oval nuclear material attached to nuclear lobes of the neutrophils by a stick like nuclear thread (stalk).
4. Examine 100–200 neutrophils (at least 100 neutrophils).

Result: In normal females, 5–7 drumsticks/100 neutrophils are visualised.

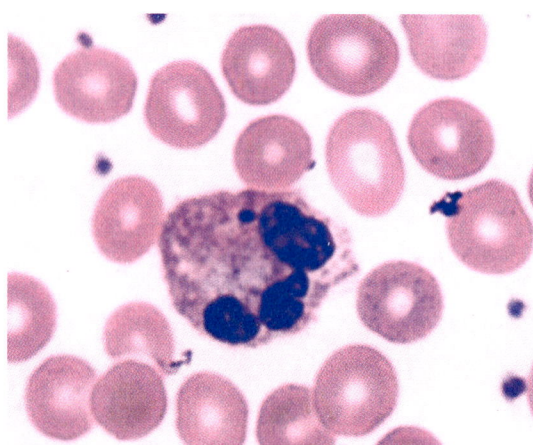

Fig. 14.4: Neutrophil of normal female (XX) showing Barr body (drumstick) in peripheral smear

Fixatives used in Cytology (Cytological Smears or Cytosmear)

In order to prevent distortion of cells as the smears dries up, the specimen must be immediately fixed in Koplin jar while the smears are moist. Common fixatives are:

1. Alcohol–ether fixative: Most commonly used. Absolute or 95% ethyl alcohol and ether in 1:1 volume (say 50 ml of alcohol and 50 ml of ether).
2. 95% ethyl alcohol
3. Carnoy's fluid: It permits good nuclear staining and has the advantage of lysing red blood cells. But it is more expensive and cannot be reused.
4. Spray fixatives: Fix it at least 30 minutes. But preferably >2 hours. But can be done up to 1 week.

Air-dried smears: MGG (May-Grünwald Giemsa) and LG (Leishman Giemsa) stains are used.

Wet-fixed smears: Papanicolaou (Pap) and/or H and E (haematoxylin and eosin) stains are used.

Fixation time: 30 minutes to 2 hours (minimum 15 minutes). Can also be fixed overnight.

Table 14.1: Papanicolaou stain (regressive method)

Staining steps	Papanicolaou laboratory	Memorial Solan Kettering
1. Fixation	95% ethyl alcohol	95% ethyl alcohol
2. Hydration	80%, 70%, 50% ethyl alcohol—six to eight dips each	70%, 50% ethyl alcohol—five dips each
	Distilled water—six to ten dips each	Distilled water—five dips
3. Nuclear stain (DNA specific)	Harris haematoxylin (without acetic acid)—6 minutes	Harris haematoxylin (without acetic acid)—6 minutes
4. Rinse	Distilled water (× 2, i.e. two times)	Distilled water—five dips
5. Removal of haematoxylin	0.25% HCl—six dips	0.5% HCl aqueous solution—three to five dips slowly
6. Rinse	Running tap water (lukewarm)—6 minutes	Running tap water—6 minutes
7. Dehydration	50%, 70%, 80%, 95% ethyl alcohol—six to eight dips each	50%, 70%, 80%, 95% ethyl alcohol—five dips each
8. Cytoplasmic stain	OG 6—1.5 minutes	OG 6—3 minutes
9. Rinse	95% ethyl alcohol (× 2)—rinse gently, do not keep in alcohol, otherwise cells will be discoloured	95% ethyl alcohol (× 2)—five dips each (slowly)
10. Cytoplasmic and nuclear stain (RNA specific)	EA 36 (EA 50 or EA 36)—1.5 minutes	EA 50—3 minutes (drain or paper towel)
11. Rinse	95% ethyl alcohol (× 3), rinse gently but thoroughly	95% ethyl alcohol (× 3)—five dips each (slowly)
12. Dehydration	Absolute ethyl alcohol (× 2)—six to eight dips each	Absolute ethyl alcohol (× 2)—five dips each (slowly)
13. Clearing	Absolute ethyl alcohol and xylene—six to eight dips each	Absolute ethyl alcohol and xylene (1:1)—five dips
	Xylene (× 4)—six to eight dips each	
14. Mounting	Permount (DPX or Canada balsam)	Histoclear (× 7)—five dips each (slowly)

Results in cervical smear
- Nucleus: Blue
- Superficial squamous cells (cytoplasm): Red to orange
- Intermediate and parabasal cells (cytoplasm): Green to greenish blue
- Red blood cells: Orange to orange—green

Cervical Smear
Currently three types of squamous cells are given importance during cervical smear reporting—superficial cells, intermediate cells and basal–parabasal cells.

1. **Superficial squamous cells:** These cells are mature, usually polygonal, squamous epithelial cells. The cytoplasm stains

either cyanophilic or eosinophilic and nucleus is pyknotic. All nuclei with diameter smaller than 6 µm (less than that of a RBC diameter for comparison) should be called pyknotic. Many superficial cells exhibit an eosinophilic, orange-yellow or orangeophilic cytoplasmic staining due to presence of intracellular cytoplasmic keratin.

2. **Intermediate squamous cells**: Intermediate cells are also mature but they contain nonpyknotic vesicular nuclei, i.e. nuclei which exhibit structural details.

The most important feature which distinguishes a superficial cell from an intermediate cell is the nuclear appearance. The former has pyknotic nuclei (compressed, smaller nuclei with condensed chromatin), whereas the intermediate cell has vesicular (large, oval or rounded non-pyknotic nuclei).

Intermediate cells usually have folding, and these cells are present in small or large clusters. However, most mature intermediate cells are flat and lie discretely. In presence of *Bacillus vaginalis* Döderlein, these cells tend to show cytolysis of the cytoplasm due to peptolytic but normal process (not seen in superficial cells).

3. **Basal–parabasal cells**: These cells are small, round or oval, immature (no keratin) squamous epithelial cells. These cells usually contain relatively large

Table 14.2: Different types of squamous epithelial cells seen in cervical/vaginal Pap (Papanicolaou) smear

Cell type	Size	Nuclei	Cytoplasm	Morphology
1. Superficial	30–60 µm	<6 µm, clear and pyknotic	Polyhedral, either cyanophilic or eosinophilic. Keratinising cells have keratohyaline granules in cytoplasm and are orange-yellow or orangeophilic. No cytoplasmic fold	Pyknotic nuclei
2. Intermediate	20–40 µm	6–9 µm vesicular	Polyhedral or elongated, cyanophilic. Cytoplasmic folds	Cytoplasmic folds; Vesicular nonpyknotic nuclei
3. Parabasal	15–25 µm	6–12 µm vesicular	Oval to round cells, well defined cytoplasmic border. Basophilic with occasional small vacuoles	Large, vesicular nuclei
4. Basal	14–20 µm	8–12 µm hyperchromatic, may have small nucleoli	Oval to round, deeply basophilic	Large, hyperchromatic nuclei

nuclei. The staining pattern is cyanophilic or indistinct.

Ayre's Spatula

Ayre spatula is a device used to collect Pap smear. It is a wooden spatula with U-shaped openings on one side and a flat surface on another. The broad end is for vaginal sample collection, whereas narrow end is used for cervical sample collection. It is rotated 360° (clockwise or anticlockwise) to obtain exfoliated cells from all quadrants.

Recent studies have shown that long-tipped spatulas **(Aylesbury device)** cervical brush or a **cytobrush** along with an extended tip spatula are better than Ayre's spatula in collecting endocervical cells.

However, Ayre's spatula is still popular in developing (less-income) countries. Ayre's spatula is introduced into the cervix after visualizing the external os using a vaginal speculum. The cervical cells are collected by rotating (360°) the spatula firmly over the ectocervix and quickly transferring the cells onto slides or jar for wet fixation (alcohol or ether-alcohol mixture).

Another device which is popular for cervical sample collection is **Szalay cytospatula** with extended tip. The advantage of this spatula is, it can collect endocervical cells as it has extended tip (longer) compared to Ayre's spatula. Ready to use Pap smear kit (CMB-2020) is also available in market which contains microscope slides, wooden spatula, cervical cytobrush and plastic Maller tray. The UK screening programmes changed their cervical screening method from the **Pap (Papanicolaou) test** to liquid-based cytology (LBC) in 2008.

New Technologies in Cervical Smear

Over the years, several methods have been proposed to improve the cytological specimens. Neubauer et al in 1981 described a **sedimentation velocity separation method**; and Naslund proposed a **pulse wash method**. Then Steven et al suggested **chemical depolymerization of cervical mucin** to help produce monolayers.

But in practice, new technology which is most useful is **liquid-based cytology (LBC)**. But automated scanning devices and computer assisted microscopy are also helpful.

Liquid-based cytology: Liquid-based cytology (LBC) technique involves rinsing all the materials collected on the sampling device into a preservative fluid, creating a cell suspension. This specimen in fluid is sent to laboratory rather than a glass slide presmeared with cellular material. In the laboratory, the cell suspension can be processed to remove excess blood and inflammatory cells and to get only representative epithelial (cervical) cells. The technique allows more accurate result.

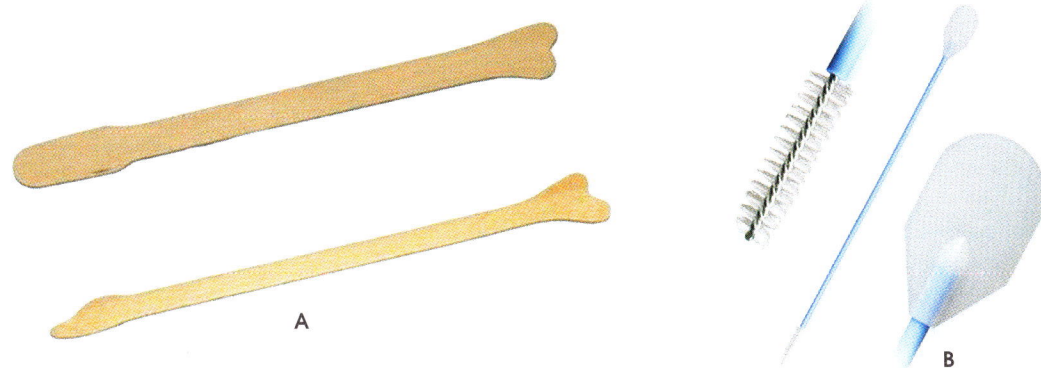

Fig. 14.5A and B: (A) Ayre's spatula (normal and the other with extended tip); (B) Cytobrush with handle

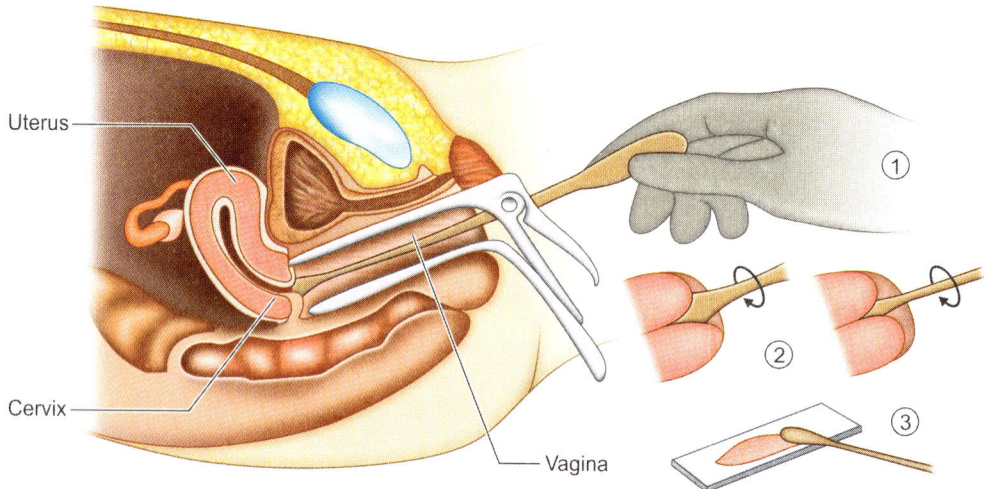

Fig. 14.6: Collection of cervical Pap smear by using Ayre's spatula (different steps, 1, 2 and 3)

Automated scanning devices: Screening of cervical smears manually is a very laborious and monotonous method. Due to tiredness and monotony of job, rare abnormal cells may be overlooked. Automated primary screening devices have been tried over the years. Two systems were eventually approved by the FDA in USA in 1990s. One is AutoPap 300 (Neopath, Seatle, USA) and another is PAPNET (Neuromedical Systems Inc., New York, USA).

Computer assisted microscopy: In the 1990s, there was a practice to attach microscope with the computer which would support cytotechnologists with conventional microscopy. One of the most successful was **Pathfinder**, manufactured by **Compucyte**. The system connected sensors to the microscope stage to a computer and monitor display. Zeiss microscopes produced a similar system called the Highly Optimized Microscope Environment (HOME). Another company Acumed had a system called ACcell.

Unfortunately those systems were very costly and commercially unsuccessful. Most are no longer being developed nowadays.

SurePath and **ThinPrep 2000 system** are two such systems currently approved by the US Food and Drug Administration (FDA) for cervicovaginal testing.

1. **SurePath method:** In the SurePath method, the sample is vortexed, stained, layered onto a density gradient and is centrifuged. Instruments required are a computer-controlled robotic pipette and a centrifuge. The cells form a **circle of 12.5 mm in diameter.**

2. **ThinPrep method:** This method requires an instrument and special polycarbonate filters. After the instrument immerses the filter into the vial, the filter is rotated to homogenize the sample. Cells are collected on the surface of the filter when a vacuum is applied. The filter is then pressed against a glass slide to transfer the processed cells into a **20 mm diameter circle.**

Both methods (SurePath and ThinPrep) result in a well-preserved approximate monolayer of cells, with a background devoid of blood, mucus or parasites. But current high cost of these patented, commercial systems required of trained cytotechnologists and pathologists to interpret the ThinPrep slides, leads to search for alternative, less costly newer methods.

One such method is **SpinThin method**, developed by Khalbuss et al in 2000. It uses a modified electric toothbrush to release the cells into suspension from the collecting device. The cell are then spun directly onto a (20 × 10 mm) area of glass slide using a Cytospin II centrifuge with mega-funnel. Results correlate well with conventional smears and follow-up histology.

Another method has been developed by Johnson et al in 2000. It places the cervical collection device into 15 ml of **CytoRich red** (Tripath Imaging Inc.), a proprietary formula of buffering agents, emulsifiers, formaldehyde and alcohol. After it comes to laboratory, cell suspensions are vortexed, poured through tulle (oridal veil fabric) and centrifuged. After that, the supernatant is discarded and the sediment is vortexed. A drop of sediment is placed into an 8 ml of Hettich cytocentrifuge chamber which is filled with 2 ml of **CytoRich yellow** (Tripath Imaging Inc.), a fixative that prevents dehydration and collapse of three-dimensional structures when slides are air-dried and then spun onto adhesive-coated slides.

Abnormal Cells in Cervical Smear

Nuclear characteristics are the main determinants for the grading of an epithelial abnormality although cytoplasmic features may provide additional inflammation.

Nuclear atypia should be classified as mild, moderate and severe. Cytoplasmic changes should be classified according to quantity, staining pattern/quality, density and shape.

Papanicolaou introduced the term dyskaryosis in cervical smear. He described dyskaryotic cells as follow, "The nuclei show distinct abnormal features such as enlargement, hyperchromasia, anisokaryosis, bi- or multinucleation, etc."

Mild dysplasia/cervical intraepithelial neoplasia (CIN) grade 1 or low grade SIL (squamous intraepithelial lesion): These cells have plentiful clear, translucent cytoplasm with well-defined angular borders. Cells resemble superficial and intermediate type squamous cells and a slightly enlarged nucleus, occupying less than one-third of the total area of the cell. Nuclear chromatin is evenly distributed, finely granular and slightly hyperchromatic. Cells are distributed singly.

Moderate dysplasia (CIN grade II, high grade SIL): The size of abnormal cells varies. Abnormal cells of the superficial squamous cell type as well as smaller cells of intermediate and parabasal cells are usually found. Cytoplasm is cyanophilic but a few cells may show eosinophilia. Nuclei are enlarged and round to oval, sometimes irregular in shape. The nucleus usually occupies less than half of total area of the cell. Nuclear chromatin is evenly distributed and slightly to moderately hyperchromatic. Nucleoli are either absent or inconspicuous. Cells are distributed singly and in small loose aggregates.

Severe dysplasia (CIN grade III, high grade SIL): These abnormal cells look like parabasal cells. Cytoplasm is usually sparse and represents a small rim around the nucleus. Cells are distributed singly as well as in aggregates. The nucleus usually occupies more than two-thirds of the total area of the cell. Nuclei have hyperchromatic, irregularly distributed, coarsely granular chromatin. Nucleoli are usually seen in actively proliferating lesion which is eosinophilic. But may be obscured by dense hyperchromatic chromatin.

Carcinoma *in situ*

Cells occur singly but predominantly in syncytial (tight) aggregates. In a syncytial group, cells are arranged irregularly and have indistinct cell borders and overlapping nuclei. The latter two features are absent in dysplastic cells. The neoplastic cells are relatively small. Nuclei vary in size and shape. Nuclear chromatin is hyperchromatic, irregularly distributed and coarsely

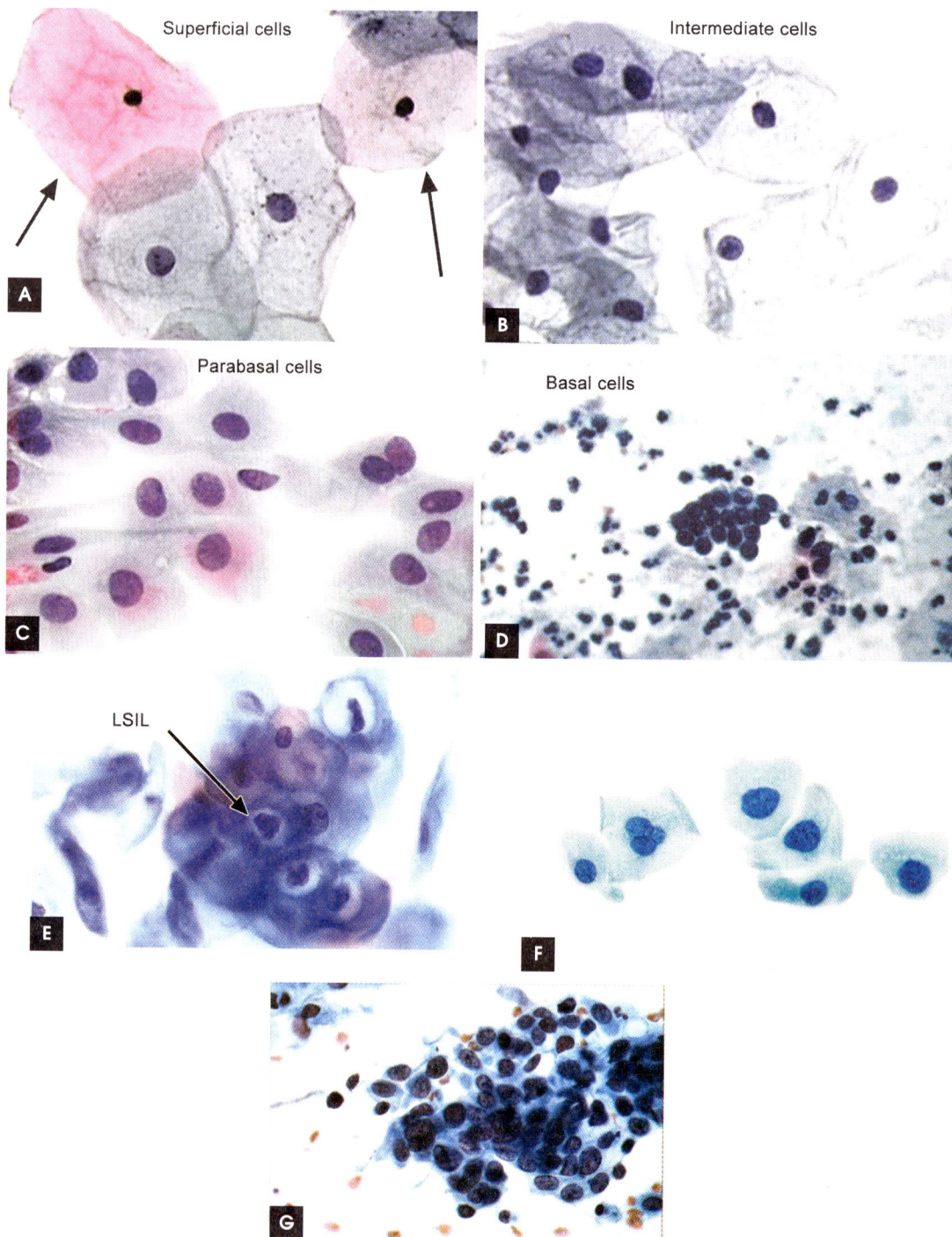

Fig. 14.7: Cervical Pap smear. A to D: Normal smear showing superficial, intermediate, parabasal and basal cells; (E) Mild dysplasia/cervical intraepithelial neoplasia (CIN) grade I or low grade SIL (squamous intra-epithelial lesion); (F) Moderate dysplasia (CIN grade II, high grade SIL); (G) Serve dysplasia (CIN grade III, high grade SIL)

granular. Nuclear grooves may be seen occasionally. It is rare to find eosinophilic nucleoli. Macronucleoli which are found in invasive carcinomas, are very rarely seen in *in situ* carcinomas.

Invasive squamous cell carcinoma: This may be of two types—nonkeratinizing and keratinizing.

Nonkeratinizing squamous cell carcinoma: High power view (Pap smear) tadpole cell

Syncytial aggregates of tumour cells with indistinct cell border and moderate amount of cytoplasm. Nuclei are round to oval or irregularly shaped. Nuclear chromatin is moderately hyperchromatic, coarsely granular, and irregularly distributed. Nucleoli are conspicuous. "Tadpole" like malignant squamous epithelial cell in the background.

Keratinizing squamous cell carcinoma: Tumour cells frequently appear singly. Elongated caudate, bizarre cells or binucleated cells are seen. Cells have relatively large amount of cytoplasm. Cytoplasmic orangeophilia is characteristic of keratinizing cancer. Nuclei may be round to oval but most of the times elongated or irregular. Nuclear chromatin is hyperchromatic and coarsely granular. Occasionally "keratin pearl" may be observed.

Adenocarcinoma (Endocervical or Endometrial)

Sometimes adenocarcinoma arising from endocervix or from endometrium may also be diagnosed by cervical smear.

These malignant cells are arranged in sheets, in papillary pattern and in glandular pattern. Discretely arranged cells are also found. The cells have high nucleocytoplasmic ratio and oval to round nuclei. The nuclear chromatin is vesicular. Prominent nucleoli and macronucleoli are also seen.

Cytology of Body Fluids (Effusions)

The intrathoracic and intraperitoneal organs are covered by a single layer of mesothelial cells (flattened cuboidal epithelium), which is continuous with the lining of the thoracic

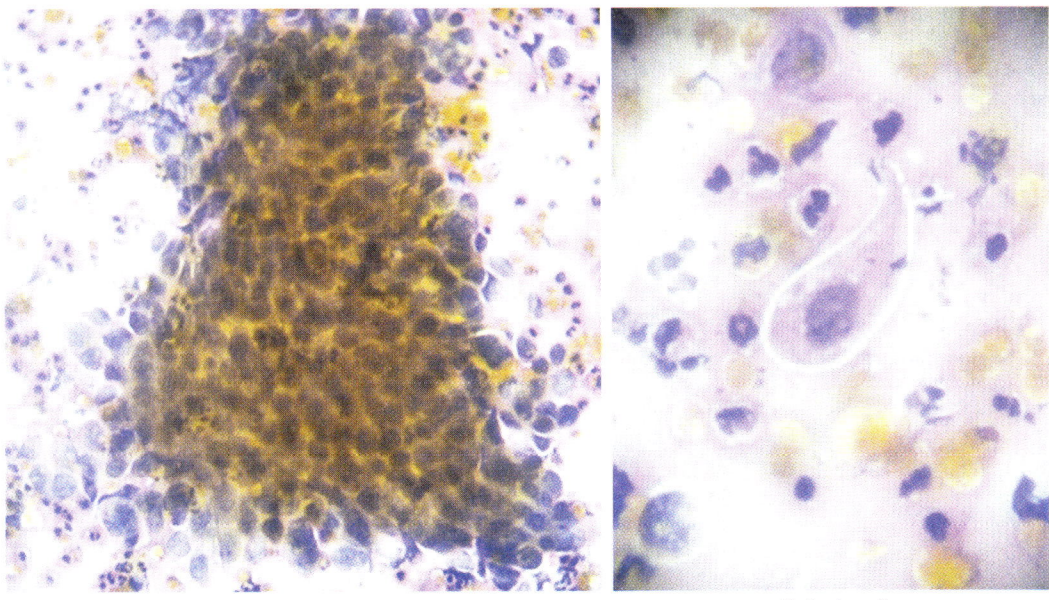

High power view (Pap smear) Tadpole cell

Fig. 14.8: Non-keratinising squamous cell carcinoma

and peritoneal cavities. The potential space between the two layers of epithelium (visceral and parietal) contains a small amount (few ml) of lubricating fluid, known as serous fluid.

An accumulation of fluid, called an effusion, results from an imbalance of fluid production and reabsorption. This fluid accumulation in the pleural, pericardial, and peritoneal cavities is known as serous effusion. These effusions may be infectious effusions, noninfectious inflammatory effusions and malignant effusions.

Infectious effusions: It is due to direct effects of infective organism or as by-product of inflammation. Varying types of inflammatory cells may be present. Cultures and/or Gram and AFB stains may be useful to identify an organism.

Noninfectious inflammatory effusions: This is due to conditions or reaction to a stimulus like autoimmune conditions (rheumatoid arthritis or SLE) or reactive conditions (tissue necrosis, radiation therapy).

Malignant effusions: It is due to a primary tumour of mesothelium (mesothelioma) or a metastatic tumour (most commonly metastatic adenocarcinoma). The fluid may be cloudy, bloody or partially clotted.

The fluid is aspirated from body cavities and is centrifuged. The deposit is smeared on glass slides and stained with Papanicolaou's stain and examined microscopically. Sometimes, MGG and H and E stains are also used.

Normal Cells in Fluid Cytology

- Lymphocytes
- Mesothelial cells
- Histiocytes/monocytes
- Occasional neutrophils or eosinophils
- Reactive mesothelial cells

Mesothelial cells: Bland cells forming a monolayer covering serous surfaces of body cavities. It is 20–40 µm in diameter.

Nuclei
- Single or binucleated
- Centrally located but can be eccentric
- Round to oval with well defined, smooth nuclear borders
- Fine chromatin
- Inconspicuous nucleoli

Cytoplasm
- Dense centre with pale periphery
- Lacy "skirt" cell borders
- Blunt cytoplasmic process due to degeneration

The mesothelial cells appear in smears as broad and flat sheets. There is gap between cells called **'window'**.

Histiocytes: They have smaller nuclei than mesothelial cells and nuclei are vesicular often with nuclear indentation. The cytoplasm is abundant and may be vacuolated or granular.

Abnormal findings
- Lymphocytes (>50%)
- Neutrophils (>50%)
- Eosinophils (>10%)
- Presence of microorganisms, LE cells, sickle cells, Charcot-Leyden crystals, psammoma bodies, collagen balls.

Reactive mesothelial cells: Varying cell size and increased number of mesothelial cells. Central or paracentral nuclei are enlarged. Coarse chromatins which are evenly distributed. Binucleation or multinucleation may be seen. Nuclear membrane is regular.

Mesothelioma: One cell population of malignant mesothelial cells. Larger clusters with irregular, knobby flower-like borders. Dense endoplasm with delicate, lacy ectoplasm. Central enlarged nucleus with macronucleoli and irregular borders. Abnormal mitotic figures may be seen.

Metastatic adenocarcinoma: Most adenocarcinoma cells in serous fluids originate in neoplasms of the breast, lung or ovary. The cells may show the classic feature of adeno-

Table 14.3: Suggested immunocytochemistry (ICC) markers

	Reactive mesothelial cells	Mesothelioma
• Calretinin	+	+
• CK 5/6	+	+
• p53	–	+
• Desmin	+	–
• EMA	–	+

Table 14.4: Tumours causing malignant effusions

Primary	Secondary/metastatic
• Malignant mesothelioma • Effusion lymphoma	• Metastatic adenocarcinoma • Metastatic squamous cell carcinoma • Neuroendocrine tumours • Lymphoma/leukaemia • Melanoma • Sarcoma • Other cancers/neoplasm

vacuolated cytoplasm. However, there may be great variation in adenocarcinoma cells in effusions.

Differences between adenocarcinoma and mesothelioma: Adenocarcinoma cells may be single or may form clusters composed of only few cells or large papillary fragments or cell balls/spheroids. Such cell balls may also be seen in mesothelioma. But the mesothelial cells have irregular knobby border and they have windows (intercellular gaps). The N–C ratio is more in adenocarcinoma cells and nuclei are more vesicular. The nuclear outline of adenocarcinoma cells are more angulated than mesothelioma which are smoothly round or oval. Prominent nucleoli though seen in both the cases, but macronucleoli are seen in adenocarcinoma.

Immunocytochemistry: Adenocarcinoma cells express GLUT 1, CA 19–9, CEA (carcinoembryonic antigen) which is negative in mesothelioma cells. On the other hand, calretinin, WT-1, D2-40 are positive in mesothelial cells but negative for adenocarcinoma cells. Acid mucopolysaccharide is also positive in mesothelial cells.

Electron microscopy: Adenocarcinoma cells are characterized by short, plump microvilli

carcinoma: A tendency to form smoothly contoured cohesive group composed of large cells with eccentric, malignant-appearing nuclei, prominent nucleoli and

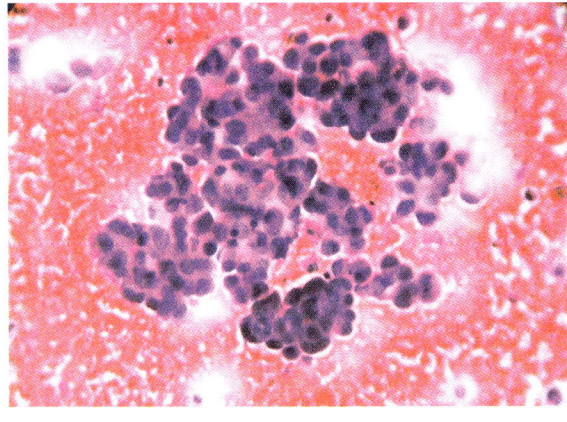 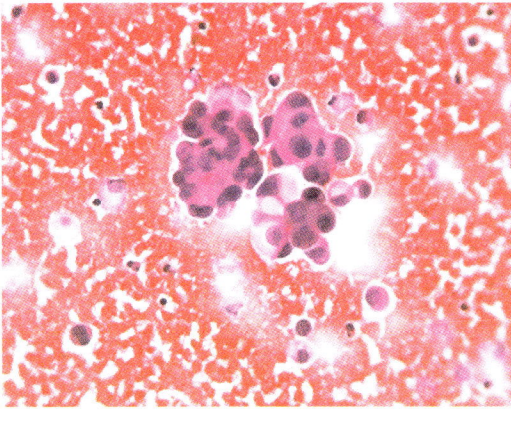

A   B

Fig. 14.9A and B: Adenocarcinoma in peritoneal fluid cytology. (A) Malignant cells arranged in papillary configuration (MGG, 400X); (B) Malignant cells arranged in acinar/pseudoglandular pattern. Also some tumour cells showing cytoplasmic mucin vacuoles (Pap, 400X)

in contrast to mesothelial cells which have numerous, long and slender microvilli.

FINE NEEDLE ASPIRATION CYTOLOGY (FNAC)

Equipment

i. *Needles fitted in syringes:* Standard disposable 20–23 gauge needles are commonly used. For highly vascular (thyroid) and/or highly cellular tissue (lymph node) 24–25 gauge needle are preferred. For very hard tissue (bone) 20 gauge needle is recommended.

ii. *Syringes:* Good quality disposable plastic syringes, 5–20 ml of strong rigid material with a good negative pressure is used. Routinely 10 ml syringe is used. For fibrotic and hypocellular lesion 20 ml syringe may be used. For highly vascular and/or cellular lesion 5 ml syringe may be used.

iii. *Syringe holder:* Made of stainless steel, commercially available (Cameco syringe pistol).

iv. *Glass slides:* Thoroughly cleaned, dry and grease free.

v. *Fixative:* For wet fixation of smears, 70–90% ethanol in Coplin jars. Alternatively, Carnoy's fixative is used.

vi. *Stains:* For wet fixed smears Papanicolaou (Pap) stain and/or H and E stain are used. For air-dried smear MGG (May Grunwald-Giemsa) or LG (Leishman-Giemsa) stain is used.

FNAC Technique

The syringe (with needle) is fitted with a syringe holder which permits a single hand operation during aspiration. Then follow these steps:

1. Skin overlying the lesion is properly cleaned with antiseptic solution.
2. Immobilize the site to aspirated (breast, thyroid, lymph node, soft tissue, etc.) with thumb and index finger of left hand. Then insert the needle to the target area/lesion while holding the syringe holder by right hand.
3. Once the needle is in the mass, retract the piston of syringe holder to create a negative pressure in the syringe.
4. Move the needle back and forth several times (usually 3–4, up to 6 passes) in various directions for a few seconds.
5. Withdraw the needle slowly while maintaining a negative pressure until the subcutaneous tissue is reached. Then the piston of the syringe is released to equalize the pressure.
6. Withdraw the needle completely and disconnect from the syringe.
7. Fill the syringe with air and reconnect to the needle.
8. The content of the needle is expressed on glass slides and smears are prepared (air dried and wet fixed).

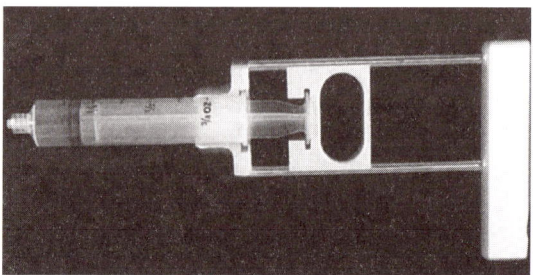

Fig. 14.10: Syringe fitted in a syringe holder before doing FNAC

Indications of FNAC

- In the rapid diagnosis of neoplastic conditions especially cancers and metastasis.
- In the diagnosis of inflammatory, infectious and degenerative conditions.
- Also, useful in the diagnosis and monitoring of graft rejections in transplantation surgery.

MGG Stain

Reagents: (i) May-Grunwalds's stain, (ii) Giemsa stain, (iii) methanol, (iv) phosphate buffer (pH 6.8), (v) conical flask (200–250 ml).

Cytology: Exfoliative and FNAC

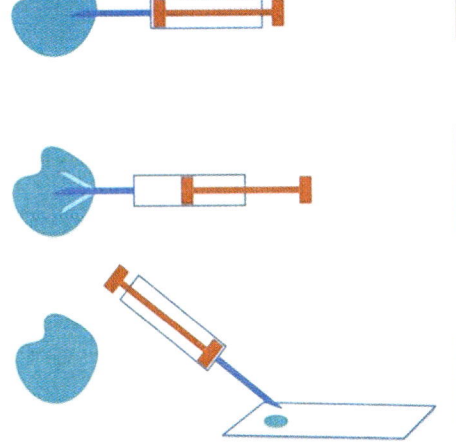

Fig. 14.11: Steps in FNAC

The lesion is pierced with a thin gauge (21–25) needle

The plunger is withdrawn. Without exiting the lesion and without releasing the plunger, the needle is moved in an out in different directions

The needle is withdrawn and the material aspirated smeared onto a slide, stained and examined

Table 14.5: Advantages and disadvantages of FNAC

Advantages	Disadvantages
• The diagnosis is rapid (few minutes) compared to conventional histological (biopsy) diagnosis	• Rare chances of needle tract seedling and possibility of cancer cells being disseminated along the needle tract
• This procedure is easy and cost effective	• Preoperative FNA (fine needle aspirate) may cause changes in the tissue which may cause subsequent histological diagnosis difficult
• Modern imaging techniques like USG and CT scan allowed guided FNAC for deep-seated lesions, lung, mediastinum, abdominal, retroperitoneal and pelvic organs. Surgical biopsy may not be easily accessible	• Changes like haematoma, infarction, capsular pseudoinvasion, and pseudomalignant reparative reactions may occur
• No need of hospital stays and paying hefty bills	• Complications like pneumothorax, air emboli and internal bleeding may occur rarely
• Less traumatic than usual knife biopsy.	
• The samples can be used for microbiological and biochemical analysis in addition to cytological preparations	

Preparation of May-Grunwald stain: 0.3 gm of powdered dye and 100 ml of methanol is mixed in a conical flask. The mixture is warmed to 50° C. The flask is allowed to cool at room temperature and mixture is shaken several times during the day. After standing for 24 hours, the solution is filtered.

Staining procedure
- Air-dried smears are fixed in methanol in a Coplin jar for 5 minutes.
- Stain with diluted May-Grunwald stain (1:1 dilution with phosphate buffer) for 5 minutes.
- Stain with diluted Giemsa stain (1:9 dilutions with buffer) for 15–20 minutes.

Table 14.6: Comparison between wet-fixed (Pap) and air-dried (MGG) smears

	Wet-fixed (Pap stain) smear	Air-dried smear (MGG stain)
• Cell and nuclear size	Comparable to tissue fragments	Size more than tissue
• Cytoplasmic detail	Poorly demonstrated	Well demonstrated
• Nuclear detail	Excellently demonstrated	Different and not well demonstrated
• Nucleoli	Well demonstrated	Not demonstrated always
• Stromal components	Poorly demonstrated	Well demonstrated and differently stained often
• The 'wet' smear	Good fixation	Artefacts common
• The 'dry' smear	Drying artefacts seen	Good fixation

- Wash with phosphate buffer (pH 6.8).
- Dried in air
- Mount in DPX or Canada balsam.

Some Common FNAC Findings (Microscopic)

Reactive Hyperplasia of Lymph Node

- Smears show high cellular yield (hypercellular)
- A mixed population of lymphoid cells with a predominance of small mature lymphocytes.
- Centrocytes, centroblasts and immunoblast are present but in "logical" proportions.
- The ratio of small lymphocytes and other large cells are approximately 80:20.
- Plasma cells are increased.
- Tingible body macrophages (scattered histiocytes with intracytoplasmic nuclear debris) are seen.
- Background reveals lymphoid globules or lymphoglandular bodies (pale-blue rounded cytoplasmic fragments up to 8 µm (in Giemsa/MGG stain).

Granulomatous Lymphadenitis

- Clusters of cohesive epithelioid histiocytes surrounded by lymphocytes.

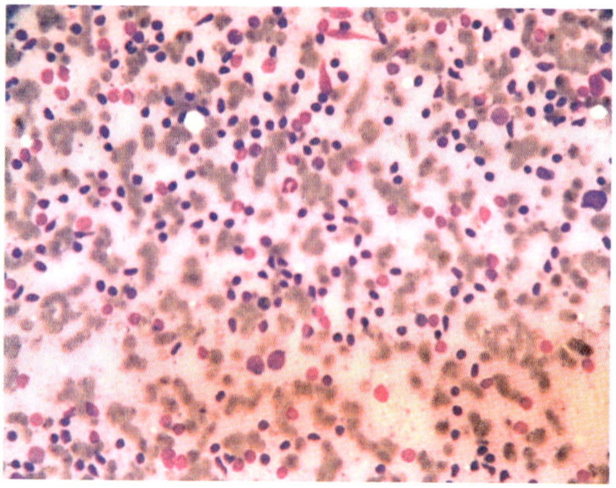

Fig. 14.12: Reactive hyperplasia of lymph node (MGG, 100X)

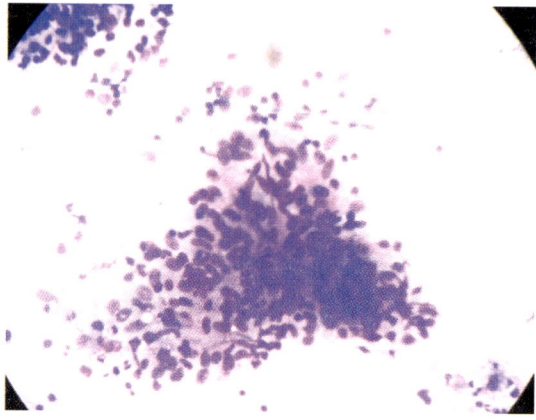

Fig. 14.13: Low power view of granulomatous lymphadenitis (MGG stain)

- These epithelioid histiocytes (cells) have elongated nuclei like the sole of a shoe. The nuclear chromatin is finely granular and pale with a small nucleolus. The cytoplasm is pale and lacks distinct cell border.
- Multinucleated giant cells of both Langhans and foreign body types are found with typical arrangement of nuclei.
- Caseation (necrosis) may or may not be present.
- Background reveals mixed population of lymphoid cells of lymph node.

Nodular Colloid Goitre

- Abundant colloid material (usually thin colloid).
- Follicular epithelial cells (benign type) present in monolayered sheets and in cohesive groups.
- Many bare nuclei of benign follicular epithelial cells (lymphocyte like) in a background of thin colloid.
- Cyst macrophages in the background when there is colloid goitre with cystic degeneration.

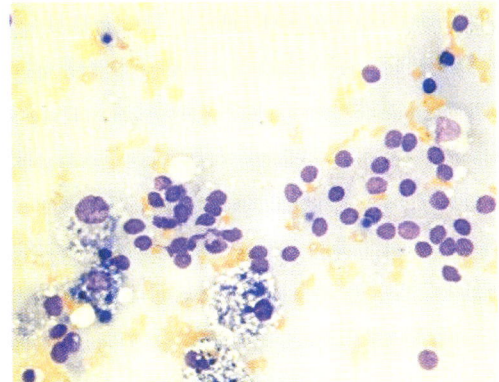

Fig. 14.14: High power view of nodular colloid goitre with cystic degeneration (MGG stain)

Papillary Carcinoma of Thyroid

- Highly cellular smear.
- The epithelial cells are arranged in papillary, in monolayered sheets or dispersely.
- Finger-like papillae have anatomical borders, nuclear crowding and overlapping. Vascular core may or may not be present in the papillae.
- Nuclei are enlarged, ovoid with finely granular, powdery chromatin (Pap stain).
- Nucleoli are small and inconspicuous.
- Nuclear cytoplasmic inclusions and longitudinal grooves/folds are frequently present. The cytoplasmic inclusions are present in more than 5% of cells and in 90% of cases.
- Dispersed cells (single cells) have dense cytoplasm and distinct cell borders.

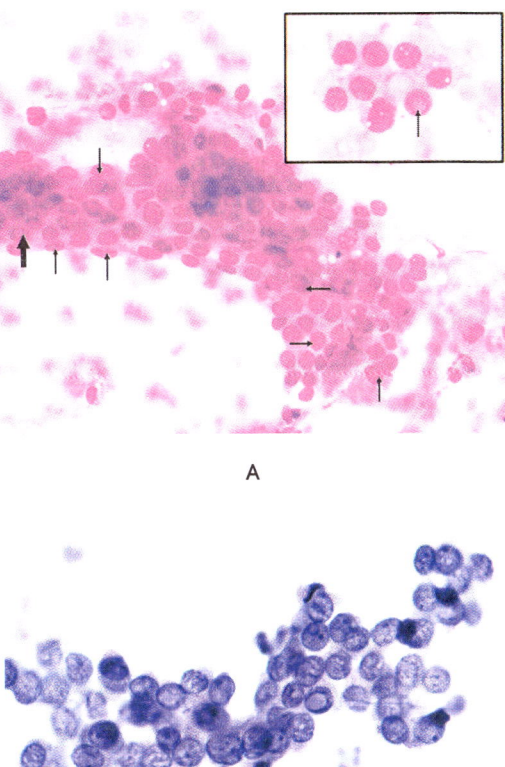

Fig. 14.15A and B: (A) FNA smear showing many nuclear grooves (thin arrow), whereas thick arrow and inset showing intranuclear cytoplasmic inclusions (MGG, 400X); (B) Papillary structure, intranuclear grooves, intranuclear cytoplasmic inclusions and granular, powdery chromatin (Pap, 400X).

- Scanty, viscous, stringy colloid (chewing gum colloid).
- Macrophages, giant cells and psammoma bodies may be present.

Fibroadenoma of Breast

- Moderate to high cellular yield (depending upon the fibrosis).
- Large, branching, monolayered sheets of benign ductal epithelial cells. Smaller, darker nuclei of myoepithelial cells are present in between the ductal epithelial cells.
- Numerous, single bare bipolar nuclei of benign type in the background.
- Scanty fragments of fibromyxoid stroma. They stain pink to magenta with MGG stain, have fibrillary appearance and contain spindle fibroblasts.

Note

In fibrocystic disease (FCD) or fibroadenosis, apocrine changes in the epithelial cells and macrophages in the background are seen in addition to above finding.

Duct Carcinoma of Breast

- Highly cellular smears (high cellular yield).
- Loosely cohesive and individual scattered malignant cells.
- Malignant epithelial cells arranged in three dimensional clusters, syncytial groupings and occasional acinar/glandular patterns.

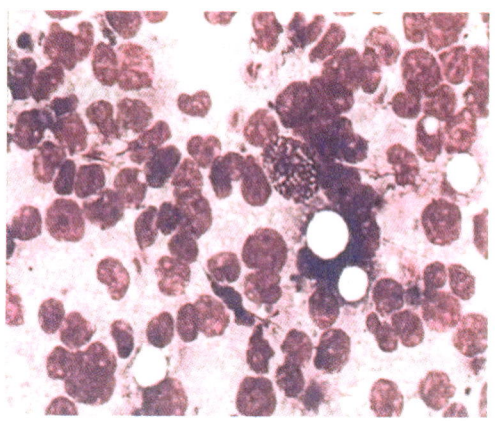

A

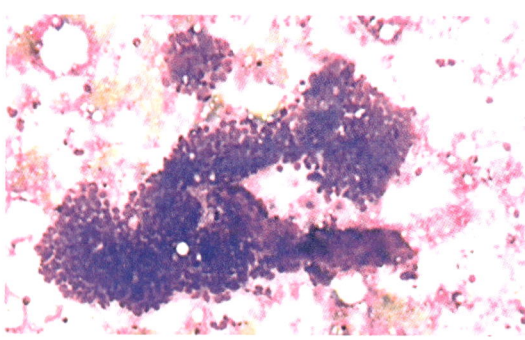

A

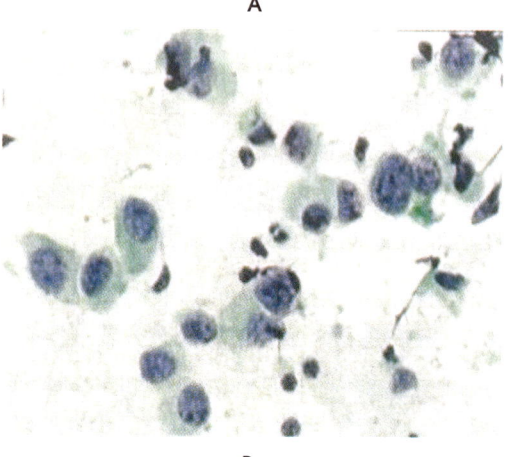

B

Fig. 14.17A and B: Invasive duct carcinoma of breast. (A) MGG stain, high power view; (B) Pap stain, high power view

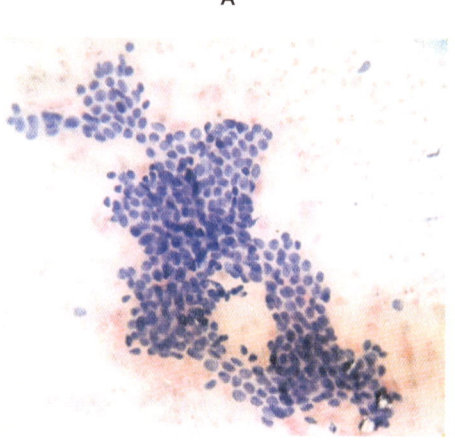

B

Fig. 14.16A and B: (A) Fibroadenoma of breast (MGG × 100); (B) Fibroadenoma of breast (Pap × 100)

- Absence of single bare nuclei of benign type.
- Nuclear atypia like irregular shape, irregular contours (buds, indentations, sharp angles, folds, etc.) and chromatin irregularities are present.
- Necrosis if present is important clue.
- Tumour diathesis may be seen.

Lipoma

- Fragments of mature adipose tissue, a few single fat cells (adipocytes) and fat droplets.
- These fat cells (adipocytes) are large and have abundant empty cytoplasm with eccentrically placed small, dark nucleus.
- Few strands of anastomosing or branching capillary vessels are seen.

Neurofibroma/Benign Peripheral Nerve Sheath Tumour

- Slender spindle cells within fibrillary mesenchymal tissue fragments.
- These spindle cells have long hair like cytoplasmic processes and pale nuclei with pointed ends. The nuclei are pyknotic.
- The cytoplasmic processes of several cells may form bundles and can be tangled.
- The nuclei often form a parallel row or palisade (in case of neurilemmoma or schawannoma).

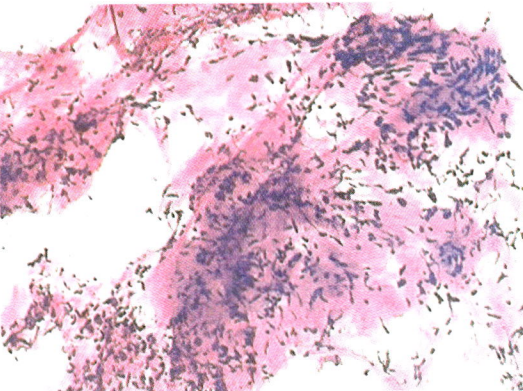

Fig. 14.19: Neurofibroma (MGG, 100X)

Ganglion (Ganglion Cyst)

- Abundant amorphous mucoid material.
- A few pale histiocyte-like cells.

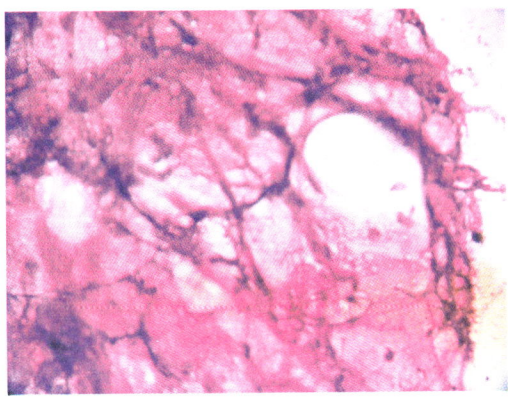

A

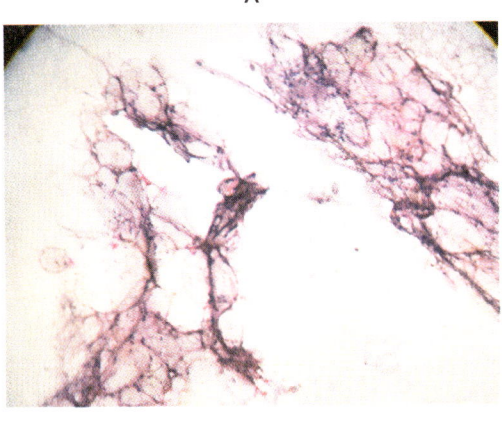

B

Fig. 14.18A and B: (A) Lipoma (MGG × 400); (B) Lipoma (Pap × 100)

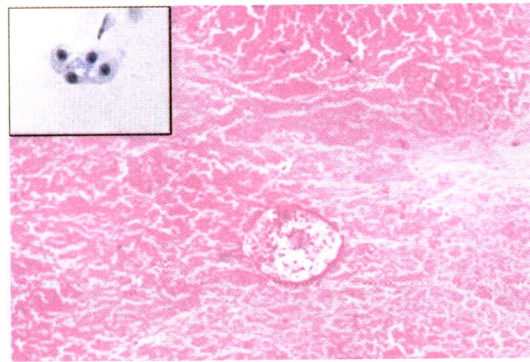

Fig. 14.20: Ganglion cyst, MGG × 400 (inset shows Pap stain)

Pleomorphic Salivary Adenoma of Salivary Gland

- Fibrillary chodromyxoid or myxoid stromal substance.
- In MGG stained smears, this stromal substance appears as an intensely red to dark purple, fibrillar material.
- Rounded, monomorphic epithelial cells with a well defined sometimes eccentric cytoplasm are seen together with spindled myoepithelial cells.
- These epithelial and myoepithelial cells are seen single and in poorly cohesive clusters and sheets.
- Nuclei of these cells are oval with bland nuclear chromatin.

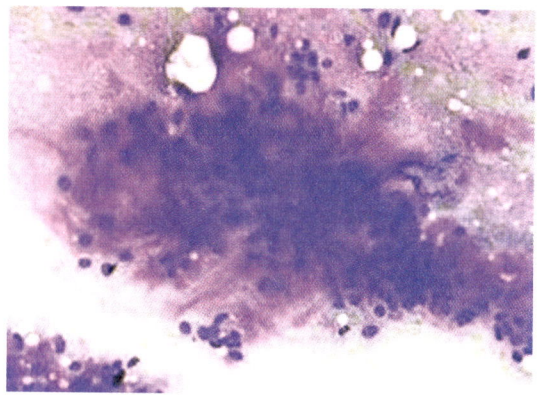

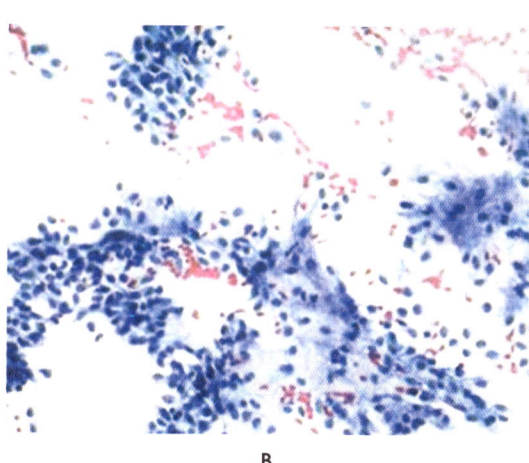

Fig. 14.21A and B: (A) MGG stain, low power view; (B) Pap stain, low power view

VIVA VOCE

Q. 1. What are the other names of FNAC?
Ans:
i. The terminology FNAC or fine needle aspiration cytology was popular among some British and American workers. They also called **needle biopsy cytology (NBC).**
ii. Other terminologies are **aspiration biopsy cytology (ABC)** and **fine needle aspiration biopsy (FNAB)** which were used by Scandinavian and American workers.

Q. 2. What is usual fixative for Pap smears?
Ans: Usually 95% ethyl alcohol, 100% methanol or 85% isopropyl alcohol are used as fixative. A mixture of ether and ethyl alcohol (1:1 v/v) is also used.

Q. 3. What are the indications for Barr body detection in buccal smear?
Ans:
i. To determine the genotypic sex in children who have ambiguous external genitalia (phenotypic sex) like male or female pseudohermaphrodites.
ii. In Turner's syndrome (45, XO), Klinefelter syndrome (47, XXY) or super females (47, XXX).

Q. 4. What are the different stains used for buccal smear staining?
Ans: Orcein stain, basic fuchsin stain and Shorr's stain.

Among these first two stains are commonly used.

Q. 5. What is F body or Y chromatin?
Ans: The fluorescent dye, quinacrine, binds strongly to the Y chromosome and only to a lesser extent to the other chromosome in cells of humans. A bright fluorescent spot (F body), which is presumed to be the Y chromosome, is clearly visible in quinacrine stained interphase cells from various tissues and spermatozoa of human males.

Spermatozoa bearing one F body (~ 45% of total) are taken to be Y spermatozoa. Spermatozoa having two F bodies (about 1.3% of the total) are YY spermatozoa. If number of YY spermatozoa is high, then there is high non-disjunction rates during spermatogenesis.

The intensely fluorescent F body is seen under fluorescent microscope in about 60% of interphase nuclei in human males and <8% in nuclei of females. This F body is also observed in the nuclei of lymphocytes in blood smears if stained with quinacrine mustard.

Q. 6. What are interventional cytology and exfoliative cytology? What are their differences?

Ans: In **interventional cytology**, materials are obtained by aspiration technique or surgical biopsy. These include FNAC, imprint cytology, crush smear cytology and biopsy sediment cytology.

In **exfoliative cytology**, cells which are shed off from epithelial surfaces into body fluids or body cavities are used. Beside the representative cells are also obtainable from scraping, brushing or washing mucosal surfaces (abrasive cytology) (*see* table below).

Q. 7. What is biopsy sediment cytology?

Ans: First the sample deposit of the fixative (neutral buffered formalin or 10% formalin) in which the biopsy specimen has been sent is centrifuged. Then smear is prepared.

It is used in some causes of bone tumours and diagnostic criteria are same as in exfoliative cytology.

Q. 8. What are the contraindications of doing FNAC?

- Bleeding diathesis: coagulopathies like haemophilia, von Willebrand's disease
- Testis: Acute epididymo-orchitis as FNAC is extremely painful.
- Pancreas: Acute pancreatitis
- Prostate: Acute prostatitis
- Lung: Elderly patients with emphysema or pulmonary hypertension
- Adrenal: Suspected pheochromocytoma because of fluctuations in blood pressure.
- Liver: Prothrombin time should be checked
- Malignant melanoma: Extreme precautions should be taken, because some fear that there is chance of needle seedling and spread of tumour through needle tract.

Q. 9. What is the ideal needle size for doing FNAC?

Ans: Usually for most of the sites (soft tissue, breast, etc.), needle size of 21 gauge or

Needle gauge	Outer diameter in inch	Outer diameter in mm
• 18 Gauge	0.050	1.270
• 19 Gauge	0.042	1.067
• 20 Gauge	0.03575	0.9081
• 21 Gauge	0.03225	0.8192
• 22 Gauge	0.02825	0.7176
• 23 Gauge	0.02525	0.6414
• 24 Gauge	0.02225	0.5652
• 25 Gauge	0.02025	0.5144

Parameters	Interventional cytology	Exfoliative cytology
1. Smears	Abundant cellular material in clumps, aggregates and discrete.	Cells are discrete. Particular cell has to be find out by screening
2. Method of sample collection	Obtained by aspiration/intervention	Cells are exfoliated from epithelial cells.
3. Basis of diagnosis	Cellular pattern and morphologic evaluation of groups of cells	By evaluating particular cell of interest
4. Morphologic evaluation for diagnosis	Though nuclear features are very important, cytoplasmic features are also important	Nuclear features more important than cytoplasmic features

22 gauge needle is used. For highly vascular tumours like thyroid, lymph node and in children; 24 gauge or 25 gauge needles are suitable. For very hard tissue like bone 18 gauge or 20 gauge needles are used.

The standard 21 gauge needle has a length of 38 mm while 24 to 25 gauge needle has a length of 25 mm.

For guided FNAC longer needles (80–160 mm long) are needed.

For guided FNAC of abdominal organs and lung, Chiba spinal needle of 20–22 gauge needles are used. For transrectal FNAC of prostate and transvaginal FNAC of ovary needles of up to 200 mm length are employed.

Q. 10. What are the infective organisms that can be detected in Pap smears?

Ans:
- Bacteria: *Neisseria gonorrhoeae, Gardnerella vaginalis, Mycobacterium tuberculosis.*
- Virus: Cytomegalovirus, herpes simplex, human papillomavirus (HPV)
- Fungus: Candida, Aspergillosis
- Parasites: *Trichomonas vaginalis, Entamoeba histolytica.*

Part IV
Museum Techniques and Mounted Surgical Specimens

15. Museum Specimens

15

Museum Specimens

CARDIOVASCULAR SYSTEM SPECIMENS

Mitral Stenosis

Description: Mounted specimen of heart in a jar which is cut transversely showing following features:
- Ventricles, atrium and valves of the heart.
- Left ventricle is recognized by its thick wall compared to right ventricle.
- Mitral valve is seen in-between left ventricle and left atrium which has become thickened, puckered, fibrosed and deformed.
- Focal dystrophic calcification is noted in mitral valve.
- Commissures are fused resulting in stenosis and having **'fish-mouth' appearance**.
- Left atrium is dilated.
- Left ventricle is slightly smaller in size compared to normal left ventricle.

Diagnosis: Mitral stenosis

Q. What are the clinical features of mitral stenosis and what is the most common cause?

Ans: Rheumatic fever is the most common cause. Clinical features are pulmonary hypertension, left atrial and left ventricular hypertrophy, opening snap and diastolic murmur.

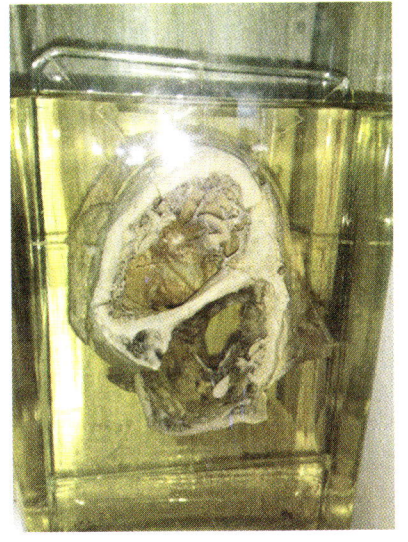

A

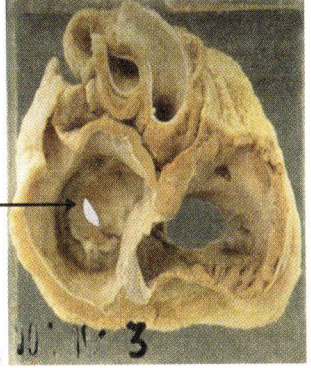

The transverse section shows the "funnel-shaped" mitral valve orifice due to thickening and fusion of the valve cusps B

Fig. 15.1A and B: Button hole; (B) Fish mouth

Q. What are the complications of mitral valve stenosis?
Ans: Congestive cardiac failure, atrial fibrillation, recurrent haemoptysis, subacute bacterial endocarditis and embolism.

Q. What are the consequences of mitral valve stenosis?
Ans: Mitral valve stenosis hampers normal blood flow from left atrium to left ventricle during diastolic period. This leads to hypertrophy of left atrium, pulmonary congestion, brown induration of lungs and right ventricle hypertrophy (cor pulmonale).

Atheroma of Aorta

Description: Mounted specimen of a large artery (abdominal aorta) in a jar showing following features:

- Intimal surface which is identified by many small holes which are actually ostia of branch vessels.
- Elevated white to yellowish fibrous or fibrofatty patchy or plaques (0.3–1.5 cm to long in size) are seen close/surrounding to the opening of ostia of branch vessels.

Diagnosis: Atheroma of artery (aorta)

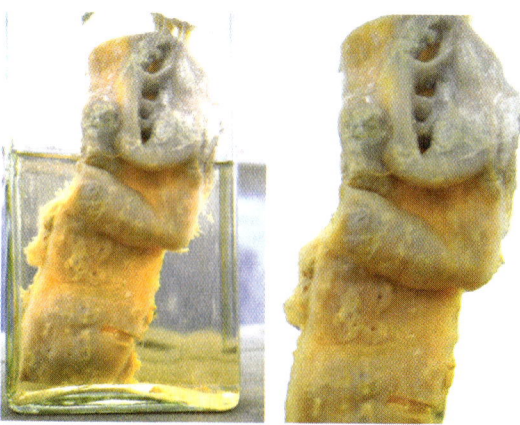

Fig. 15.2A and B: (A) Mounted specimen of atheroma; (B) The lesions

Q. What are the arteries commonly affected by atheroma?
Ans:
i. Large elastic arteries (abdominal aorta, carotid, iliac).
ii. Large to medium-sized muscular arteries (coronary, popliteal, anterior and posterior tibial, mesenteric, renal and circle of Willis).

Q. Which vessels are spared by atherosclerosis?
Ans: Internal mammary arteries and arteries of upper extremities are spared. As internal mammary arteries are not affected, these are used as graft in coronary bypass surgery.

Q. What are the different stages in the evolution?
Ans: Fatty streaks are the earliest lesions in atherosclerosis. Then formation of **atheromatous plaques** occurs in which there are intimal thickening and lipid accumulation. Plaques vary from 0.3 to 1.5 cm in diameter but may from larger masses when they coalesce.

Complications like erosion, ulceration and rupture may occur which may lead to thrombosis. Other complications are aneurysm formation.

Q. What are the components of atheromatous plaques?
Ans: They have three layers or zones. Inner layer contains **necrotic core** (lipid, cholesterol clefts, fibrin, foam cells or foamy macrophages, cell debris). Outer layer is **fibrous cap** composed of smooth muscle and collagen. In-between is the **cellular layer** (smooth muscle, lymphocytes, macrophages with less connective tissue).

Left Ventricular Hypertrophy (LVH)

Description: Mounted specimen of heart in a jar and has following features:

- Thickness of left ventricular wall is increased (>1.5 cm) and decreased in size of left ventricular chamber. Normal

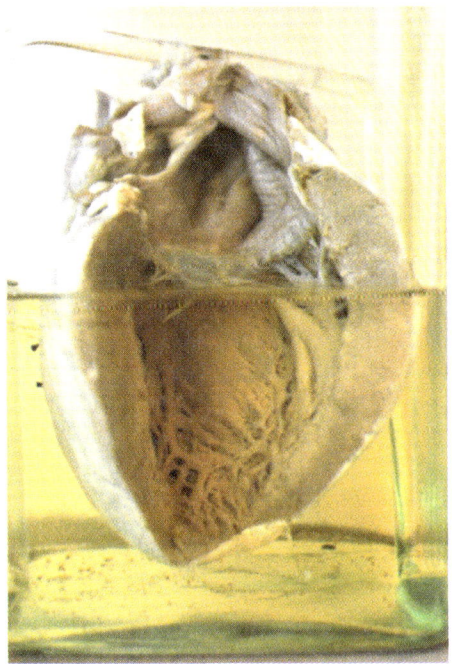

Fig. 15.3: Left ventricular hypertrophy

thickness of left ventricular wall is 1.2–1.5 cm.
- Papillary muscles and trabeculae carneae are prominent
- Heart may be massively enlarged sometimes (corbovium).

Diagnosis: Left ventricular hypertrophy

Q. What are the common causes of LVH?
Ans: It occurs due to systemic hypertension and aortic valvular disease. The overall weight of heart increases >375 gm in males and >350 gm in females. Congestive heart failure is the most common cause of death in untreated patients.

Q. What are the light microscopic features?
Ans: Microscopically, hypertrophic myocardial cells (cardiac myocytes) exhibit an increased in diameter with enlarged, hyperchromatic, **rectangular (boxcar) nuclei**.

Also, there are focal interstitial fibrosis and myofibre degeneration.

Fibrinous Pericarditis

Description: Mounted specimen of heart in a jar showing following features:
- There is deposition of fibrin over pericardium and it ranges from barely visible fibrin ridges to massive, velvety deposit.
- Fibrin deposited in-between two layers of pericardium (viscreral and parietal layers) exhibits **bread and butter** appearance.
- At places, mesothelium below fibrin is destroyed. In these areas, fibrinous coating is adherent so firmly that it becomes progressively difficult to pull off fibrinous coating.
- The surface is dry, with a fine granular roughening.

Diagnosis: Fibrinous pericarditis

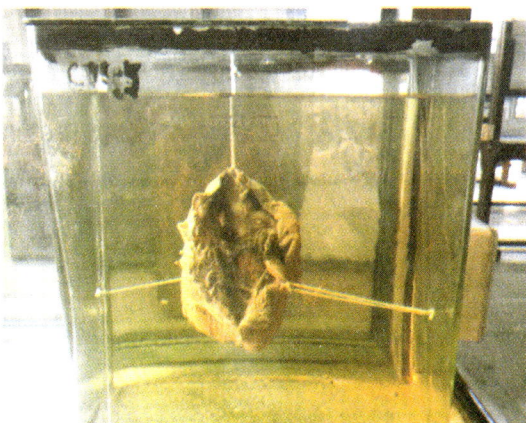

Fig. 15.4: Fibrinous pericarditis

Q. What are the causes of fibrinous pericarditis?
Ans: Fibrinous or serofibrinous pericarditis is characterized by a fibrin-rich exudate due to increased vascular permeabilility. Causes are chronic renal failure (uraemia), myocardial infarction, acute rheumatic fever, SLE, postinfarction (Dressler) syndrome, chest radiation and trauma.

Q. What are the clinical features?
Ans: Development of a loud pericardial friction rub is very characteristic of fibrinous pericarditis. Also, there are pain, systemic febrile reactions and signs of cardiac failure.

Q. What are the components of fluid in serofibrinous pericarditis?
Ans: There is accumulation of larger amounts of yellow to brown turbid fluid, which is made brown and cloudy by the presence of leukocytes and red cells (may be bloody in appearance) and fibrin. Over time, fibrin may be lysed with resolution or it may be organized.

Verrucous Lesions Mitral Valve in Rheumatic Heart Disease (RHD)

Description: Mounted specimen of heart in a jar showing following features:
- There are many small, warty, vegetations along the lines of closure of mitral valve leaflets (arrow on right side picture). Also seen on the rest of the valvular surface.
- These verrucae (actually small thrombi and composed of fibrin and platelets) are greyish or reddish-brown.

Diagnosis: Verrucous lesions of mitral valve.

Q. What are the differences of vegetations, seen in RHD, infective endocarditis, nonbacterial thrombotic endocarditis, Libman-Sacks endocarditis of SLE?
Ans: In RHD, vegetations are small (1–2 mm) warty and seen mainly along the lines of closure of the valve leaflets. In infective endocarditis, vegetations are large, irregular masses which are seen on the valve cusps that can extend onto the chordae. In nonbacterial thrombotic endocarditis, vegetations are small, bland and attached at the line of closure of valve leaflets. In SLE, vegetations are small or medium-sized which are seen on both sides of valve leaflets.

Q. Which valve is most commonly involved in RHD?
Ans: The mitral valve is affected most commonly (65–70%) followed by aortic valve involvement (25% of cases). Tricuspid valve involvement is uncommon and involvement of pulmonary valve is very rare.

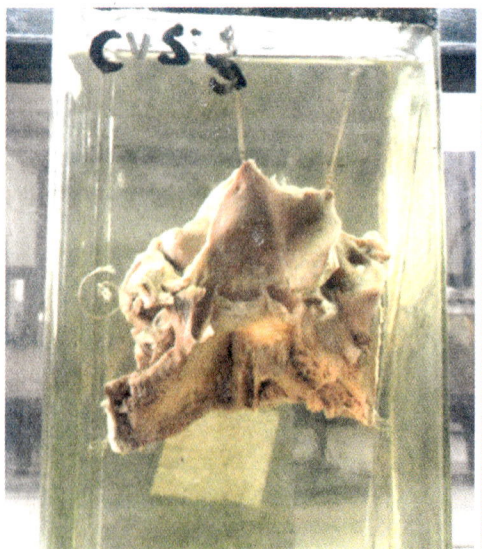
A

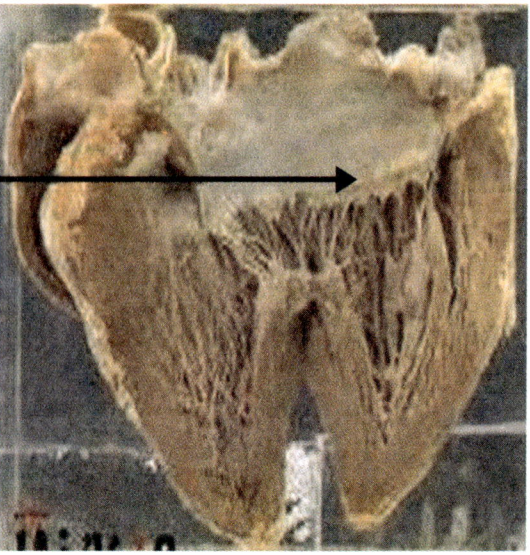
B

Fig. 15.5A and B: Rheumatic heart disease (verrucous lesions)

RESPIRATORY SYSTEM SPECIMENS

Lobar Pneumonia

Description: Mounted specimen of cut section of lung in a jar showing following features:
- Solidification of a lobe of lung (diffuse homogenous consolidation).
- This area of consolidation, looks gray brown or yellowish-gray in colour.
- The pleura is thickened and covered by fibrinosuppurative exudate.
- Other portion of the lung is unaffected and appears normal.

Diagnosis: Lobar pneumonia (gray hepatization)

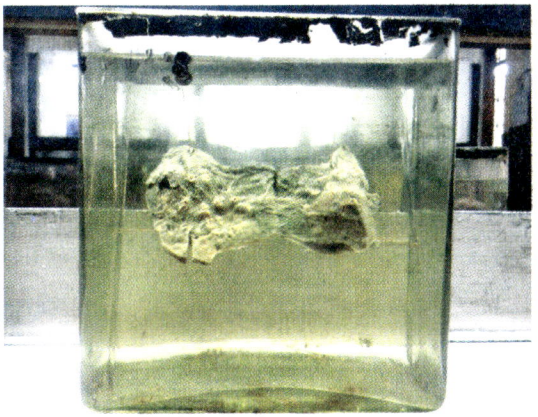

Fig. 15.6: Lobar pneumonia

Q. What are the different stages of lobar pneumonia?
Ans:
i. Stage of **congestion** (12–24 hours)
ii. Stage of **red hepatization** (2–4 hours)
iii. Stage of **gray hepatization** (4–8 days)
iv. Stage of **resolution** (8–10 days)

Q. Why has it been named as hepatization, though it is a lung tissue?
Ans: During autopsy, the affected lobe/portion of lung feels like hepatic tissue (liver) in consistency. Also, the affected lobe sinks in water unlike unaffected lung tissue which floats in water due to entrapped air within it.

Q. Why the lower lobes of lung are commonly affected?
Ans: This is because of the tendency of secretions to gravitate into the lower lobes.

Q. Why the affected portion looks gray during gray hepatization?
Ans: In this stage, there is progressive disintegration of red cells and the persistence of a fibrinosuppurative exudate (neutrophil rich), giving the gross appearance of grayish brown, dry surface.

Q. What do you mean by the term "consolidation"?
Ans: Consolidation literally means the process of becoming or the condition of being solid. In lobar pneumonia this means replacement of alveolar air by neutrophil-rich fibrinosuppurative exudate and to became solidified or consolidated.

Q. Why is it not a case of broncho-pneumonia (lobular pneumonia)?
Ans: The lesion is patchy in broncho-pneumonia and does not involve an entire lobe unlike lobar pneumonia. Also, broncho-pneumonia is associated with area of emphysaema and collapse.

Q. What are the complications of lobar pneumonia?
Ans: Lung abscess, empyema, septicaemia (bacterial dissemination), pleuritis and delayed resolution.

Bronchiectasis

Description: Mounted specimen of cut section of lung in a jar showing following features:
- Marked dilatation of bronchi and bronchioles with fibrosis in the adjoining areas.
- Dilated airways take various shapes, i.e. cylindrical, fusiform, varicose (numerous constriction and dilation) and saccular (bead-like bulge on one side). But it is predominantly cylindrical.

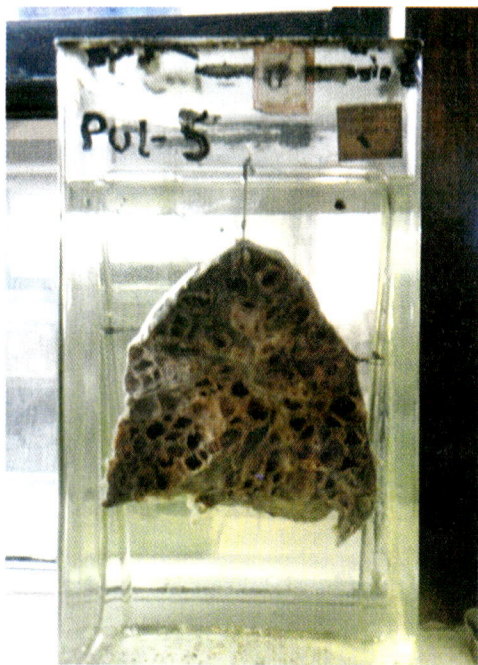

Fig. 15.7: Bronchiectasis

- These dilated airways are easily visible up to <3 mm from the pleural surface (normally, bronchioles are traceable up to 2–3 cm from pleural surface).
- Dilated bronchi and bronchioles are filled with pus.
- Unaffected lung parenchyma is compressed.

Diagnosis: Bronchiectasis.

Q. What is bronchiectasis?
Ans: Bronchiectasis is a disease characterized by permanent dilation of bronchi and bronchioles caused by destruction of the elastic tissue, resulting from or associated with chronic necrotizing infections.

Q. What are different types of bronchiectasis?
Ans: Obstructive (tumour, foreign body, etc.) and non-obstructive (postinfectious, congenital or hereditary, others).

Obstruction and infection are the major conditions associated with bronchiectasis.

Q. What are the complications of bronchiectasis?
Ans: Lung abscess, pneumonia, bronchopleural fistula, cor pulmonale, necrotizing brain abscess, meningitis, squamous cell carcinoma, and amyloidosis.

Emphysema

Description: Mounted specimen of cut section of lung in a jar showing following features:

- Central or proximal area shows marked dilatation of respiratory bronchioles surrounded by relatively spared alveolar spaces.
- The lesion is more severe in the upper lobes, particularly in the apical segments.
- The walls of emphysematous spaces contain large amount of black pigment (due to heavy smoking nicotine and other).

Diagnosis: Centriacinar (centrilobular) emphysema

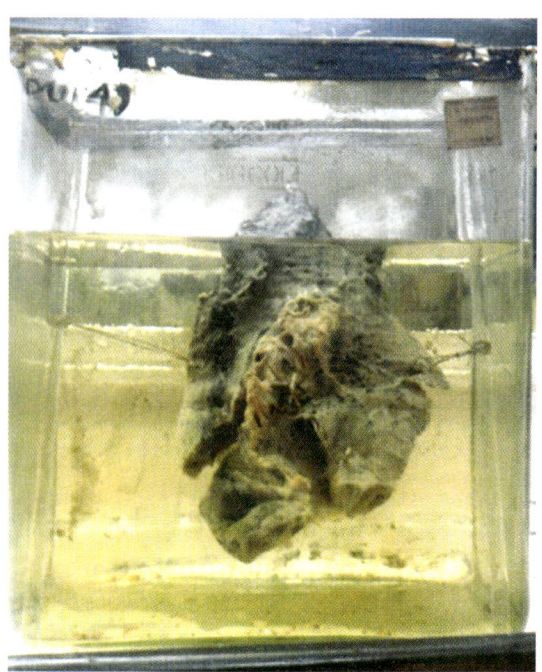

Fig. 15.8A

Museum Specimens

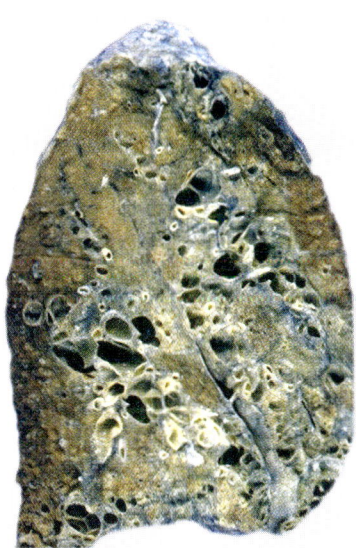

Fig. 15.8B

Fig. 15.8A and B: Emphysema

Q. What are the different types of emphysema?

Ans:
i. **Centriacinar (centrilobular) emphysema:** Respiratory bronchioles are dilated. Cause is heavy smoking, often associated with chronic bronchitis.
ii. **Panacinar (panlobular) emphysema:** Alveoli and alveolar ducts are dilated. Cause α_1-antitrypsin (antiprotease) deficiency.
iii. **Paraseptal (distal acinar) emphysema:** Proximal portion of the acinus is normal, but distal portion of acinus is dilated. Seen adjacent to areas of fibrosis, scarring or atelectasis.
iv. **Irregular emphysema:** Acini are irregularly involved and are almost invariably associated with scarring. Seen along with scars from a healed inflammatory process.
v. **Interstitial emphysema:** It occurs as a result of entrance of air into the connective tissue of lung, subcutaneous tissue or mediastinum in settings of penetrating chest injury, chronic bronchitis or obstruction. Also seen in children with whooping cough.

Q. What are the light microscopic findings of emphysema?

Ans:
- Abnormally large alveoli separated by thin septa.
- Adjacent alveoli become confluent, creating large airspaces.
- As alveolar walls are destroyed, there is decrease in the capillary bed.

Fibrocaseous Tuberculosis of Lung

Description: Mounted specimen of lung in a jar showing following features:
- Yellowish caseous necrosis area of variable size.
- Foci of caseous necrosis accompanied by fibrosis
- Acute cavities have irregular, ragged yellowish-gray walls.
- Chronic cavities have regular, smooth and thick wall lining.
- Fibrosis of lung accompanied by thickened pleura, thickened wall of bronchi and thickening of blood vessels.

Diagnosis: Fibrocaseous (cavitating) tuberculosis of lung.

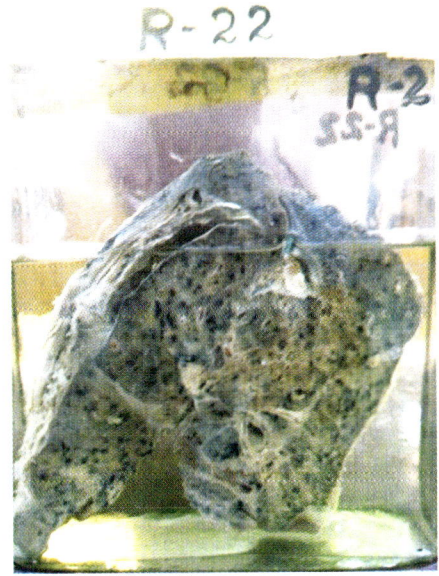

Fig. 15.9: Fibrocaseous tuberculosis of lung

Q. What is primary tuberculosis?
Ans: Primary infection may occur in any organ such as lung, intestine or skin. But in children, the usual site is lung and is called primary tuberculosis. Exposure to AFB occurs first time and consolidation is usually solitary. There is formation of **Ghon's focus** in subpleural location and midzone of lung is involved. Lymphadenopathy is common. Cavitation is rare.

Q. What is secondary tuberculosis?
Ans: It is usually caused by reinfection or reactivation of an old infection. Any age group may suffer. Multifocal lesions (consolidations) are seen. Upper lobes or apical regions are usually affected. Cavitation is common but lymphadenopathy is rare. **Simon's focus** (2 cm gray white to yellowish well circumscribed consolidation in apical regions) may be seen.

Q. What are Ghon's focus and Ghon's complex?
Ans: Ghon's focus: 1–1.5 cm area of gray-white inflammation with consolidation. Seen in lower part of upper lobe and upper part of lower lobe. The centre of this focus undergoes caseous necrosis.

Ghon's complex: Combination of parenchymal lung lesion of tuberculosis and regional hilar lymph nodes involvement is referred to as Ghon's complex.

Q. What are the different types (morphological) of pulmonary tuberculosis?
Ans:
  i. Fibrocaseous
 ii. Cavitary (ulcerative)
iii. Tuberculous bronchopneumonia
 iv. Miliary tuberculosis with haematogenous infection

Miliary Tuberculosis of Lung
Description: Mounted specimen of longitudinal section of lung in a jar showing following features:

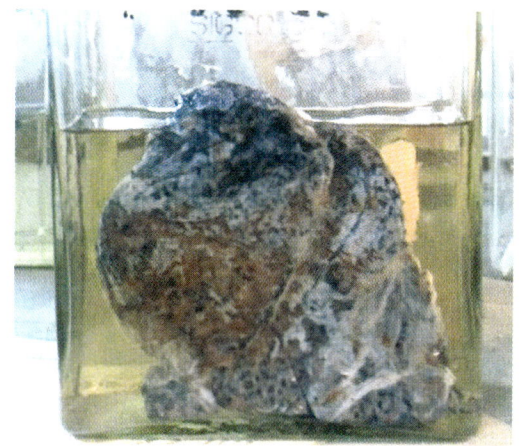

A

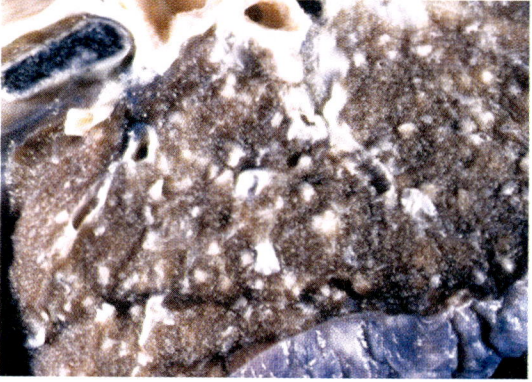

B

Fig. 15.10A and B: Miliary tuberculosis of lung

- The lung is studded with numerous uniform small **millet-size white spots (tubercles)** surrounded by intense congestion.
- These small spots (1–3 mm in diameter) are seen both in subpleural location and in section.

Diagnosis: Miliary tuberculosis of lung

Q. Why does miliary tuberculosis occur?
Ans: This is due to rupture of caseous parenchymatous or glandular lesion and when organisms draining through lymphatics enter the venous blood organisms enter systemic circulation and dissemination occurs.

Q. What are light microscopic features of miliary tuberculosis of lung?
Ans:
- Tubercles are usually located in interalveolar septa and usually no change is seen in the alveoli.
- In the granulomas, giant cells are a few in number.
- Peripheral fibrotic zone is absent.
- Vessels present in septa undergo dilatation.

Bronchogenic Carcinoma

Description: Mounted specimen of a section of lung in a jar showing following features:
- Gray-white growth arising from major bronchus, spreading both within and outside the bronchus and in the walls. Also, the tumour is infiltrating the lung substance.
- Focal areas of haemorrhage and necrosis which produce red or yellow-white mottling and softening.
- The tumour is arising from the hilum.
- Uninvolved lung tissue is compressed.

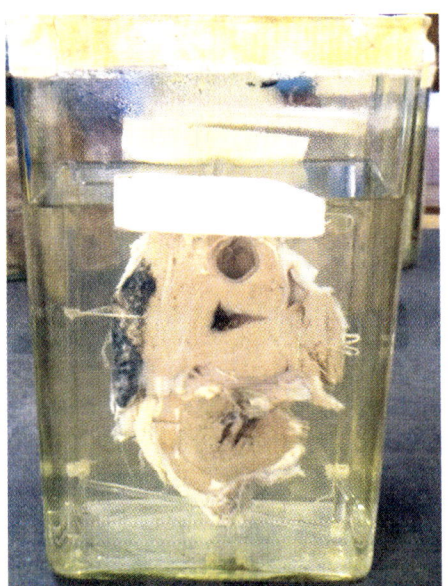

Fig. 15.11: Bronchogenic carcinoma

Diagnosis: Bronchogenic carcinoma (squamous cell carcinoma)

Note
Most lung carcinomas arise in and about the hilus of the lung. About three-fourths of the tumours originate from first-order, second-order, and third-order bronchi.

As most of the carcinomas of lung arise from bronchi, the term 'Cancer lung' and bronchogenic carcinoma are used synonymously.

Q. What are the different types of lung carcinomas?
Ans:
- Adenocarcinoma (males 37%, females 47%)
- Squamous cell carcinoma (males 32%, females 25%)
- Small cell carcinoma (males 14%, females 18%)
- Large cell carcinoma (males 18%, females 10%)

Q. What are the risk factors of bronchogenic carcinoma?
Ans: Tobacco smoking accounts from 80 to 90% of lung cancers. High-dose ionizing radiation, uranium, asbestos and air-pollutants are other risk factors. Genetic predisposition and p53 mutation also play an important role.

Q. What are precursor lesions of lung cancers?
Ans: Four types of epithelial precursor lesion:
- Squamous dysplasia and carcinoma *in situ*
- Atypical adenomatous hyperplasia
- Adenocarcinoma *in situ*
- Diffuse idiopathic pulmonary neuroendocrine hyperplasia

Q. Lepidic pattern of growth is seen in which lung carcinoma?

Ans: It is seen in bronchoalveolar carcinoma during light microscopic examination. The tumour grows along preexisting structures without destruction of alveolar architecture. This pattern of growth is known as **lepidic**, and the neoplastic cells resembling butter flies sitting on a fence. Bronchoalveolar carcinomas have two subtypes: Mucinous and nonmucinous.

GASTROINTESTINAL SYSTEM SPECIMEN

Peptic Ulcer

Description: Mounted specimen of stomach in a jar showing following features:
- Stomach is cut open along greater curvature.
- An ulcer is seen in lesser curvature with the antrum.
- The ulcer is <2 cm in diameter, oval to round and sharply delineated
- Edge is thickened and overhanging
- Margin of ulcer sharply punched out.
- Base of ulcer is smooth and clean.

Diagnosis: Chronic peptic ulcer

Q. What are the common sites of peptic ulcer?

Ans: It occurs in duodenum, stomach, lower end of oesophagus, Meckel's diverticulum and jejunum after gastrojejunostomy. Gastric peptic ulcers are usually located along the lesser curvature near the interface of the body and antrum. Duodenal ulcers usually occur within few centimeters of the pyloric valve and involve the anterior duodenal wall. Peptic ulcers are four times commoner in proximal (1st part) of duodenum than in the stomach.

Q. What are the risk factors of peptic ulcers?

Ans: *Helicobacter pylori* infection, bile reflux and delayed gastric emptying, alcohol and spicy food, use of NSAIDs, tobacco smoking, hyperparathyroidism, multiple endocrine neoplasia 1, genetic factors (blood group O

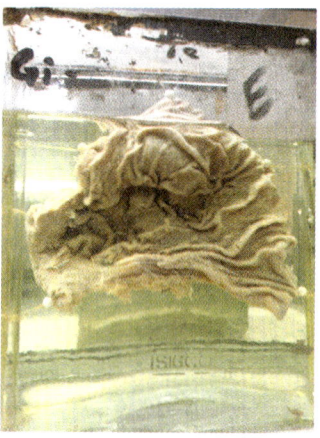

Fig. 15.12A and B: (A) Peptic ulcer; (B) Peptic ulcer with perforation

for duodenal ulcer and blood group A for gastric ulcer).

Q. What are the complications of peptic ulcers?

Ans: Perforation, hourglass deformity and pyloric stenosis, pancreatitis and rarely malignant transformation.

Gastric Carcinoma

Description: Mounted specimen of stomach in a jar showing following features:
- A large ulceroproliferative growth projecting in the lumen from the mucosa. The growth is situated body of stomach.

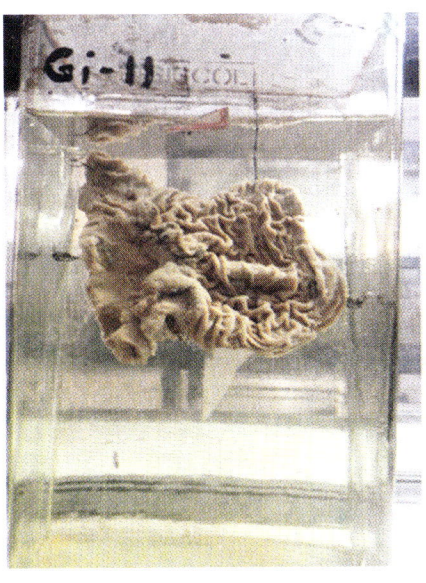
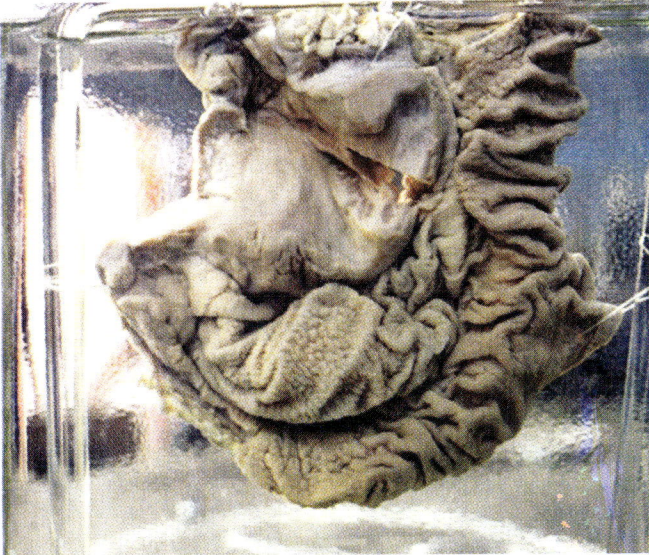

Fig. 15.13A and B: Gastric carcinoma

- There is also a large ulcer (>3 cm in diameter)
- Margin of ulcer is heaped up and irregular.
- Base of ulcer is haemorrhagic and necrotic. Also, it is hard and indurated.

Diagnosis: Gastric carcinoma

Q. What are the common sites of gastric carcinoma?
Ans:
- Pylo-antrum region (lesser curvature): 50–60%
- Cardiac region of stomach: 25%
- Body and fundus: 25%
- Greater curvature of stomach: 12%

Q. What are the different types of gastric carcinomas?
Ans: It may be classified on the basis of depth of invasion (e.g. early and advanced carcinoma); macroscopic growth pattern (e.g. flat mucosal lesions, exophytic, ulcerative and diffuse infiltrative type) and histologic types (intestinal type and diffuse type). Signet-ring carcinoma and linitis plastica are variants of diffuse type of gastric adenocarcinoma.

Q. What are the primary tumours of stomach?
Ans: They may be benign and malignant. These include adenocarcinoma (95%), lymphoma (3%), carcinoid and neuroendocrine carcinoma (1%), stromal tumour and leiomyoma (1%).

Leiomyoma is the most common benign tumour and adenocarcinoma is the most common malignant tumour.

Typhoid Ulcer of Small Intestine

Description: Mounted specimen of stomach in a jar showing following features:
- Multiple small ulcers on the mucosa of small intestine.
- Long axis of ulcers oriented parallel to the long axis of the intestine.
- Margins are regular and well circumscribed. Edges are of undermined.
- Ulcers are round to oval with foci of haemorrhage.
- The Peyer's patches are prominent.

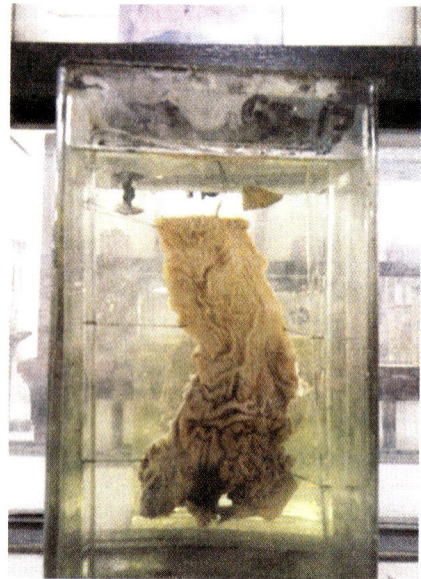

Fig. 15.14: Typhoid ulcer

Diagnosis: Typhoid ulcer of small intestine

Q. What are the stages of intestinal pathology in typhoid infection?
Ans: There are **four stages** and usually terminal ileum and caecum are involved. Four stages last for 4 weeks:
  i. Hyperplasia of Peyer's patches (first week)
  ii. Necrosis of Peyer's patches (second week)
  iii. Ulceration of intestinal mucosa (third week)
  iv. Healing of ulcers (fourth week)

Q. What are the extraintestinal lesion?
Ans: Proliferation of reticuloendothelial cells (monocytes/histiocytes) seen in spleen (sinus histiocytes), liver (Kupffer's cells), lymph nodes and bone marrow. So, patients develop splenomegaly, hepatomegaly and lymphadenopathy.

Q. What are the complications of typhoid ulcer?
Ans: Haemorrhage and perforation may occur at the end of 2nd week. Septicaemic complications like pneumonia, myocarditis, meningitis, arthritis and cholecystitis may be noticed.

Q. Describe briefly intestinal pathogenesis of typhoid infection?
Ans: Intestinal pathogens (*Salmonella typhi* bacilli invade the intestinal mucosa, engulfed by macrophages and transported to reginal lymph nodes. In the lymphoid tissue multiplication of pathogen occurs resulting in bacteremia. These pathogens reinfect lymphoid tissue and liberate endotoxin leading to delayed hypersensitivity reaction. After a few days of bacteremia, the bacteria localize in lymphoid tissue of small intestine, mesenteric nodes, gall bladder, spleen and liver. Typically, lesions are seen in Peyer's patches and follicles.

Tubercular Ulcer of Small Intestine

Description: Mounted specimen of small intestine in a jar showing following features:
- Multiple large ulcers on the mucosa of small intestine

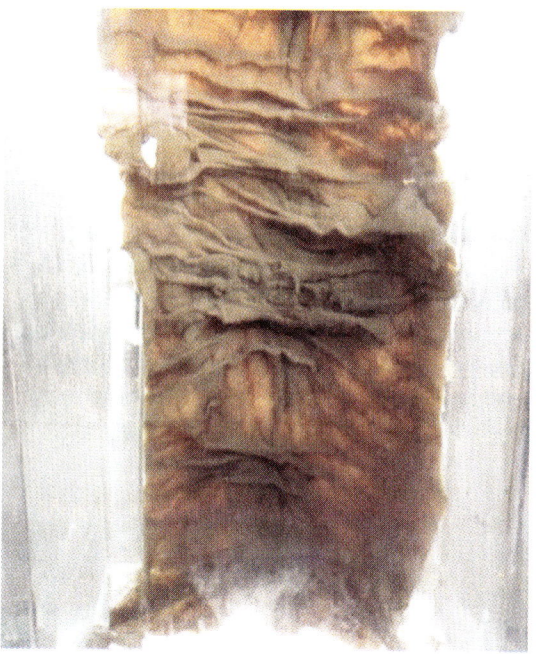

Fig. 15.15: Tubercular ulcer of small intestine

- Long axis of ulcers oriented transversely to the intestinal axis.
- Margins are irregular and may encircle the intestine (circumferential).
- Size of ulcers are large.
- Stricture formation and narrowing of intestinal lumen seen.
- Peyer's patches are not prominent.

Diagnosis: Tubercular ulcer of small intestine.

Q. What are the different ulcerative lesions of small intestine?
Ans: Peptic ulcer in duodenum, typhoid ulcer, tubercular ulcer, Crohn's disease and bacillary dysentery ulcers.

Q. What are the differences between typhoid ulcer and tubercular ulcer of small intestine?
Ans:

Q. What are the different types of intestinal tuberculosis?
Ans:

i. **Primary intestinal tuberculosis**: Mycobacterium tubercle bacilli (bovis strain) reach the intestine due to ingestion of unpasteurized milk. Draining lymph nodes of small intestine are enlarged which may be matted with caseous necrosis, known as **tabes mesenterica**. Most of them heals by fibrosis and dystrophic calcification.

ii. **Secondary tuberculosis**: The pathogens (*M. tuberculosis*) enter the intestine by swallowing of infected sputum in a case of pulmonary tuberculosis. Intestinal lesions are prominent compared to draining lymph nodes.

Parameters	Typhoid ulcer	Tubercular ulcer
• Causative organism	*Salmonella typhi*	Mycobacterium tuberculosis bacilli
• Site of involvement	Terminal ileum (most common), also jejunum or colon	Ileo-caecal region
• Axis of ulcer	Longitudinal axis of intestine	Transverse axis of intestine
• Size of ulcer	Small	Large
• Base of ulcer	Black due to sloughing of mucosa	Creamy white due to presence of caseous material
• Margin	Regular well circumscribed	Irregular and may encircle gut (circumferential)
• Bleeding from ulcer	Common	Absent
• Stricture formation	Absent	Present due to fibrosis
• Perforation of ulcer	Common	Absent
• Light microscopy	Erythrophagocytosis and presence of pathogens in macrophages. Absence of neutrophils	Epithelioid granulomas, Langhans and foreign body type giant cells, caseous necrosis. Zn stain shows AFB
• Lymphoid involvement	Peyer's patches—follicles and regional lymph nodes	Lymph nodes in primary and Peyer's patches in secondary tuberculosis

Q. What are the complications of tubercular ulcer?

As: Stricture, peforation and fistula are known complications.

Q. What is hyperplastic ileocaecal tuberculosis?

Ans: It is variant of intestinal TB characterized by thickening of terminal ileum, caecum and ascending colon along with mucosal ulceration. Clinically, a mass is papable and may be misdiagnosed as ileocaecal carcinoma.

Colorectal Cancer (Rectosigmoid)

Description: Mounted specimen of cut open sigmoid colon and rectum in a jar showing following features:
- A circumferential annular/napkin ring configuration mass is seen in the rectosigmoid region.
- Tumour is firm with gray-white appearance.

Diagnosis: Carcinoma of rectosigmoid

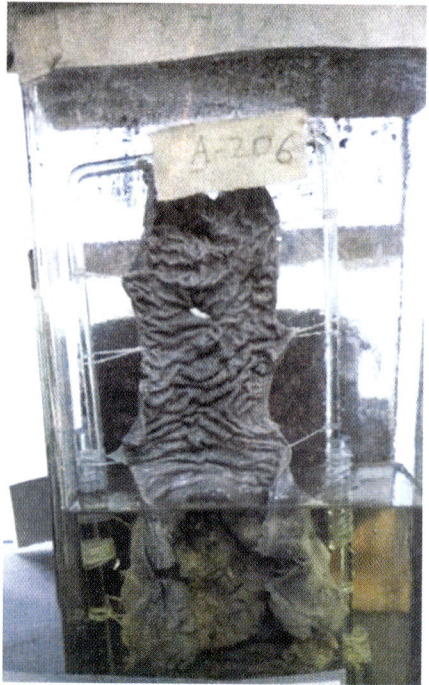

Fig. 15.16: Rectosigmoid cancer

Colorectal Cancer (Colon)

Description: Mounted specimen of cut open ascending colon and part of transverse colon in a jar showing following features:
- An ulceroproliferative, exophytic polypoid mass is seen in the ascending colon.
- Crater-like ulcerations with raised margins are noted.
- The mass is cauliflower-like, soft and friable projecting into the lumen.

Diagnosis: Carcinoma of colon

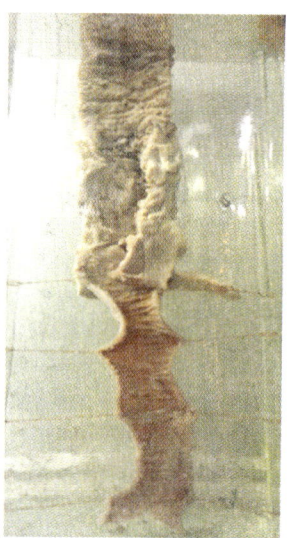

Fig. 15.17: Colon cancer

Q. What are the risk factors for colorectal cancer?

Ans: Elderly persons, familial adenomatosis polyposis, inflammatory bowel disease; dietary factors (consumption of excessive red meat, animal fat, refined carbohydrate), NSAIDs, obesity, tobacco smoking and chronic alcoholism.

Q. What are the common sites of colorectal cancer?

Ans: Rectosigmoid is the commonest site (38%) followed by sigmoid colon (20%), descending colon (10%), caecum (8%), hepatic flexure (8%), transverse colon (5%), ascending colon (3%) and anus (3%).

Q. What are the differences between right-sided and left-sided colorectal carcinoma?
Ans:

Parameters	Right-sided colorectal carcinoma	Left-sided colorectal carcinoma
• Site	Caecum and ascending colon	Rectosigmoid area and descending colon
• Growth pattern	Ulceroproliferative, exophytic, polypoid soft to firm mass	Circumferential, napkin-ring firm mass
• Invasiveness	More invasive	Less invasive
• Involvement of other structures	Common like mesentery, lymph nodes, distant metastasis	Lesson common
• Clinical presentation	Silent and diagnosed late	Obstructive features, so diagnosed early
• Prognosis	Poor	Good

KIDNEY (RENAL) SPECIMENS

Granular Contracted Kidney

Outer surface showing granularity and inner surface (cut section)

Description: Mounted specimens of cut section of kidneys in a jar showing following features:

- Kidneys are symmetrically contracted.
- Surface is finely granular.
- Capsule is adherent to cortex.
- Cortex is thin with an increase in peri-pelvic fat.
- Consistency seems to be firm.

Diagnosis: Granular contracted kidney

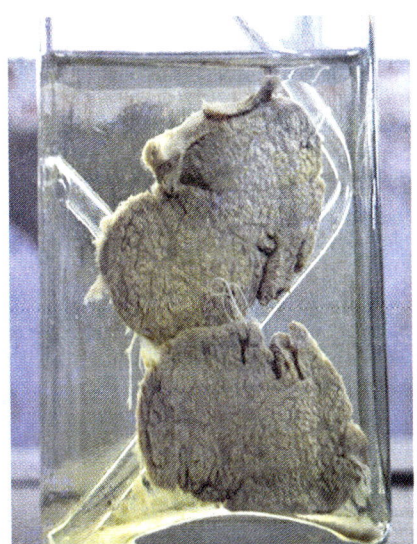
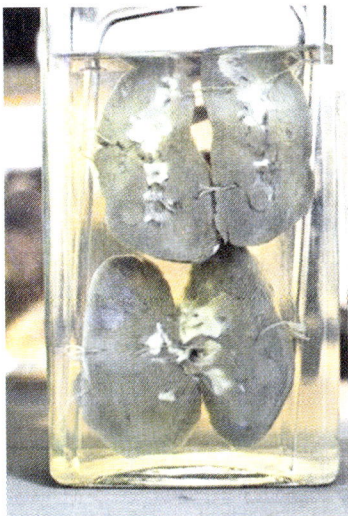

A — Outer surface showing granularity
B — Inner surface (cut section)

Fig. 15.18A and B: Granular contracted kidney

Q. What are the causes of granular contracted kidney?
Ans:
i. Chronic glomerulonephritis
ii. Chronic pyelonephritis (U-shaped scar)
iii. Benign nephrosclerosis (benign hypertension, V-shaped scar)
iv. Less common causes are diabetic nephropathy, myeloma kidney and amyloid kidney.

Q. What are the differences between chronic glomerulonephritis and chronic pyelonephritis?
Ans:

Large White Kidney (RPGN)
Description: Mounted specimen of kidney in a jar showing following features:
- Kidney is enlarged, pale and soft
- Surface is smooth
- Capsule is thin
- Petechial (pin-point) haemorrhages seen or cortical surface

Diagnosis: Large white kidney (rapidly progressive glomerulonephritis)

Q. What are the causes of large white kidney (RPGN)?
Ans: RPGN may be classified into 3 groups as per causes

Parameters	Chronic glomerulonephritis	Chronic pyelonephritis
• Causes	Different types of glomerulonephritis	Reflux nephropathy or chronic obstructive pyelonephritis
• Pathogenesis	End stage glomerular disease due to specific glomerulonephritis	Chronic tubulointerstitial inflammation and fibrosis associated with renal disease
• Gross appearance of kidney surface	Diffusely, granular, cortical surfaces	Depressed area on dilated and blunted calyx
• Nature of scar	Fine and symmetrical	Coarse and asymmetrical
• Glomeruli	Reduced in number and atrophic	Normal; may show periglomerular fibrosis
• Tubules	Atrophied	Atrophy in some and hypertrophy in others. Filled with colloid casts (thyroidisation)
• Interstitial and periglomerular fibrosis	Mild	More severe
• Renal calyx and pelvis	Normal	Dilated
• Clinical features	Onset is insidious. Proteinuria, oedema, azotemia, hypertension	May be asymptomatic. Some present with back pain, fever, pyuria, polyuria, nocturia, bacteria, with gradual onset of hypertension and renal insufficiency

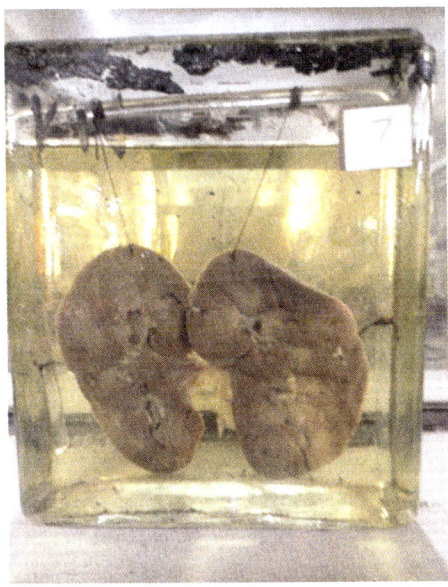

Fig. 15.19: Large white kidney

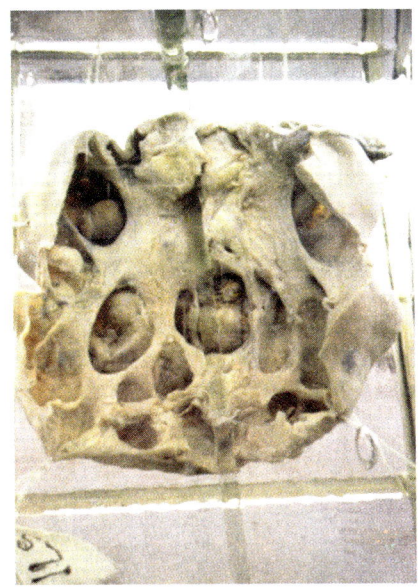

Fig. 15.20: Hydronephrosis

i. Idiopathic RPGN: Nearly half of all cases
ii. Glomerulonephritis (GN) associated with systemic disease such as SLE, diabetes, polyarteritis nodosa and Goodpasture's syndrome.
iii. Postinfectious (post-streptococcal GN)

Other causes of large white kidney (uncommon): Membranous GN, membranoproliferative GN, amyloidosis.

Q. What are light microscopic features of RPGN?

Ans: Depending on underlying cause, the glomeruli may show diffuse or focal endothelial proliferation, mesangial proliferation and focal necrosis.

But the important finding is distinctive **crescents**. Crescents are formed by proliferation of parietal cells and migration of macrophages and monocytes into Bowman's (urinary) space. Fibrin strands are frequently seen between cellular layers of crescents.

Hydronephrosis

Description: Mounted specimen of cut section of kidney in a jar showing following features:

- Kidney is enlarged and outer surface is irregular.
- Multiple cystic cavities are seen in the cut surface which is present in the renal pelvis and calyces.
- Wall of these cystic spaces communicate with renal pelvis.
- Cyst wall is thin and devoid of congestion.
- Many of these cystic spaces contain whitish stones.
- Cortex and renal tissue are compressed and atrophic.

Diagnosis: Hydronephrosis with renal stones.

Q. What is hydronephrosis?

Ans: It is the permanent dilation of the renal pelvis and calyces associated with progressive atrophy of the kidney due to obstruction to the outflow of urine.

Q. Why these multiple cysts are not part of polycystic kidney?

Ans: Here, these cysts communicate with renal pelvis. But in polycystic kidney, the cysts do not communicate with renal pelvis.

Also, here stones within cystic spaces are found, which are the cause of obstruction and leading to hydronephrosis.

Q. What are the causes of hydronephrosis?
Ans:
i. Renal pelvis: Calculi, tumours, ureteropelvic stricture
ii. Intrinsic ureter: Calculi, tumours, blood clot, inflammation
iii. Extrinsic ureter: Tumour compression (e.g cervix), pregnancy, retroperitoneal fibrosis
iv. Urinary bladder: Vesicoureteral reflux, calculi, tumours, neurogenic
v. Prostate: Hyperplasia (BHP), carcinoma, prostatitis
vi. Urethra: Posterior valve stricture, rarely tumours

Q. What is flea-beaten kidney? What are the causes?
Ans: Kidney is enlarged. The cortex shows tiny petechial haemorrhage visible through capsule giving the characteristic appearance of flea-bitten kidney. Cut surface also shows this haemorrhage.

Causes are: Acute post-streptococcal glomerulonephritis, malignant nephrosclerosis, rapidly progressive GN (RPGN), haemolytic-uraemic syndrome, thrombotic thrombocytopenic purpura and Henoch-Schönlein purpura.

Polycystic Kidney

Description: Mounted specimen of cut section of kidney in a jar showing following features:
- Kidney shows marked multicystic nodulations with transparent walls, visible on surface.
- Both small and large cysts are seen resembling bunches of grapes.
- In cut section, almost entire renal parenchyma (both cortex and medulla) is replaced by multiple smooth-walled dilated cysts.

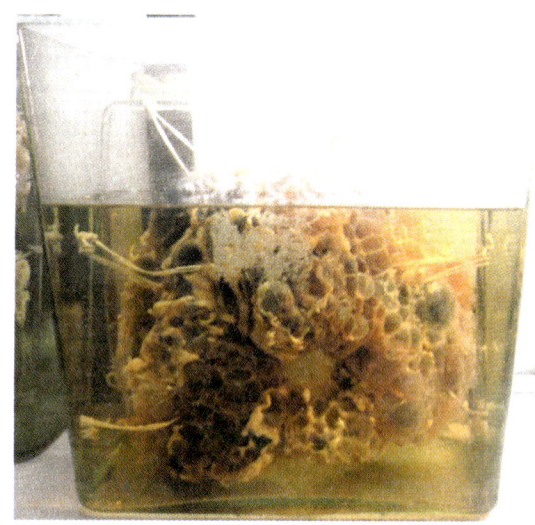

Fig. 15.21: Polycystic kidney

- All these cysts fail to communicate with renal pelvis and renal pelvis is not dilated.
- Occasional cysts communicate with each other producing a larger cyst.
- Renal tissue presents in-between the cysts is compressed and atrophic.

Diagnosis: Polycystic kidney: Adult type

Q. What are the different types of cysts in kidney?
Ans: Polycystic kidney disease, renal dysplasia, medullary cystic disease, acquired (dialysis-associated) cystic disease, simple renal cyst, renal cysts in hereditary malformation syndrome (e.g. tuberous sclerosis), glomerulocystic disease.

Q. What are differences between adult and childhood polycystic kidney disease?
Ans: Adult polycystic kidney disease (ADPKD) is autosomal dominant and mutations in gene located on chromosome 16p13.3 (PKD1) and 4q21 (PKD).

Childhood polycystic kidney disease (CHPKD) is autosomal recessive and mutations seen on chromosome region 6p21–p23 (PKHD1 gene).

Also, in CHPKD, the cysts are smaller which give the kidney a sponge-like appearance. Dilated elongated channels seen in CHPKD which are present at right angles to the cortical surface replacing the cortex and medulla.

Renal Cell Carcinoma (Hypernephroma)

Description: Mounted specimen of cut section of kidney in a jar showing following features:
- A solitary large well circumscribed rounded tumour is seen in the upper pole.
- The tumour has a variegated appearance due to areas of haemorrhage necrosis and cystic spaces (solid-cystic).
- Cut surface of the tumour is yellowish-gray or golden yellow in colour.
- Peripherally kidney tissue is compressed to form an incomplete capsule.

Diagnosis: Renal cell carcinoma (hypernephroma, Grawtiz's tumour)

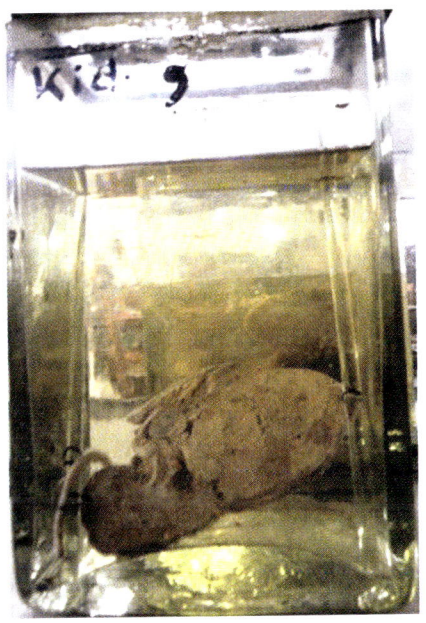

Fig. 15.22: Renal cell carcinoma

Q. What are the light microscopic features of renal cell carcinoma?

Ans: The most common variant is clear cell variant RCC (70–80%). Other variants are RCC papillary (chromophil) type (10–15%), RCC chromophobe type (5%), Bellini duct carcinoma (rare) and Xp11 translocation RCC (rare).

In clear cell carcinoma the tumour cells are arranged in sheets to trabecular (cord like) or tubular (resembling tubules) pattern. The tumour cells are round or polygonal in shape. They have abundant clear cytoplasm, which contains glycogen and lipid. The tumour has delicate branching vasculature. Centrally placed round nuclei with nucleoli seen with vasculature. Centrally placed round nuclei with nucleoli seen within tumour cells.

Q. What special stains may be used to demonstrate constituents in clear cytoplasm of carcinoma cells?

Ans: Tumour cells are rich in glycogen which may be demonstrated by PAS (Periodic acid–Schiff) stain on formalin-fixed paraffin-embedded (FFPE) tissue sections.

Lipids (fats) are dissolved during processing of tissue in paraffin-embedded tissue sections. Hence, cannot be demonstrated in FFPE. Lipids can be identified by frozen section technique by applying fat stains (Sudan III, Sudan IV, Sudan black or Oil red O). There is no mucin in the cytoplasm of the tumour cells.

Q. What are the classic diagnostic features of RCC?

Ans: There are three classic diagnostic features: Haematuria, palpable renal mass and costovertebral pain. But these features combinedly seen only in 10% of cases. Haematuria which is intermittent in nature is the most reliable feature of these triads.

Renal Tuberculosis

Description: Mounted specimen of cut section of kidney in a jar showing following features:
- Kidney is slightly enlarged
- Cut section shows foci of caseous with formation of cavities in some. The caseous

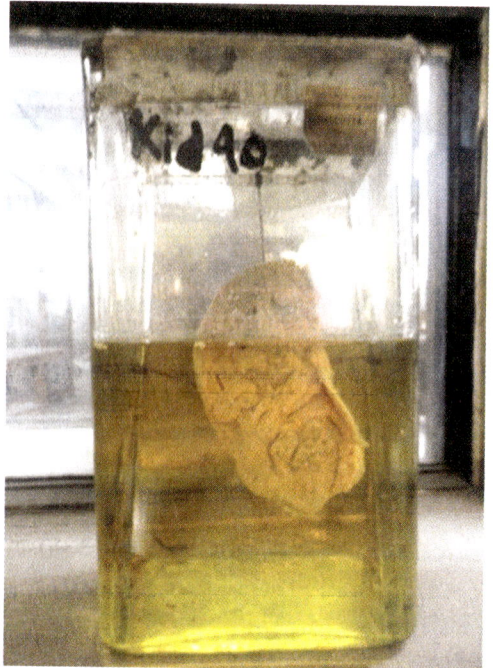

Fig. 15.23: Renal tuberculosis

areas are seen specially near base of pyramid. Wall of the cavities is irregular and caseous.
- Caseous material present within the cavities.
- Renal capsule and perinephric fat are adherent.

Diagnosis: Renal tuberculosis (caseous type)

Q. What are the different morphological types of renal tuberculosis?
Ans:
- Acute miliary tuberculosis
- Chronic ulcerative and caseous type
- Tuberculous pyonephrosis

Q. What is the pathogenesis of renal tuberculosis?
Ans: It is usually blood-borne and almost always secondary to an active tuberculosis lesion elsewhere. Infection starts at renal cortex and then it spreads to glomeruli. Later on, tuberculosis bacilli may progress to the adjacent tubules and peritubular tissues.

Q. What are urinary findings in renal tuberculosis?
Ans: Urine analysis reveals acidic pH, proteinuria and pus cells. It can cause asymptomatic pyuria or it may produce **sterile pyuria** (no organism detected in ordinary culture medium). LJ media or Bactec culture media will demonstrate *M. tuberculosis*.

BONE

Osteomyelitis and Sequestrum

Description: Mounted specimen of tibia in a jar showing following features:
- Tubular tibial bone with fragile bone and a large hole (**cloaca**).
- Dry, irregular piece of dead bone with granular surface (**sequestrum**) is seen through cloaca.
- Also seen sheath of living reactive oven or lamellar bone deposited around sequestrum. This is **involucrum**.

Diagnosis: Osteomyelits with sequestrum

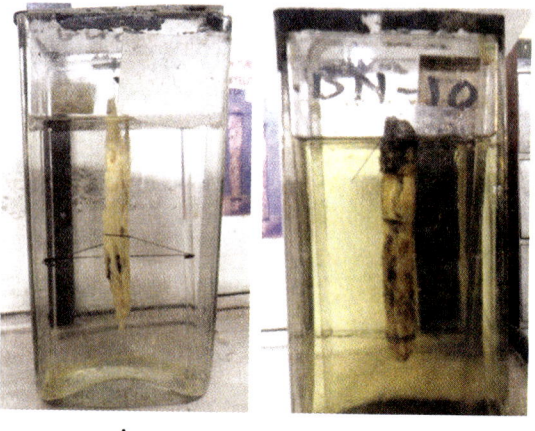

Fig. 15.24A and B: Chronic osteomyelitis and sequestrum

Q. What is sequestrum?
Ans: Due to rigid structure and limited space with bone, inflammatory exudates in bone cavity compress the endosteal blood vessels and impair the blood flow to the bone.

As a result erosion, thinning and infarction necrosis of cortical bone occurs which is known as **sequestrum**. Frequently, this dead bone detaches from main bone and floats inside the abscess cavity due to action of lytic enzymes.

Q. What is involucrum?
Ans: With passage of time, there is new bone formation beneath the periosteum over the infected bone which is known as **involucrum**. This involucrum has irregular surface and has perforations through which discharging sinus tract pass.

Q. What is Brodie's abscess?
Ans: Sometimes, acute osteomyelitis may be contained (limited) to a localized area and walled off by fibrous tissue and granulation tissue. This is known as Brodie's abscess.

Q. What are the causative organisms of osteomyelitis?
Ans: Pyogenic osteomyelitis is caused by *Staphylococcus aureus* (commonly), *E. coli*, Pseudomonas, Klebsiella and anaerobes. Tuberculous osteomyelitis is caused by *Mycobacterium tuberculosis*. Osteomyelitis also may occur in systemic infectious diseases like enteric fever (typhoid), actinomycosis, mycetoma (Madura foot), syphilis and brucellosis.

Q. What are the common sites of osteomyelitis?
Ans: It primarily affects the metaphyseal area of long bones of extremities around knee, hip and ankle joints. Tuberculous osteomyelitis usually involves vertebral column and less commonly hip bone, long bones (femur, tibia) and small bones of hands and feet.

TB (Tuberculosis) Spine

Description: Mounted specimen of a portion of spine (hemisection) in a jar showing following features:
- Destruction of a part of vertebral body and intervertebral disc.

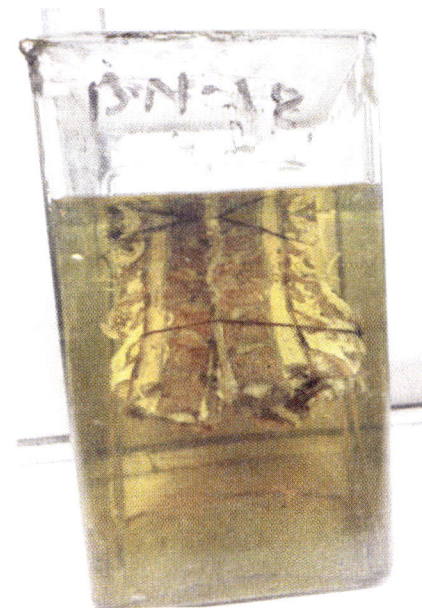

Fig. 15.25: TB spine

- The lesion starts in the bodies and spread through medullary cavity and breaks through intervertebral discs involving multiple vertebrae.
- It also extends into soft tissues forming cold abscess.
- The affected vertebrae are weak and tend to collapse, producing an acute anteflexion or angular kyphosis.
- Intervertebral space is diminished.

Diagnosis: Tuberculosis of spine (Pott's disease) with kyphosis.

Q. What is Caries spine or Pott's disease?
Ans: Tuberculosis of spine is known as Pott's disease. It often commences in the vertebral body and may be associated with compression fractures and destruction of intervertebral discs, producing permanent damage and paraplegia.

Q. What is cold abscess?
Ans: Extension of caseous material and pus from vertebrae (commonly lumbar) to the sheaths of psoas muscle produces cold abscess or psoas abscess.

Osteogenic Sarcoma

Description: Mounted specimen of lower end of femur in a jar showing following features:
- A bulk gray-white solid mass is seen at the lower end of femur.
- Cut surface is grayish-white with areas of haemorrhage and necrosis.
- The cortical bone is involved and destroyed. The tumour involves the medullary cavity.
- The tumour looks fleshy with irregular fusiform shape and located at the end of a long bone (femur) gives the lesion so-called **'leg of mutton' appearance**.
- Periosteum is elevated due to pressure of growth producing a triangle—**Codman's triangle**.

Diagnosis: Osteogenic sarcoma of femur (conventional intramedullary)

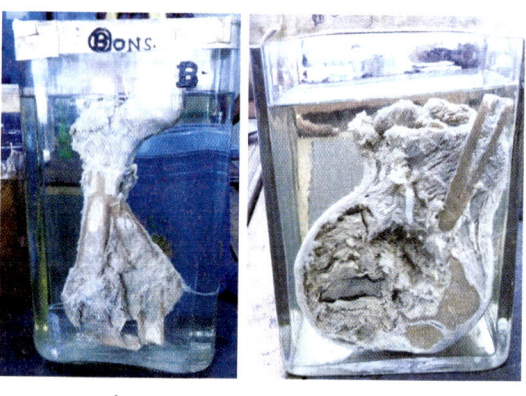

A B

Fig. 15.26A and B: Osteogenic sarcoma

Q. What are the types of osteosarcoma as per site of origin?

Ans: Osteosarcomas are classified into 3 types: Intramedullary, intracortical, surface.

Q. What are the different histologic variants?

Ans: Conventional type (osteoblastic, chondroblastic, fibroblastic); telangiectatic, small cell, giant cell, fibrohistiocytic, anaplastic and well differentiated osteosarcoma.

Q. What are the sites of osteosarcoma?

Ans: Most common sites, in descending order of frequency, lower end of femur and upper end of tibia (i.e. around the knee joint about 80%); the upper end of humerus (10%), pelvis and upper end of femur (i.e. around hip joint about 15%); and less often in jaw bones, skull and vertebrae.

Q. What is secondary osteosarcoma?

Ans: It develops following pre-existing bone disease, e.g. Paget's disease of bone, fibrous dysplasia, chronic osteomyelitis, multiple osteochondromas, bone infarcts and prior irradiation.

Giant Cell Tumour of Bone (Osteoclastoma)

Description: Mounted specimen of lower end of radius and ulna in a jar showing following features:
- A fusiform growth involving lower end of radius and ulna (epiphysis).
- The growth is red-brown, friable mass with areas of cystic degeneration due to necrosis.
- Foci of haemorrhage and necrosis seen.
- Due to presence of many small cystic spaces (degeneration), it has a honey-comb appearance.
- Cortex is thinned and eroded.

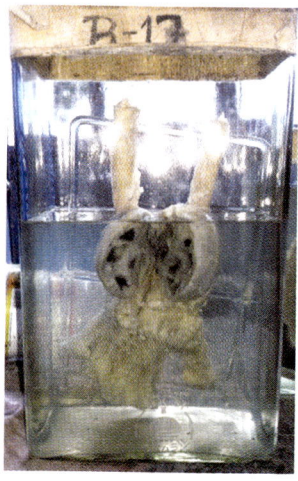

Fig. 15.27: Giant cell tumour of bone (osteoclastoma)

Diagnosis: Giant cell tumour of bone (osteoclastoma)

Q. What are the light microscopic features of GCT?
Ans: It is a biphasic tumour-composed of mononuclear stromal cells and multi-nucleated giant cells. The mononuclear stromal cells (tumour cells) are round to oval in shape, uniform with indistinct cell membrane. Multinucleated giant cells of osteoclastic type (>100 nuclei) are uniformly scattered among mononuclear stromal cells. The nuclei of stromal cells have identical features to that of the mononuclear cells.

Q. What are the common sites of GCT?
Ans: GCT arises in the epiphysis of long bones close to the articular cartilage. Most common sites are lower end of femur, upper end of tibia, lower end of radius and upper end of fibula.

Q. What are the other giant cells containing benign bone tumours?
Ans: Aneurysmal bone cyst, chondroblastoma, metaphyseal fibrous defect (non-ossifying fibroma), simple bone cyst, brown tumour of hyperparathyroidism, giant cell reparative granuloma and chondromyxoid fibroma.

Q. What are the radiographic findings?
Ans: On radiography, GCT gives **soap-bubble appearance**. It shows a large osteolytic eccentric lesion, which erodes into the subendosteal bone plate.

FEMALE GENITAL AND BREAST SPECIMENS

Fibroid Uterus (Leiomyoma)

Description: Mounted specimen of uterus in a jar showing following features:
- Hemisection of uterus and cervix showing one large nodular growth.
- These growths are well-circumscribed, whitish, glistening and encircled by fibrous capsule.

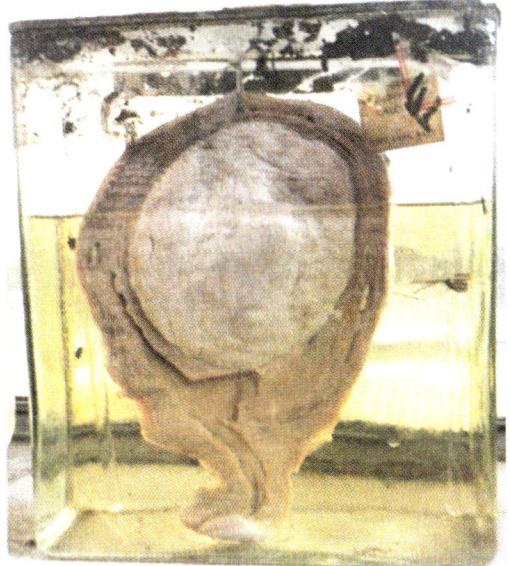

Fig. 15.28: Fibroid uterus

- These nodules have a typical whorled or so-called **'watered silk' appearances**.
- This growth is found within myometrium (intramural).
- Rest of the uterine muscle appears to be reddish-brown.

Diagnosis: Fibroid (leiomyoma) of uterus

Q. What are the common sites of leiomyoma?
Ans: Most commonly it occurs in the uterus. It also occurs in the cervix, broad-ligament, ovary, gastrointestinal tract, retroperitoneum, skin, etc.

Q. What are the light microscopic features?
Ans: Leiomyoma (fibroid) comprised of whorled bundles of well differentiated smooth muscle cells. Individual smooth muscle cells are uniform in size and shape containing oval nucleus and long slender bipolar cytoplasmic processes. Mitotic figures are sparse (rare).

Q. What are the other histological variants apart from common form?
Ans: Cellular leiomyoma or apoleptic leiomyoma, symplastic (bizarre) leiomyoma,

epithelioid leiomyoma, lipoleiomyoma, benign metastasizing leiomyoma and disseminated peritoneal leiomyomatosis.

Q. What are the secondary changes in leiomyoma (fibroid)?

Ans: These are hyaline change/degeneration, yellow-brown to red softening (cystic degeneration), atrophy, fatty change, red degeneration, dystrophic calcification and chondroid/osseous metaplasia.

Hyaline degeneration is the commonest secondary change in leiomyoma.

Carcinoma of Cervix

Description: Mounted specimen of uterus and cervix in a jar showing following features:

- A gray-white exophytic solid mass which projects above the surrounding mucosa.
- The surface is irregular
- The tumour involves the ectocervix and also lower part of endocervix.

Diagnosis: Carcinoma of cervix.

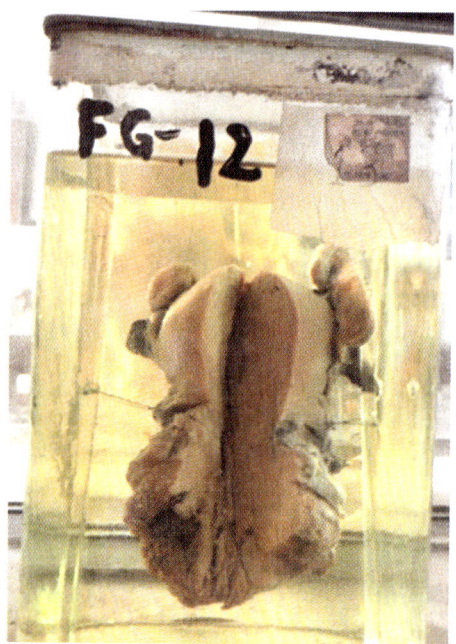

Fig. 15.29: Carcinoma of cervix

Q. What are the histologic variants of carcinoma of cervix?

Ans: Squamous cell carcinoma (80–90%), adenocarcinoma (10–20%), adenosquamous carcinoma (4%) and small cell carcinoma (rare).

Q. What are the risk factors for cervical carcinoma?

Ans:
i. Early sexual activity <16 years of age with multiple sexual partners.
ii. Human papillomavirus (HPV), type 16, 18, 31, 33; oncoproteins E6 and E7.
iii. Herpes simplex virus II and HPV: Synergetic.
iv. Molecular genetics: Mutation of p53 and RB tumour suppressor gene by HPV (16, 18, 31, 33) oncoproteins E6 and E7.
v. Cigarette smoking, immunosuppression, multiple pregnancies and oral contraceptive use.

Q. What are the modes of spread of cervical carcinoma?

Ans:
i. Lymphatic route: To pelvic lymph nodes (paracervical, obturator, external iliac, internal iliac, common iliac and aortic lymph nodes).
ii. Direct invasion: To parametrium. Compression of ureter.
iii. Haematogenous route: Distant metastases to lung, liver, bones and brain.

Dermoid (Teratoma) Tumour of Ovary

Description: Mounted specimen of already cut open ovarian cyst in a jar showing following features:
- External surface is smooth and ovary is enlarged.
- Already cut open ovary, showing a multilocular cyst containing sebaceous, greasy pultaceous/chessy material and tufts of hairs.
- Teeth are present in a well-defined nipple-like structure covered with hair, known as **Rokitansky's protuberance**.
- One firm to hard bony area is also present.

Museum Specimens

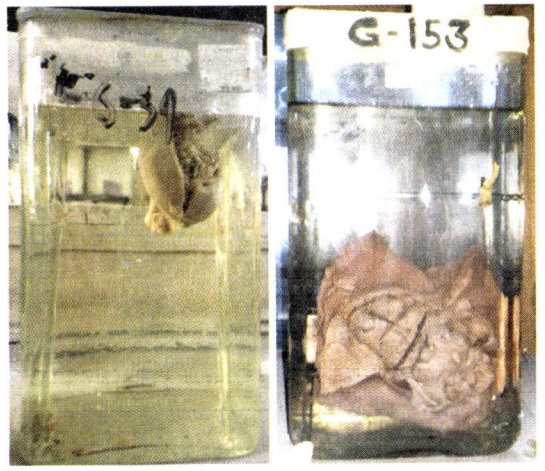

Fig. 15.30A and B: Dermoid (teratoma) of ovary

Diagnosis: Mature cystic teratoma (dermoid cyst) of ovary.

Q. What are the light microscopic features of mature cystic teratoma?
Ans: The cyst is lined by stratified squamous epithelium, sebaceous glands, hair shaft and other adnexal structures. Many tumours also exhibit cartilage, bone, teeth, smooth muscles and respiratory epithelium.

Q. What is immature teratoma?
Ans: This teratoma is composed of a mixture of embryonal and adult tissues derived from all three germ layers. Embryonal component of the tumour resembles tissues from an embryo or fetus. Immature cartilage, glands, muscle, bone and neural rosettes are present.

Q. What is malignant transformation of mature cystic teratoma?
Ans: Rarely (<1%) mature cystic teratoma may undergo malignant transformation. Malignancy is usually squamous cell carcinoma followed by carcinoid tumour, adenocarcinoma, thyroid carcinoma, melanoma, osteosarcoma, carcinosarcoma or glioblastoma multiforme.

Q. What are the other sites of teratoma?
Ans: Sacrococcygeal teratoma is the commonest site for embryonal teratoma and single most common tumour found in newborns of humans. Other sites are mediastinum, retroperitoneum, floor of mouth, urinary bladder, kidney, nasopharynx and base of skull.

Carcinoma of Breast

Description: Mounted specimen of breast (mastectomy) in a jar showing following features:

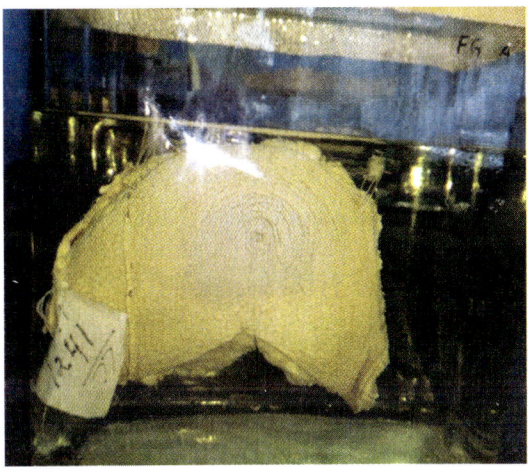

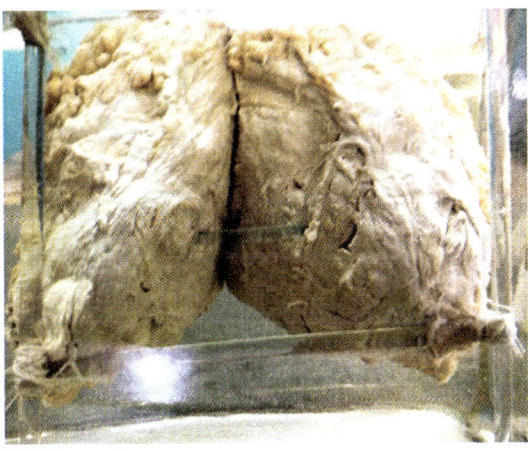

Fig. 15.31A and B: Carcinoma of breast

- A solid grayish-yellow growth is seen.
- The growth is irregular, poorly circumscribed and poorly defined margins.
- Foci of haemorrhage and necrosis are present.
- The growth extends or radiates through surrounding parenchyma into fat (crab-like configuration)
- Nipple is retracted.

Diagnosis: Carcinoma of breast

Q. What are the different histologic types of breast carcinoma?
Ans: It can be classified into two broad groups:

i. **Carcinoma *in situ* (15–30%):** Ductal carcinoma *in situ* (80%) and lobular carcinoma *in situ* (20%)

ii. **Invasive carcinoma (70–85%):** No special-type carcinoma (79%), lobular carcinoma (10%), tubular/cribriform carcinoma (6%), mucinous (colloid) carcinoma (2%), medullary carcinoma (2%), papillary carcinoma (1%), metaplastic carcinoma (<1%).

Q. What are the common locations of breast carcinoma?
Ans: In decreasing frequency it is located in upper outer quadrant (50%), central region beneath nipple (20%), lower outer quadrant (10%), upper inner quadrant (10%) and lower inner quadrant (10%) respectively.

Q. What are the risk factors of breast cancers?
Ans: Older age (>50 years), family history of breast cancer, genetic mutations (such as BRCA1 and BRCA2), early menarche (<12 years), late menopause (>55 years), late or no pregnancy, taking oral contraceptive pills, using combination therapy as hormone replacement, drinking alcohol, smoking, physical inactivity, obesity after menopause, etc.

Q. What are the major prognostic factors?
Ans:
i. Tumour size: <1 cm good prognosis, >2 cm bad prognosis
ii. Invasive carcinoma has worse prognosis than *in situ* carcinoma
iii. Involvement of axillary lymph nodes is associated with worse prognosis.
iv. Distant metastasis indicates bad prognosis.
v. Inflammatory carcinoma carries poor prognosis
vi. Local invasion into adjacent skeletal muscle carries poor prognosis.

Q. What are the good prognostic factors?
Ans: Age group 30–50 years, early diagnosis, early treatment, certain histologic types (ductal carcinoma *in situ*, lobular carcinoma *in situ*, low grade invasive ductal carcinoma (NOS)—luminal type A, cribriform carcinoma—luminal type A, tubular carcinoma—luminal type A, papillary carcinoma, colloid carcinoma), negative expression of C-erB2, p53, Srp27, cathepsin D and EGFR, tumor size <2 cm, estrogen and progesterone receptor positivity.

MALE GENITAL SPECIMENS

Carcinoma of Penis

Description: Mounted specimen of penis in a jar has following features:

- A large cauliflower-like fungating mass having rolled out and everted margin.
- The mass arises from the glans penis and inner surface of the prepuce.
- The surface of the mass is ulcerated
- Resected margin of penis (opposite side of growth) is grossly unremarkable.

Diagnosis: Carcinoma of penis (squamous cell carcinoma)

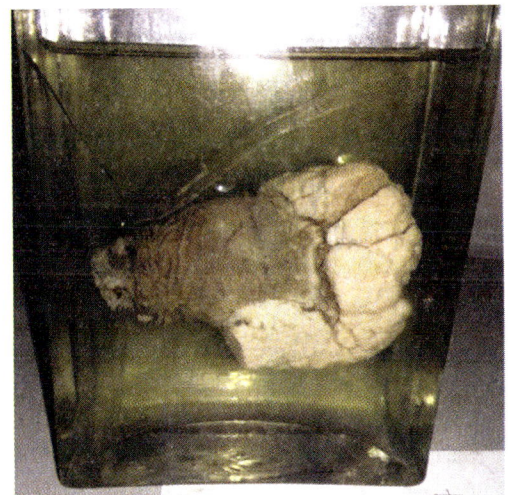

Fig. 15.32: Carcinoma of penis

Q. What are the risk factors of carcinoma of penis?
Ans: HPV type 16, type 18 and cigarette smoking are risk factors. HPV DNA can be detected in penile squamous cell carcinoma in about 50% of patients.

Males with bad genital hygiene and without circumcision have more chances to exposure to carcinogens and subsequently developing carcinoma of penis.

Q. What is verrucous carcinoma?
Ans: This is an exophytic well-differentiated variant of squamous cell carcinoma which has low malignant potential. These tumours are locally invasive but they rarely metastasize.

Q. What are the histologic subtypes of squamous cell carcinoma?
Ans: Keratinising squamous cell carcinoma (SCC), non-keratinising SCC, basaloid SCC, warty carcinoma and papillary variants of SCC.

Seminoma of Testis

Description: Mounted specimen of bisected testis in a jar has following features:
- Large homogeneous gray-white mass.
- The mass has lobulated cut surface.
- No haemorrhage or necrosis.
- Tunica albuginea is not penetrated by the tumour.

Diagnosis: Seminoma of testis

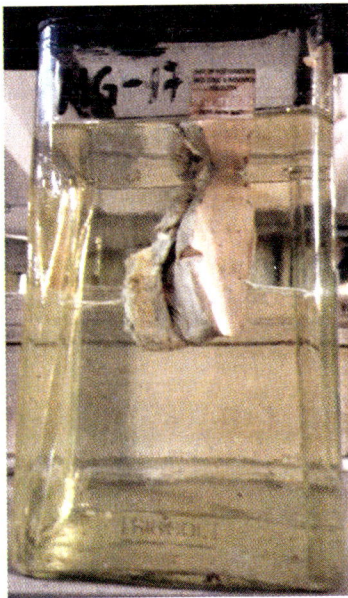

Fig. 15.33: Seminoma of testis

Q. What are the histologic variants of seminoma?
Ans: Classic seminoma is the most common variant (85–90%) of all cases. Other variants are anaplastic seminoma, spermatocytic seminoma, seminoma with syncytiotrophoblastic element and seminoma with yolk sac element.

Q. What are the light microscopic features of classic seminoma?
Ans: Monomorphic polyhedral large cells arranged in sheets and divided by fibrous septa. The tumour cells have distinct cell membrane and abundant clear cytoplasm and a large central nucleus with one or two prominent nucleoli. The fibrous septa is infiltrated by lymphocytes. Mitoses are scant.

Occasionally granulomas with giant cells may be present.

Q. What are the routes of metastasis?
Ans:
i. Lymphatic route: To retroperitoneal/para-aortic, mediastinal and supraclavicular lymph nodes.
ii. Blood or haematogenous route: To lungs, liver and brains.

Benign Hyperplasia of Prostate

Description: Mounted specimen of prostate in a jar having following features:
- Enlarged prostate with multiple gray-white rubbery nodules of variable sizes.
- Cut surface shows solid mass with a few microcysts.
- Nodules compress the urethra (prostatic) into a slit-like lumen.

Diagnosis: Benign hyperplasia of prostate (BHP) or nodular hyperplasia.

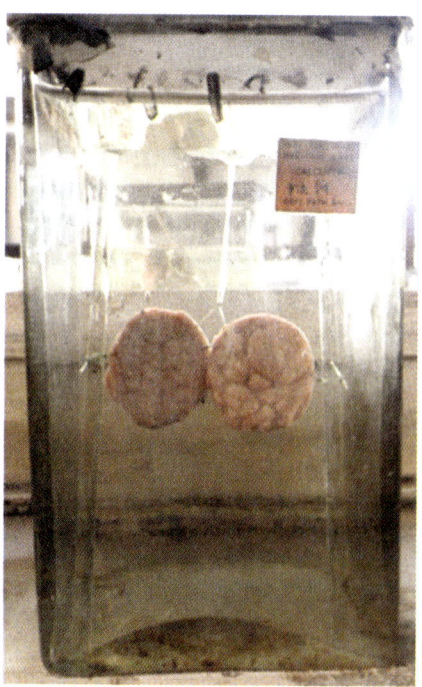

Fig. 15.34: Benign hyperplasia of prostate (BHP)

Q. What are the clinical features of BHP?
Ans: Male patients are usually elderly (>60 years). They experience increased urinary frequency, nocturia, difficulty and in starting and stopping the stream of urine, overflow dribbling, dysuria (painful micturition) and have an increased risk of developing bacterial infection of the bladder and kidney (UTI).

Q. What are the light microscopic features of BHP?
Ans: There is adenoleiomyomatous hyperplasia of prostate, i.e. hyperplasia of smooth muscles and glands. The glands are of different sizes and are lined by two layers of epithelium—inner columner and outer flattened myoepithelial cell layer (basal cell layer). Stroma is composed of fibromuscular tissue.

Q. Which zone is affected by BHP?
Ans: Prostate has 3 zones: Central zone, transition zone and peripheral zone. Transition zone is the site for BHP, whereas peripheral zone is the site for prostatic cancer.

HEPATOBILIARY SYSTEM SPECIMENS

Micronodular Cirrhosis

Description: Mounted specimen of liver in a jar has following features:
- Liver is shrunken and atrophic. Approximate weight would be 900 gm (normal 1440–1660 gm or 3.2–3.7 pounds).
- Surface is irregular and multiple small nodules of <3 mm in size are seen.
- Colour of liver is yellowish-orange.
- Consistency of liver is firm
- Gall bladder is seen in the gall bladder fossa of liver (inferior surface).

Diagnosis: Cirrhosis of liver (micronodular variant)

Q. What are the different types of cirrhosis based on morphology?
Ans: There are 3 types of cirrhosis:
i. Micronodular: Nodules measuring <3 mm in size.

Museum Specimens

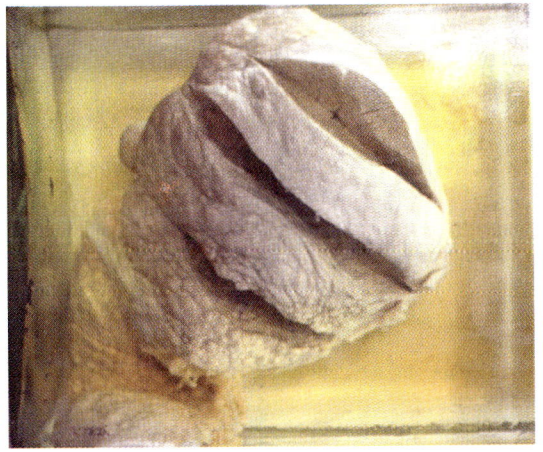

A

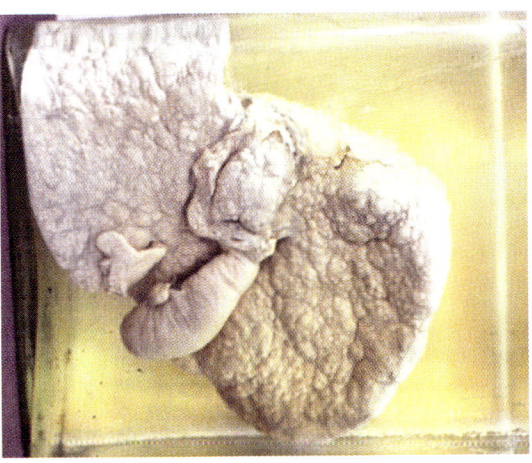

B

Fig. 15.35A and B: Micronodular cirrhosis

ii. Macronodular: Nodules measuring >3 mm in size
iii. Mixed or micro-macronodular cirrhosis: Both micronodules (<3 mm) and macronodules (>3 mm) are present.

Q. What are the causes of micronodular cirrhosis?
Ans: Alcoholic cirrhosis, primary biliary cirrhosis, hereditary haemochromatosis, hepatic venous outflow obstruction (Budd-Chiari syndrome, veno-occlusive disease), large bile duct obstruction, Indian childhood cirrhosis.

Q. What are the causes of macronodular cirrhosis?
Ans: Chronic viral hepatitis (HBV or HCV), cryptogenic cirrhosis, Wilson's disease, α_1-antitrypsin deficiency, drugs and toxins.

Q. What are the causes of mixed nodular cirrhosis?
Ans: Most common cause is alcoholic liver disease. Other causes are viral hepatitis (B, C, D), haemochromatosis, biliary disease and Wilsons's disease.

Q. What are the light microscopic features of cirrhosis?
Ans:
- Liver architecture is disrupted. Initially the developing fibrous septa are delicate and extend through sinusoids from central to portal tract or portal to portal tract.
- Regenerative activity of entrapped parenchymal hepatocytes generate uniform micronodules. Later on, these micronodules become larger and none prominent to produce macronodules. These scattered larger nodules create a 'hobnail' appearance on the surface of liver.
- Hepatocytes look normal in some nodules while they may be irregular with dysplastic changes in other nodules.

FATTY LIVER

Description: Mounted specimen of liver in a jar has following feature:
- The liver is enlarged and approximate weight is 5 kg.
- Liver is soft in consistency.
- It is yellow and greasy.

Diagnosis: Fatty liver

Q. What is microvesicular and macrovesicular hepatic steatosis (fatty liver)?
Ans: With moderate intake of alcohol, initially small droplets of lipid (triglyceride) accumulate within cytoplasm of hepatocytes and produce **microvesicular steatosis**.

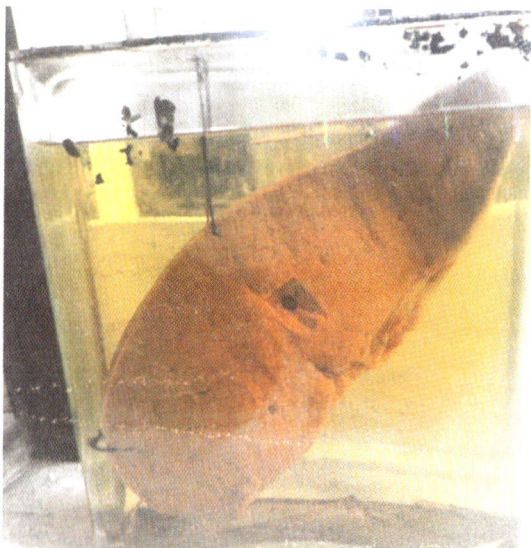

Fig. 15.36: Fatty liver

With chronic intake of alcohol, accumulated lipid droplets create large, clear globules that compress and displace the hepatocyte nucleus. These larger lipid droplets in cytoplasm produce **macrovesicular steatosis**.

Q. What are the causes of microvesicular steatosis?
Ans: Apart from alcoholism, other causes are tetracyclines, acute fatty liver of pregnancy, Reye's syndrome and hepatitis C.

Q. What are the causes of macrovesicular steatosis?
Ans: Apart from alcoholism (ethanol), other causes are obesity, diabetes, corticosteroids, methotrexate and total parenteral nutrition.

Q. What are the light microscopic features of fatty liver?
Ans: Initially there is a little or no fibrosis at the outset. But with continues alcohol intake (commonest cause) fibrous septa develop around the terminal hepatic veins and extend into the adjacent sinusoids. But this fatty change is completely reversible if the cause/injury is withdrawn (commonly alcohol intake).

Metastatic Liver

Description: Mounted specimen of cut section of liver in a jar has following features:
- Liver shows multiple nodular growths of different sizes.

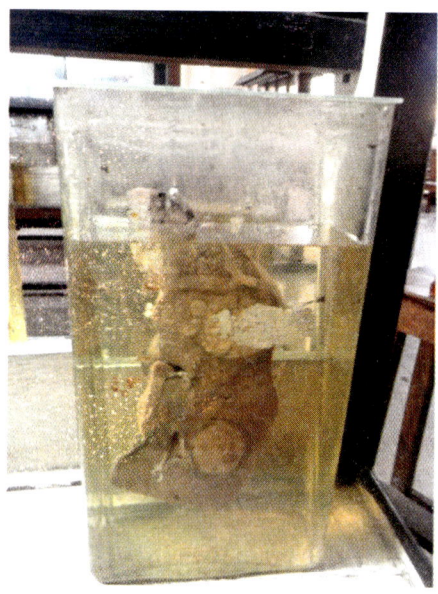

A

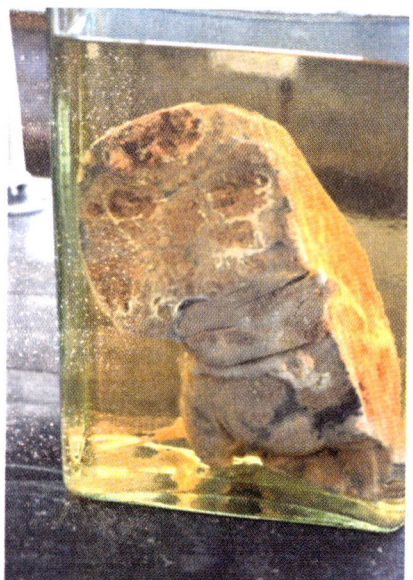

B

Fig. 15.37A and B: Metastatic liver

- These nodules are yellowish-white in colour.
- Central part of many of these nodules is depressed (umbilication).
- There are areas of haemorrhage (blackish) and necrosis.
- Cystic changes are also seen.

Diagnosis: Metastatic carcinoma of liver

Q. What are the primary sites which cause liver metastasis?
Ans:
i. **Metastasis from epithelial cancer:** Breast, lung, stomach, colon, rectum, pancreas, kidney, prostate, endometrium, thyroid.
ii. **Metastasis from mesenchymal malignancies:** Angiosarcoma, rhabdomyosarcoma.
iii. **Metastasis from round cell tumours:** Wilms' tumour, neuroblastoma, Ewing's sarcoma, bronchial carcinoid.
iv. **Haematolymphoid malignancies:** Leukaemic infiltration (common), NHL (non-Hodgkin lymphoma)

Q. How IHC (immunohistochemistry) can help for confirmatory diagnosis?
Ans:
- Epethial cancer (carcinoma): EMA (epithelial membrane antigen) and pan-CK (cytokeratin)
- Rhabdomyosarcoma: MyoD1, desmin, vimentin, myogenin
- Wilms' tumour: WT1 and WT2
- Neuroblastoma: NSE (neuron-specific enolase), synaptophysin, chromogranin, neurofilament
- Ewing's sarcoma: CD99 (MIC2), vimentin and NSE
- Bronchial carcinoid: NSE, synaptophysin, chromogranin
- NHL B cell: CD45, CD20, CD19
- NHL T cell: CD45, CD3, CD5
- Leukaemia: B or T cell markers, immunophenotyping (flow cytometry)

Gall Stones

Description: Mounted specimen of cut open gall bladder in a jar has following features:
- Multiple faceted, round to ovoid, pale yellow stones are seen.
- These stones have finely granular, hard external surface
- Gall bladder wall is thick.
- Gall bladder mucosa is reddened and irregular as a result of coexistent chronic cholecystitis.

Diagnosis: Cholesterol gall stones with chronic cholecystitis.

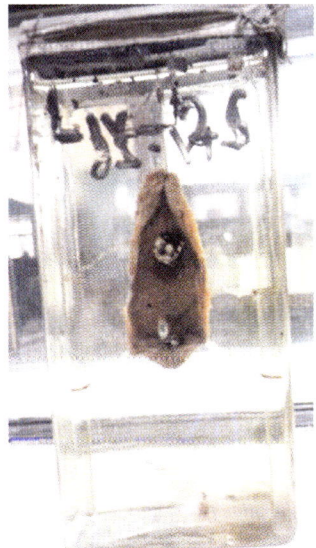

Fig. 15.38: Gall stones

Q. What are the different types of gall stones?
There are two main types—cholesterol stones and pigment stones. More than 90% are gall stones which contain >50% of crystalline cholesterol monohydrate.

The remaining are pigment stones composed predominantly of bilirubin calcium salts.

There are mixed cholesterol stones also. These mixed stones contain 50% cholesterol and rest mucoprotein, calcium and bilirubin.

Q. What are the predisposing factors for gall stone formation?

Ans: Risk factors for cholesterol stones are female sex, diabetes mellitus, pregnancy, hyperlipidaemia, estrogen therapy, bile stasis and inborn errors of bile acid metabolism.

Risk factors for pigmented stones are haemolytic syndromes, severe ileal dysfunction (or bypass) and bacterial contamination of biliary tree. Also, some parasitic infections of bilary tract like *Ascaris lumbricoides* and liver fluke O may lead to pigmented gall stone formation.

Q. Which gall stones are radio-opaque?

Ans: Black pigmented gallstones are radio-opaque due to presence of calcium carbonate and phosphates and approximately 50–75% black stones are radio-opaque.

Q. Which gall stones are radiolucent?

Ans: Pure cholesterol stones and stones composed largely of cholesterol are radiolucent. Also, brown pigmented gall stones are radiolucent.

Q. What are the complications of gall stone?

Ans: Most common complication is severe biliary colic or pain which tends to be excruciating and constant or "colicky" (spasmodic). Other complications include obstructive jaundice, ascending cholangitis and acute pancreatitis.

Less common complications are acute cholecystitis, empyema, perforation of gall bladder, porcelain gall bladder, mucocele of gall bladder, gall stone ileus and rarely squamous cell carcinoma.

Part V

Problem Cards and Discussion

16. Problem Cards

16

Problem Cards

PC 1

Q1. What is this black discolouration? 1

Q2. Define this pathological process. 1

Q3. What are the causes? 1

Q4. What are the different types of this pathological process? 1

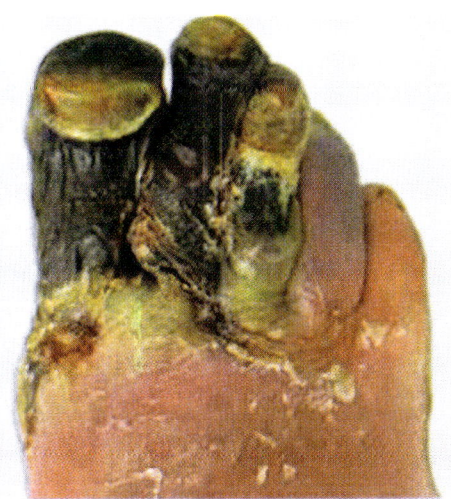

Fig. 16.1

PC 2

Q1. What is this intensely eosinophilic cell in the epidermis? 1

Q2. Give two examples of physiological conditions of this process? 1

Q3. Give two examples of pathological conditions of this process. 1

Q4. What is the most characteristic morphological feature? 1

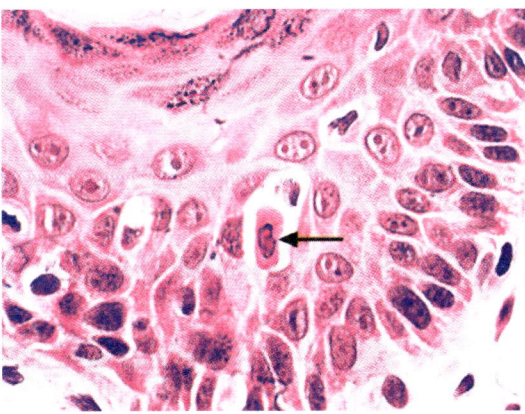

Fig. 16.2

PC 3

A 52-year-old poor man suffering from fever and cough for 2 months with cervical lymphadenopathy. Cervical lymph node shows following histological features:

Q1. What is the diagnosis of the disease? 1

Q2. What particular cells have been focused by arrows? 1

Q3. Which cytokines play an important role in pathogenesis? 2

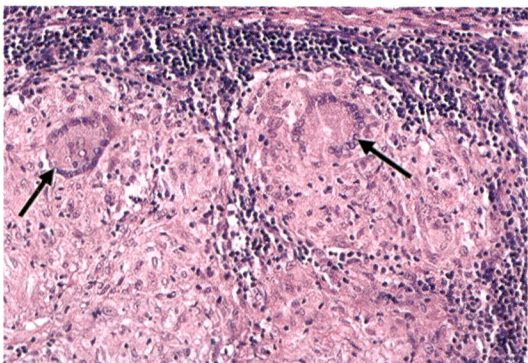

Fig. 16.3

PC 4

A 47-year-old female who had varicose veins in left leg and was on prolonged rest after hysterectomy. She suddenly developed swelling of left leg, pain and red or discoloured skin of left leg.

Q1. What is the diagnosis? 1
Q2. Name the triad and component which predisposes to the pathophysiology. 1
Q3. Name some hereditary (primary) factors which can cause it. 1
Q4. What are the microscopic features of this pathologic lesion? 1

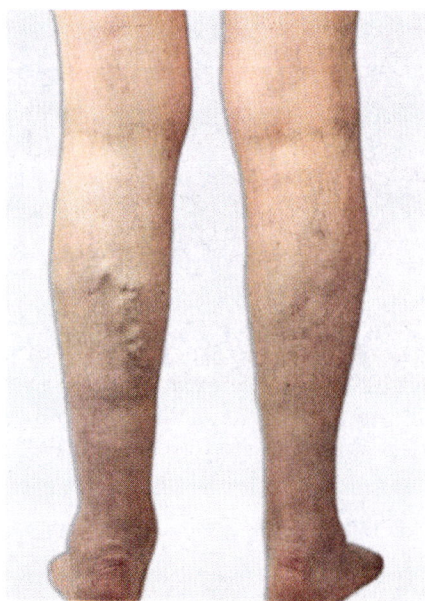

Fig. 16.4

PC 5

A patient had clinical diagnosis of splenic artery occlusion following thromboembolism. Cut section of the spleen shows following morphological features:

Q1. What is the diagnosis? 1
Q2. Why this pathologic lesions are white? 1
Q3. In which organs red-coloured lesions of same pathologic process are seen? 1
Q4. What are the properties of this pathologic lesion? 1

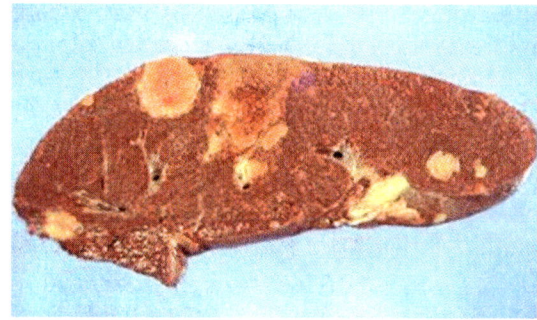

Fig. 16.5

PC 6

A baby was born with severe mental retardation (IQ 30) with flat facial profile, oblique palpebral fissures, epicanthic folds and congenital heart defects.

Q1. What is this genetic disorder? 1
Q2. What are the chromosomal changes? 1
Q3. What is the most common cause? 1
Q4. What are the future complications? 1

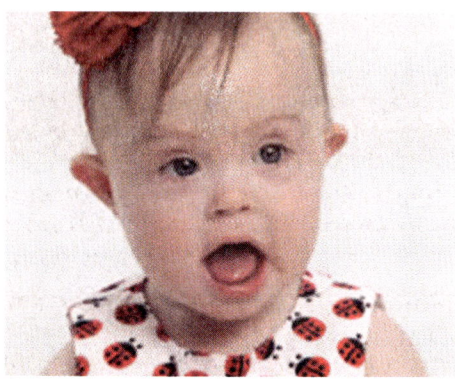

Fig. 16.6

PC 7

A person was given penicillin injection for treatment without a test dose. Within a few minutes (10 minutes) he develops mucosal secretion (nasal, conjunctival), smooth muscle contraction and oedema.

Q1. What is the diagnosis? 1
Q2. Which cell is responsible for this reaction? 1
Q3. Which chemical mediators are responsible for this? 1
Q4. Which antibody is most important to cause this reaction? 1

PC 8

An adult person presents with fever, severe weight loss, generalized lymphadenopathy and opportunistic infections. History reveals that he had unprotected sex in brothels.

Q1. What is the diagnosis? 1
Q2. How does CD4+ T cell count help to diagnose the disease? 1
Q3. What neoplasms may develop in these patients? 1
Q4. What are the most sensitive and specific tests? 1

PC 9

A patient had died of multiple myeloma and chronic inflammatory diseases. During autopsy, liver was found to be enlarged. Cut section of liver was firm and had a waxy appearance. Painting the cut surface with iodine imparts a yellow colour which transformed to blue violet after application of sulphuric acid (H_2SO_4).

Q1. What is the diagnosis? 1
Q2. What other organs may be involved? 1
Q3. Name two special stains to diagnose this disease and their colours. 1
Q4. What are the biopsy sites for microscopic examinations?

PC 10

A patient had a small firm tumour (1.5 × 1.3 cm) on arm for several years. It was surgically resected. Grossly, the tumour is well circumscribed and white-glistening. Microscopically it is found to be nerve sheath origin.

Q1. From history and gross, is it a benign tumour or malignant tumour? 1
Q2. What morphological features (microscopical) differentiate a benign and malignant tumour? 2
Q3. Mention two differences between carcinoma and sarcoma. 1

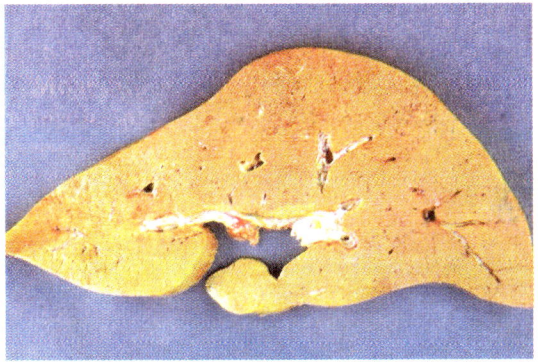

Fig. 16.7

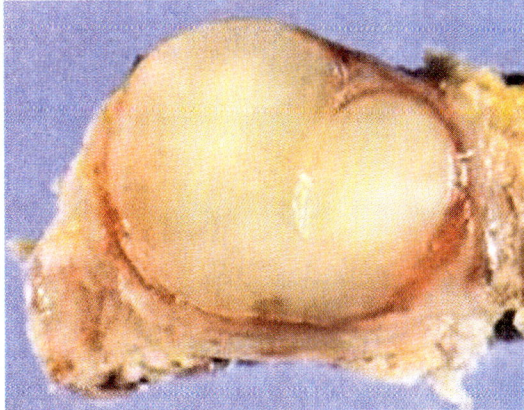

Fig. 16.8

PC 11

A 58-year-old male patient developed yellowish discolouration of conjunctiva and skin. Biochemical investigation reveals increased bilirubin, serum transaminases (SGOT and SGPT) and hepatitis viral antigens and antibodies.

Q1. What is this clinical condition?
Q2. What is the normal value of bilirubin in adults? 1
Q3. Mention some causes of unconjugated hyperbilirubinaemia. 1
Q4. Mention some causes of conjugated hyperbilirubinaemia. 1

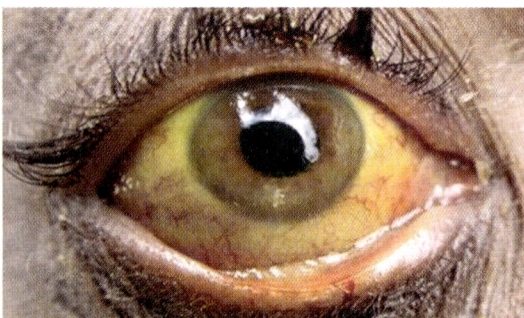

Fig. 16.9

PC 12

A 52-year-old patient had tuberculosis and chest X-ray show following features.
Q1. What is the provisional diagnosis based on chest X-ray? 1
Q2. What will be glucose and protein value in this fluid compared to plasma? 1
Q3. What will be LDH content and fluid LDH/serum LDH ratio? 1
Q4. What is anasarca? 1

PC 13

A 5-year-old girl is suffering from fever, anaemia, bone pain and generalised lymphadenopathy. Peripheral blood smear and flow cytometry reveal the following features.
Q1. What is the diagnosis? 1
Q2. What will be the bone marrow picture? 1
Q3. Which marker/markers are positive in the flow cytometry? 1
Q4. Which special stain can be used for these abnormal cells? 1

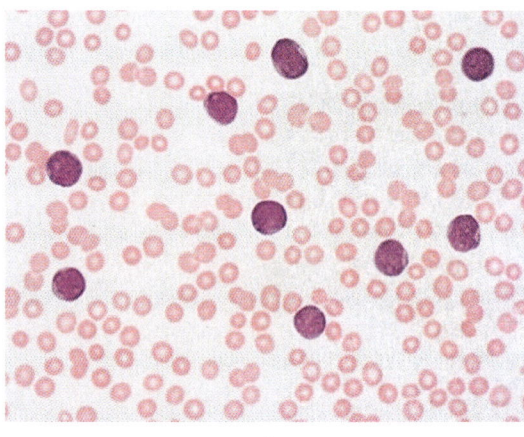

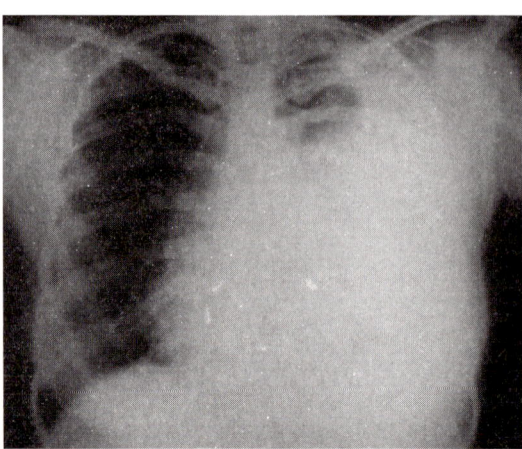

Fig. 16.10

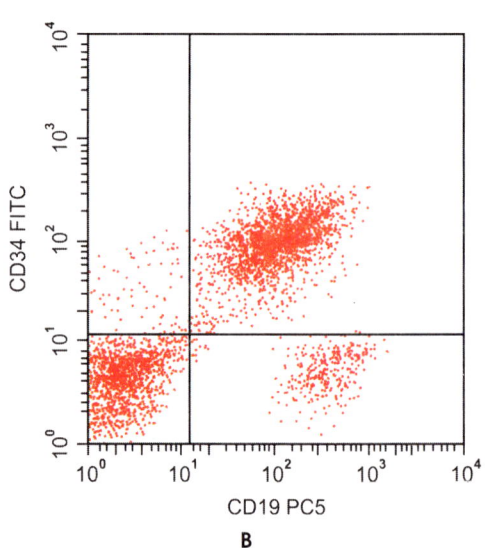

Fig. 16.11A and B

PC 14

A middle-aged man suffering from fatigue, fever and gum bleeding. His bone marrow smear shows the following features:
Q1. What is the diagnosis? 1
Q2. What is that constituent in the cytoplasm of cells indicated by arrow? 1
Q3. Why there is gum bleeding? 1
Q4 What markers are positive in flow cytometry (immunophenotyping)? 1

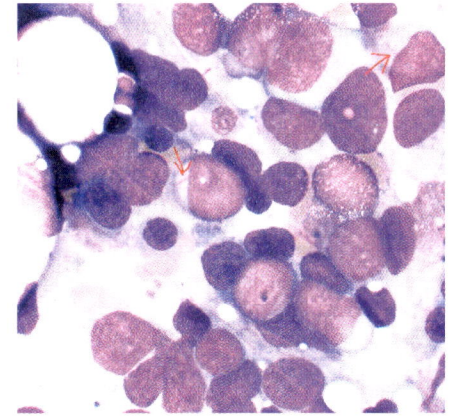

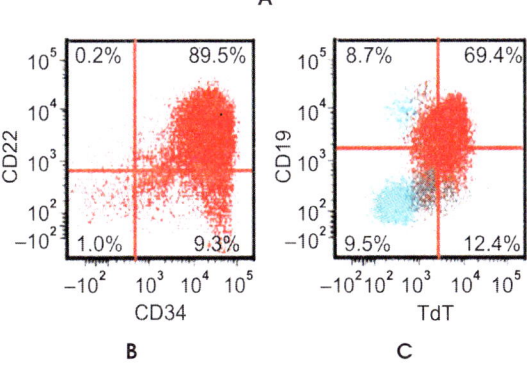

Fig. 16.12A to C

PC 15

A 56-year-old female patient is suffering from moderate anaemia, weakness, fatigability and dragging sensation in the abdomen. TLC is 108,000/mm^3.

Peripheral blood smear has following features:

Q1. What is the diagnosis? 1
Q2. Why there is dragging sensation in the abdomen? 1
Q3. Which particular chromosome can be detected in this case? 1
Q4. What will be the NAP (neutrophil alkaline phosphatase) score? 1

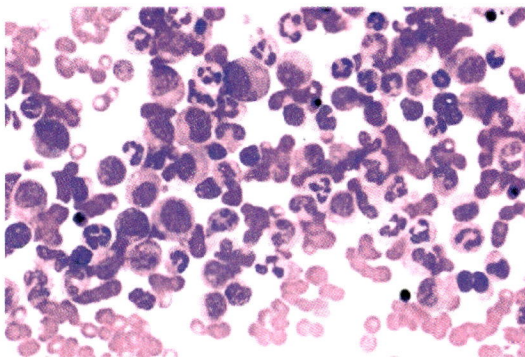

Fig. 16.13

PC 16

A 60-year-old male patient is suffering from anaemia and symmetrically enlarged, discrete and non-tender lymph nodes. Peripheral blood smear shows the following features:

Q1. What is the diagnosis? 1
Q2. Why 10–15% of these patients develop haemolytic anaemia?
Q3. What aggressive tumour may develop in these patients? 1
Q4. What immunomarkers will be positive? 1

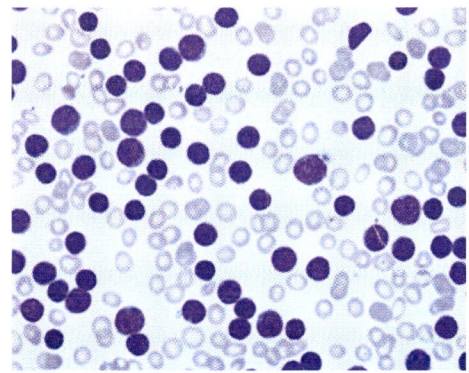

Fig. 16.14

PC 17

A young adult presented with painless lymphadenopathy (potato size cervical lymph node). He also had constitutional symptoms like fever, night sweats and weight loss. Microscopy of lymph node and IHC staining have following features:

Q1. What is the diagnosis? 1
Q2. Which variant of the disease is shown in the upper right picture? 1
Q3. Which markers are positive for the neoplastic cells (lower left)? 1
Q4. Which variant of the disease is shown in the lower right picture? 1

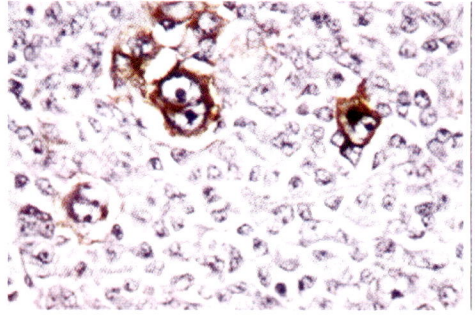

C

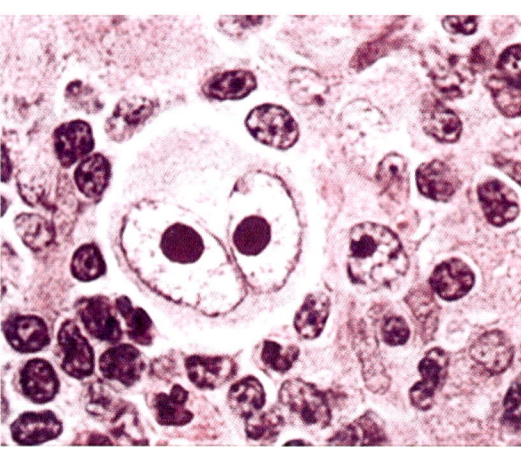

A

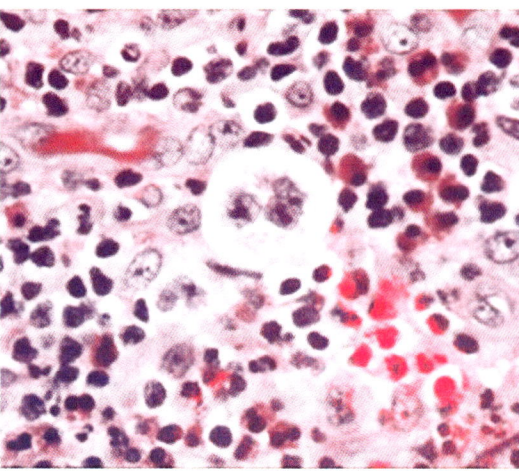

B

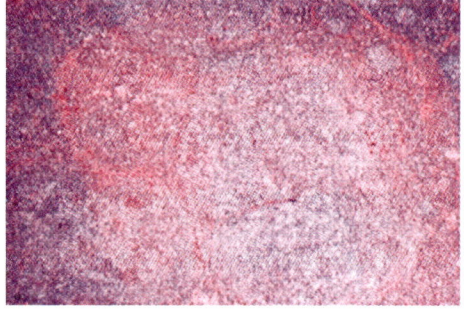

D

Fig. 16.15A to D

PC 18

An elderly woman suffering from bone pain, pathologic fractures and renal failure. Bone marrow aspirates have following microscopic features:

Q1. What is the diagnosis? 1
Q2. What will be found in serum electrophoresis? 1
Q3. What may be found in X-ray of skull? 1
Q4. What will be urinary findings? 1

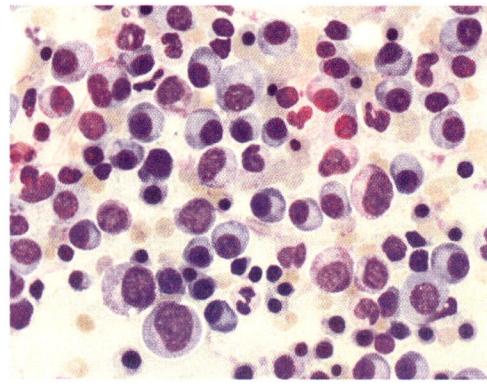

Fig. 16.16

PC 19

A 38-year-old female presented with pinpoint haemorrhages (petechiae) in the dependent areas and ecchymoses. Spleen is of normal size. But microscopy of spleen has following features:
Q1. What is the diagnosis? 1
Q2. What will be the peripheral blood picture? 1
Q3. What will be bone marrow picture? 1
Q4. Is there any antibody for the pathogenesis? 1

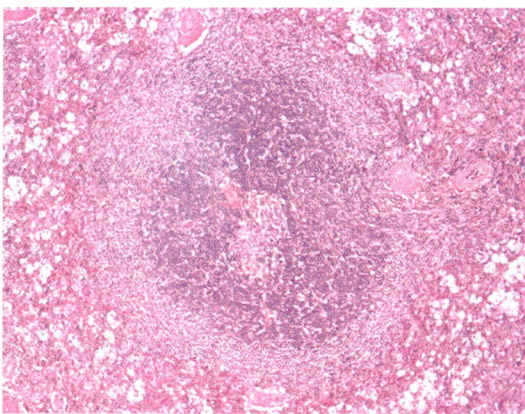

Fig. 16.17

PC 20

A pregnant lady is suffering from weakness, extreme fatigue and skin pallor. Peripheral blood smear shows the following features:
Q1. What is your diagnosis? 1
Q2. What will be bone marrow findings? 1

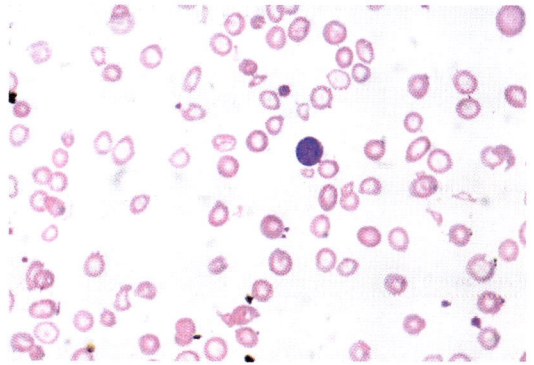

Fig. 16.18

Q3. What biochemical investigations will help to reach the diagnosis? 2

PC 21

A 62-year-old female is suffering from anaemia. Bone marrow has following features:
Q1. What is the diagnosis? 1
Q2. What are the features seen in peripheral blood? 2
Q3. Describe the particular cell in the bone marrow. 1

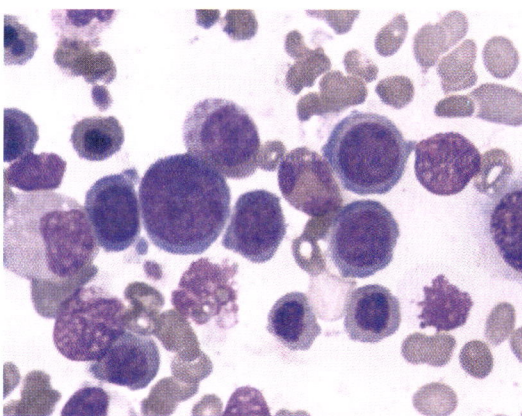

Fig. 16.19

PC 22

A 7-year-old child is suffering from anaemia, priapism and bone pain. Peripheral blood smear has the following features:
Q1. What is the diagnosis? 1
Q2. What is the molecular defect? 1

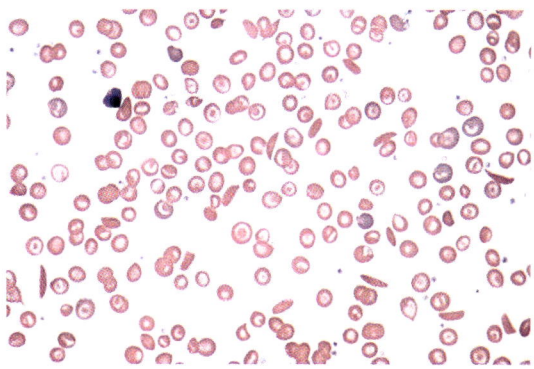

Fig. 16.20

Pathology Practicals

Q3. Which organs are affected by vaso-occlusive or pain crises? 1
Q4. What particular blood test is helpful? 1

PC 23

A patient presented with anaemia, splenomegaly and jaundice. Peripheral blood smear has following features:
Q1. What is the diagnosis?
Q2. What is the molecular defect? 1
Q3. What is the cause of aplastic crises in these patients? 1
Q4. Which particular laboratory test (simple and cost-effective) will help to diagnose? 1

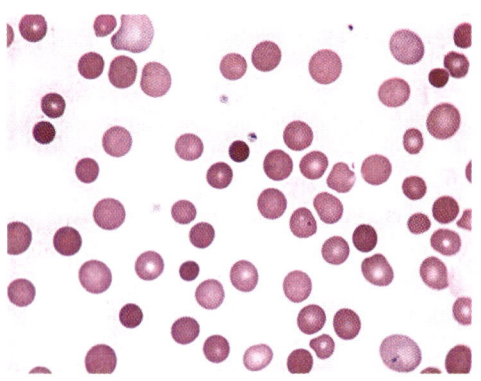

Fig. 16.21

PC 24

A child is suffering from growth retardation, severe anaemia, hepatosplenomegaly and prominent cheek bones. Mother is also known to suffer from the disease. Haemoglobin electrophoresis shows the following features:

a. Upper panel—normal control
b. Middle panel—affected mother
c. Lower panel—affected child

Q1. What is the disease in child? 1
Q2. What is the disease in affected mother? 1
Q3. What will be peripheral blood pictures? 1
Q4. Why there is crew-cut appearance on X-ray? 1

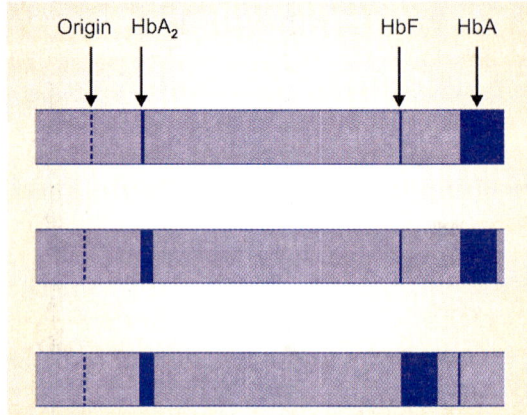

Fig. 16.22

PC 25

During marriage negotiation both the bride and groom underwent blood testing for HPLC. The groom has the following HPLC features:

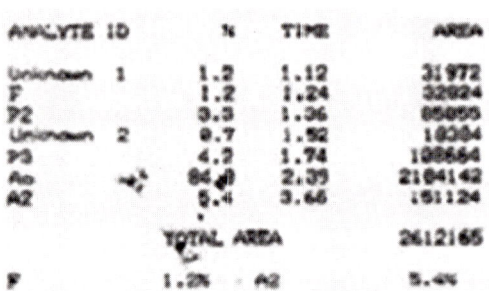

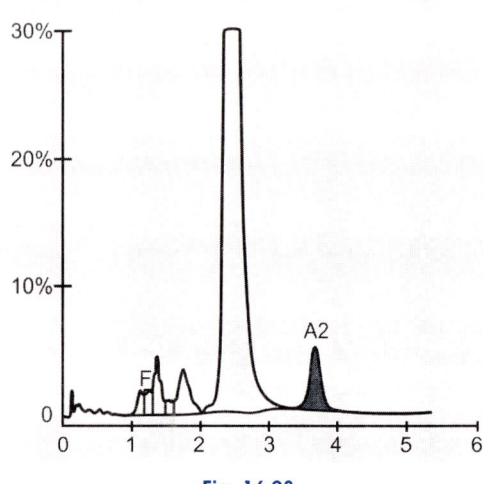

Fig. 16.23

Q1. What is your diagnosis? 1
Q2. What will be genotypic defect in this person? 1
Q3. Will there be any anaemia? 1
Q4. What will be finding in Hb electrophoresis? 1

PC 26

A 56-year-old male is suffering from fever, productive cough and chest pain. TLC is 18000/mm³ with neutrophilia. Chest X-ray shows following features:
Q1. What is your diagnosis? 1
Q2. What is the finding in air bronchogram (chest X-ray)? 1
Q3. What is the commonest organism in nosocomial form of this disease? 1
Q4. What will be histologic findings in lung biopsy? 1

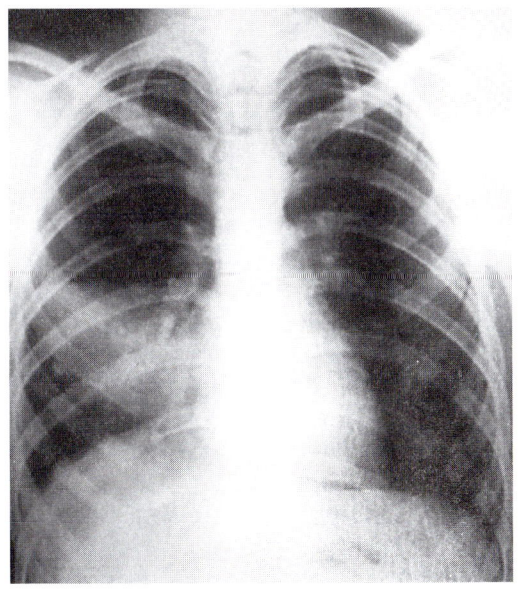

Fig. 16.24

PC 27

A 45-year-old female, a slum dweller with lower socioeconomic background presents with fever, dyspnoea, cough and haemoptysis for 3 months. Chest X-ray has the following features:

Q1. What are the radiological features and your diagnosis? 1
Q2. What is the source of haemoptysis in this patent? 1
Q3. Which special stain is commonly used to diagnose the case? Why causative organisms give positive colour with this stain? 2

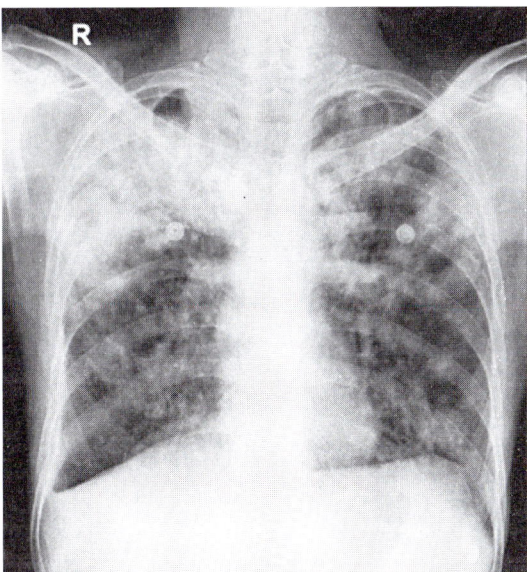

Fig. 16.25

PC 28

An elderly patient had barrel-shaped chest and presents with dyspnoea, prolonged expiration, and sits forward. Spirometry reveals the following features:

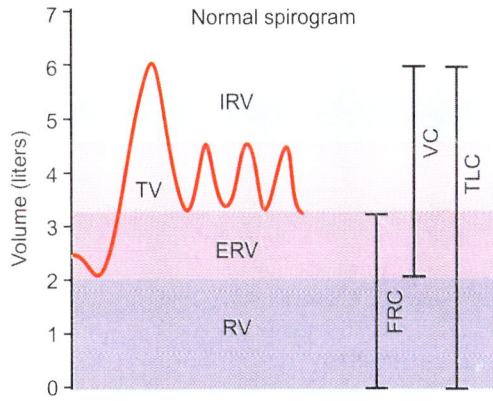

Fig. 16.26A

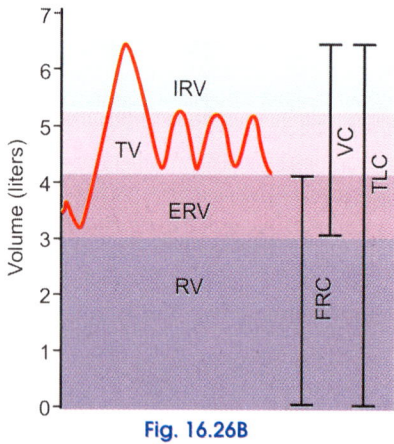

Fig. 16.26B

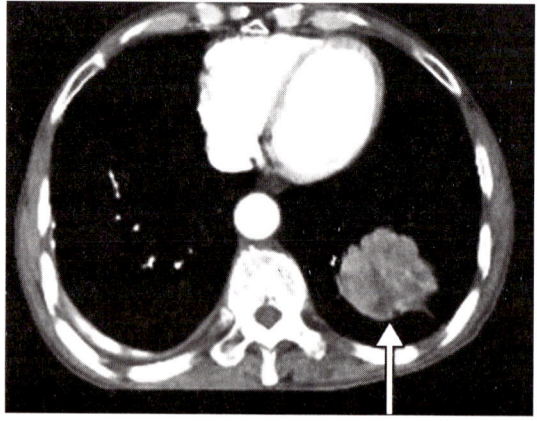

Fig. 16.27

Q1. What is your diagnosis? 1
Q2. Why these patients are called pink puffers? 1
Q3. Which hypothesis explains the pathogenesis? 1
Q4. What are the causes of death? 1

PC 29

A patient presented with chest tightness, dyspnoea and wheezing. Peripheral blood shows eosinophilia. Sputum reveals Curschmann spirals and Charcot-Leyden crystals.

Q1. What is your diagnosis? 1
Q2. If the attack remains for a prolonged time (days or week) instead of a few minutes to hour; what is that condition known as? 1
Q3. Which constituent of eosinophils causes epithelial damage? 1
Q4. What is Charcot-Leyden crystals? 1

PC 30

A 75-year-old man presented with weight loss, cough, chest pain and dyspnoea. Contrast-enhanced CT scan of lung shows a 5.5 cm, round, completely enhanced mass in left lobe of lung (arrow).

Q1. What is your provisional diagnosis? 1
Q2. How would you confirm the diagnosis? 1
Q3. What are the histologic types? 2

PC 31

An elderly woman is suffering from hypertension for years. Now she develops oedema over ankle (pedal) and pretibial. USG reveals hepatosplenomegaly and ascites. Echocardiography reveals left ventricular hypertrophy (LVH).

Q1. What is your diagnosis? 1
Q2. If there were pulmonary congestion and edema along with LVH and hypertension, then what was your diagnosis? What particular cells may be found in this case? 1+1 = 2
Q3. What particular colour change may be observed in liver? 1

PC 32

A 56-year-old man (smoker and diabetic) suddenly developed acute chest pain and presented with rapid, weak pulse, profound sweating (diaphoresis) and dyspnoea.

Q1. What is your diagnosis?
Q2. What are the most sensitive and specific biomarkers? 1
Q3. What gross features and light microscopic features will be seen in the affected organ(s) after 1–3 days? 2

PC 33

A child has mitral valve prolapse and bicuspid aortic valve. He develops fever.

Echocardiography shows irregular masses on the valve cusps. Blood culture reveals a pathogenic organism.
Q1. What is your diagnosis? 1
Q2. What is the causative organism most likely? 1
Q3. What are that irregular masses known as and what is the composition? 1
Q4. How the masses on valve differ in rheumatic heart disease (RHD)? 1

PC 34

A 38-year-old female presented with epigastric burning or aching pain. The pain tends to occur 1 to 3 hours after meals during the day and is worse in night. Pain relieves by alkali or food.
Q1. What is your diagnosis? 1
Q2. What is common organism associated in the pathogenesis? 1
Q3. What are the common locations? 2

PC 35

A 48-year-old male presented with bloody diarrhoea with stringy, mucoid material lower abdominal pain and cramps. On colonoscopy, pseudopolyps and mucosal bridges found.
Q1. What is your diagnosis? 1
Q2. What are the histologic features? 2
Q3. What are the extraintestinal manifestations? 1

PC 36

A young child suddenly develops malaise, fever, nausea and oliguria. 1–2 weeks after a sore throat. Urine is smoky or cola-coloured.
Q1. What is your diagnosis? 1
Q2. What biochemical markers you will advise for? 1
Q3. What are the light microscopic features of kidney biopsy? 2

PC 37

A 52-year-old man presented with generalised oedema. Urinary findings show massive proteinuria (>3.5 gm/day) and lipiduria.
Q1. What is your diagnosis? 1
Q2. What is the most common primary cause? 1
Q3. Why there is hyperlipidaemia in these types of patients? 1
Q4. What do you understand by selective proteinuria? 1

PC 38

A 7-year-old child presented with fever, chills, neutrophilia and marked to intense throbbing pain near upper end of femur (neck region) of right side. X-ray shows a lytic focus of bone destruction surrounded by a zone of sclerosis. Biopsy of the affected bone shows the following features:
Q1. What is your diagnosis? 1
Q2. What is the commonest organism? 1
Q3. Which area of bone is affected in neonate and children? 1
Q4. In sickle cell disease, which organism cause such lesion? 1

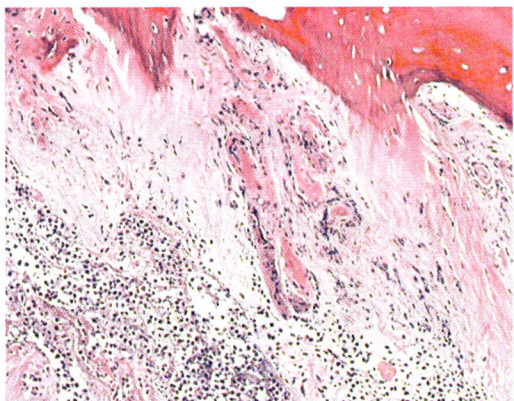

Fig. 16.28

PC 39

A 12-year-old girl child presented with painful enlarging masses at mid of left thigh and the affected site is tender, warm and swollen. X-ray shows mottled, destructive osteolytic lesion with poorly marginated edges in the diaphysis of left femur (blue circle). Sunburst periosteal reaction (red circle) and lamellated periosteal reaction in an onion-skin reaction (white arrows) also seen.

Q1. What is your diagnosis? 1
Q2. Where from does the tumour originate? 1
Q3. What are the light microscopic features? 2

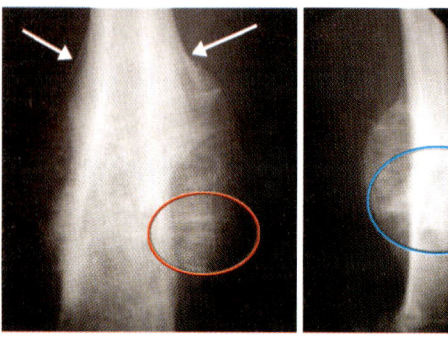

Fig. 16.29

PC 40

70-year-old man presented with urinary symptoms such as difficulty in starting or stopping the stream, dysuria. On rectal examination, a suspected nodule was found. Serum PSA level was high.

Q1. What is your diagnosis? 1
Q2. Which grading system is used for this tumour? 1
Q3. What is the cut-off value of serum PSA in normal men? 1
Q4. Name one IHC marker for this tumour? 1

PC 41

A 68-year-old female complains of tender hepatomegaly, weight loss, fatigue and upper abdominal pain. CT scan shows a large mass (red arrow).

Q1. What is your provisional diagnosis? 1
Q2. Which biochemical marker you will advise for? 1
Q3. What are the etiologic factors of this tumour? 1
Q4. How does this tumour appear grossly? 1

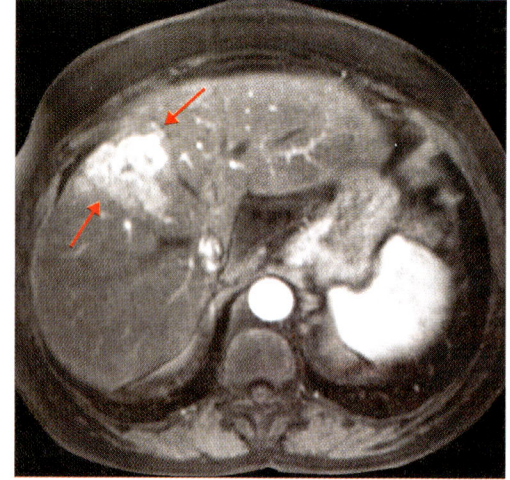

Fig. 16.30

PC 42

36-year-old female sex worker presented with low grade fever, weight loss, persistent diarrhoea and cervical lymphadenopathy for 4 months.

Q1. What is your clinical diagnosis? 1
Q2. Which one is the commonest type in India? 1
Q3. Which antigen and antibody most commonly used for detecting the disease? 1
Q4. What is the most common fungal infection associated with this disease? 1

PC 43

A 28-year-old male worker presents with raised itchy superficial chest lesion slowly developing over an old scar.

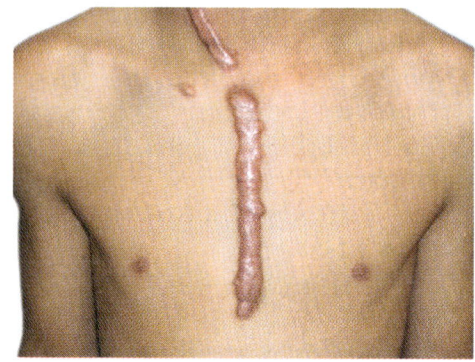

Fig. 16.31

Q1. What is this lesion? 1
Q2. What is the basic defect? 1
Q3. Name another closely related pathologic lesion? 1
Q4. How these two lesions can be differentiated? 1

PC 44

A 55-year-old female presented with irregular vaginal bleeding for 3 months.

Cervical cytology (Pap smear) shows highly dysplastic cells with degenerated round and oval nuclei and dense eosinophilic cytoplasm.

Q1. What is your provisional diagnosis? 1
Q2. Which virus is an important factor? 1
Q3. What are the histologic subtypes? 2

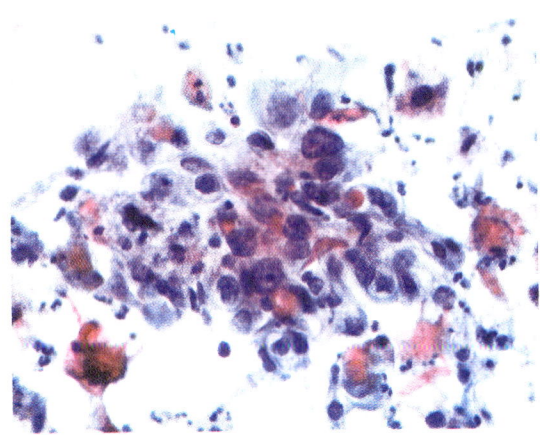

Fig. 16.32

PC 45

A 12-year-old boy presented with repeated painful knee swelling after minor trauma which leads to progressive deformities and crippling. The boy also has a tendency towards easy bruising but petechiae are absent. Aspirated from left knee joint yielded blood.

Q1. What is your provisional diagnosis? 1
Q2. What is the inheritance of the disease? 1
Q3. What are the molecular defects? 1
Q4. What will be BT, PT and PTT in this case? 1

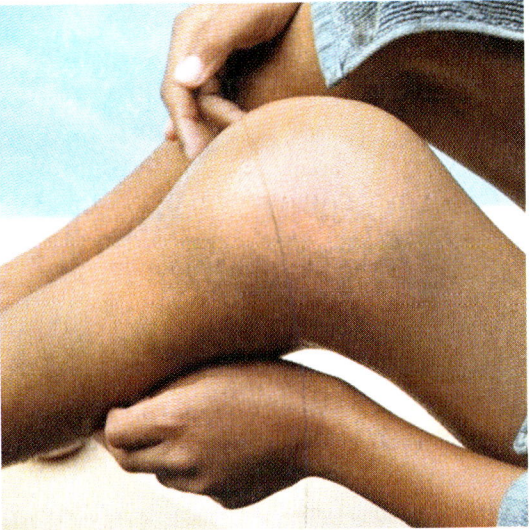

Fig. 16.33

PC 46

A 23-year-old male presented with splenomegaly, thrombocytopenia, bone pain and pathologic fractures. Bone marrow aspirates show the following features:

Q1. What is your provisional diagnosis? 1
Q2. What is the genetic defect? 1
Q3. In which organ(s), the particular cell can be found? 1
Q4. What are the different subtypes of the disease? 1

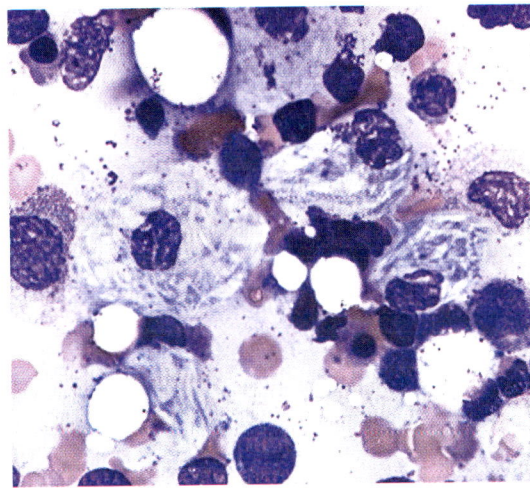

Fig. 16.34

PC 47

A female patient complains of fever, dysuria and frequency of urine.

Name: Mrs S. Tarafdar
Age: 22 years
Sex: Female
Address: 32/1 AJC Bose Road, Kolkata-14

Report on examination of urine
Physical: Appearance: Hazy
   Sp. gravity: Q. I.
   Odour: Fishy
   Sediment: Present
Chemical: Reducing substance: Nil
   Protein: Present
   Ketone bodies: Nil
Microscopical: Epithelial cells: 3–4 cells/HPF
   Pus cells: 10–15 cell/HPF
   RBC: 2–3 cells/HPF
   Casts: Nil
Crystals: Nil

Q1. What is the patient likely to be suffering from?   1
Q2. What would be the specific gravity of urine in this case and why?   1
Q3. How will you confirm the cause leading to this condition?   1
Q4. What is the appearance of the kidney, if the patient suffers for a prolonged time?   1

PC 48

Name: P. Mudi
Age: 12 years
Sex: Female

Report of examination of blood
Haemoglobin: 9 g/dl
   ESR: 12 mm at 1 hr.
   TLC: 8600/cu mm
   DLC: Neutrophil: 53%
      Lymphocyte: 39%
      Monocyte: 03%
      Eosinophil: 05%
RBC: Microcytic hypochromic
   Anisocytosis +
Poikilocytosis +
   Platelets: Adequate

Q1. What is the clinical condition of this patient?   1
Q2. Mention two common causes that may lead to such blood picture.   1
Q3. Enumerate further test you would like to come to a definite diagnosis.   1
Q4. If you examine the stool of this patient what pertinent findings may be present?   1

PC 49

Name: Hafiz Mondal
Age: 15 years
Sex: Male

Patient is referred from the ENT OPD of NRS Medical College for FNAC of neck glands

Report on examination of FNAC of cervical lymph node

Smears show necrotic material and epithelioid cells in aggregate

Q1. What is the provisional diagnosis?   1
Q2. How will you confirm the diagnosis?   1
Q3. Draw a labelled diagram of microscopic features of such lymph node.   2

PC 50

Name: T. Ali
Age: 24 years
Sex: Male

Report on examination of CSF
Physical: Appearance: Hazy
      Pressure: Coming out in jet flow
Chemical: Glucose: 20 mg/dl
      Protein: 75 mg/dl
Microscopic: Total cell count: 350 cells/cu mm

Q1. What is the condition of this patient is suffering from?   1
Q2. What type of cells do you expect in microscopical examination of CSF?   1

Q3. What are the clinical features of this condition? 1
Q4. What further examination would you find out the cause? 1

Answers to Problem Cards

PC 1

1. This is dry gangrene, a type of necrosis.
2. Necrosis is a localised area of death in living tissue and is accompanied by inflammatory reaction. This cell death is irreversible.
3. Causes are hypoxia, ischaemia and toxins (poisoning).
4. Coagulative necrosis, liquefactive necrosis, caseous necrosis, fat necrosis, fibrinoid necrosis and gangrenous necrosis (dry and wet gangrene).

PC 2

1. Apoptotic body.
2. Programmed cell death during embryogenesis and endometrial cell breakdown during menstruation.
3. Councilman bodies in viral hepatitis and graft-versus-host disease (GVHD).
4. Chromatin condensation.

PC 3

1. Tuberculosis
2. Langhans giant cells
3. i. IL-1 and IL-2: Stimulate proliferation of more T cells
   ii. IFN-γ activates macrophages.
   iii. TNF-α promotes fibroblast proliferation and activates endothelium.
   iv. Growth factors (TGF-β, PDGF) stimulate fibroblast growth.

PC 4

1. Deep vein thrombosis
2. **Virchow's triad:** Endothelial injury, alteration in the normal blood flow and blood hypercoagulability
3. • Mutation of factor V (most common)
   • Antithrombin III deficiency
   • Protein C or protein S deficiency
4. Fibrin, more enmeshed red cells and few platelets (therefore called red or stasis thrombi). Also, **lines of Zahn,** which represent pale platelet and fibrin deposits alternating with red cell layers (hence apparent laminations).

PC 5

1. Splenic infarction (white infarct)
2. Solid organs (like spleen, kidney or heart) have increased tissue density and it limits the seepage of blood from adjoining capillary beds into the necrotic area.
3. Organs with loose tissues like lung and small intestine (arterial occlusion). Organs with dual blood supply like ovary and testis (venous occlusion).
4. Red infarcts: Ill-defined haemorrhagic margins which change in colour to brown.
    White infarcts: Well defined margins and progressively pallor with time.

PC 6

1. Down syndrome
2. • In 95% of cases, there is trisomy 21 (extra copy of chromosome of 21, so total chromosome 47).
   • In 4% of cases, robertsonian translocation
   • In 1% of cases, mosaic pattern (both 46, XY and 47 chromosomes)
3. Most common cause is maternal meiotic non-disjunction.
    Meiotic non-disjunction occurs in chromosome 21 in ovum.
4. These children have 10–20-fold increased risk of developing acute leukaemia (more commonly ALL and specifically acute megakaryoblastic leukaemia, AML-M7).
   • Reduced fertility in females (males are totally infertile)
   • Increased risk of respiratory infections (RTI).

PC 7

1. Immediate (type 1) hypersensitivity; Anaphylaxis
2. Mast cell mainly. Also, TH_2 (T helper cells) play some role.
3. Histamine is responsible for early clinical features because it is preformed mediator.

    PAF is the major mediator of the late phase reaction.
4. IgE.

PC 8

1. Acquired immunodeficiency syndrome (AIDS) with human immunodeficiency virus (HIV) infection.
2. According to the Centers for Disease Control (CDC) and Prevention, US in 1993, irrespective of presence of symptoms, any HIV-infected person having CD4+ T cell count of <200/µl is labelled as AIDS.
3. Kaposi's sarcoma, primary CNS lymphoma, NHL and Hodgkin lymphoma, HPV-associated carcinoma (cervix, vagina, anus) and bacillary angiomatosis.
4. ELISA (enzyme-linked immunosorbent assay) is the most sensitive test, and Western blot is the most specific test.

PC 9

1. Amyloidosis
2. Kidney, spleen (sago spleen and lardaceous spleen), heart and oral cavity (gingiva and tongue)
3. Congo red: Pink or red colour to amyloid deposits in tissue.

    Metachromatic stains like crystal violet or methyl violet: Rose pink.
4. Biopsy from renal tissue, rectum, abdominal fat and gingiva. The rectum is the best site for taking the biopsy. The staining of abdominal fat aspirate is quite specific but has low sensitivity.

PC 10

1. Benign tumour
2. Some microscopical features are present in malignant tumour which is lacking or absent in benign tumour:
   - Pleomorphism: Both the cells and nuclei display this
   - Nuclear atypia: Hyperchromatism, irregular nuclear membrane
   - A typical, bizarre mitoses: Increased in number
   - Loss of polarity and lack of differentiation
3. i. Carcinoma arises from epithelial cells, whereas sarcomas arise from mesenchymal cells.
   ii. Carcinoma metastasizes by lymphatic route, while sarcomas prefer haematogenous route.

PC 11

1. Jaundice
2. Normal value of serum bilirubin is 0.3–1.2 mg/dl, about 80% of which is unconjugated bilirubin.
3. Physiological jaundice of newborn, haemolytic anaemia, diffuse hepatocellular disease (viral hepatitis), Criggler-Najjar syndrome, Gilbert syndrome
4. Biliary tract obstruction, primary biliary cirrhosis, Dubin-Johnson syndrome, Rotor syndrome.

PC 12

1. Left-sided pleural effusion due to accumulation of exudate.
2. Glucose content of the effusion fluid will be low (<60 mg/dl) and protein content will be high (2.5–3.5 gm/dl).
3. LDH content will be high compared to transudate and ratio will be >0.6.
4. Anasarca or dropsy is a severe and generalised oedema with widespread subcutaneous tissue swelling.

    Causes: Renal oedema, cardiac oedema and nutritional edema.

PC 13
1. Acute lymphoblastic leukaemia (ALL).
2. The bone marrow is hypercellular and shows 20–95% lymphoblasts of B or T cell origin. Megakaryocytes are reduced or absent.
3. CD34 and CD19 are positive
4. PAS +ve and acid phosphatase (focal) +ve

PC 14
1. Acute myeloid leukaemia (AML)
2. Auer rods
3. Thrombocytopenia cause spontaneous bleeding in AML patients. Also, pro-coagulants and fibrinolytic factors released by the leukaemic cells exacerbate the bleeding tendency.
4. CD34 and CD22 in the first panel. TdT and CD19 in the second panel.

PC 15
1. Chronic myeloid leukaemia (CML).
2. It is caused by splenomegaly. Splenomegaly occurs as a result of extensive extramedullary haematopoiesis.
3. Philadelphia chromosome (Ph). Ph chromosome is formed by reciprocal balanced translocation between part of long arm of chromosome 22 arm with part of long arm of chromosome 9 {t (9;22) (q34; q11)}.
4. NAP score will be reduced. (Remember, NAP score will be high in myeloid leukaemoid reactions. Also, NAP score in CML returns to normal with successful treatment, in infections and corticosteroid administration.)

PC 16
1. Chronic lymphocytic leukaemia (CLL).
2. This happens because of production of autoantibodies by non-neoplastic B cells.
3. There may be prolymphocytic transformation (15–30% of patients) or a transformation to diffuse large B cell lymphoma (DLBCL), so-called Richter syndrome (5–10% of patients).
4. CD23, CD20 and CD19 (pan B cell markers).

PC 17
1. Hodgkin lymphoma or Hodgkin disease
2. Classic form of Hodgkin lymphoma, mixed cellularity type.
3. CD30 positive in 98% of cases
   CD15 positive in 80% of cases
   CD20 positive in small subset
4. Classic form of Hodgkin lymphoma, nodular sclerosis type.

PC 18
1. Multiple myeloma (plasma cell dyscrasia).
2. Presence of M band (M protein) due to presence of **monoclonal** (hence the name M) immunoglobulin. This Ig is usually IgG (55%), followed by IgA (25% of cases).
3. Sharply punched out bone lesions.
4. Present of Bence-Jones protein (light chains of immunoglobulin). Also, increased urinary protein 6 gm/dl.

PC 19
1. Chronic immune thrombocytopenic purpura (ITP).
2. Decreased platelet count and presence of abnormally large platelets (mega thrombocytes).
3. Bone marrow reveals a modestly increased number of megakaryocytes. Some of them are immature with large, non-lobulated, single nuclei.
4. Autoantibodies directed against platelet membrane glycoprotein IIb–IIIa or Ib–IX may be found in plasma and bound to platelet surface near about 80% of patients.

Note
Usually spleen is of normal size. Typically, there is congestion of splenic sinusoids and enlargement of the splenic follicles, often associated with reactive germinal centres.

PC 20

1. Iron deficiency anaemia.
2. Mild to moderate increase in the erythroid progenitors (normoblasts). Perls'-Prussian blue reveals disappearance of stainable iron from macrophages (sideroblasts) in the bone marrow.
3. Serum iron and ferritin level are low, whereas total iron binding capacity (TIBC) is high (which is a reflection of elevated transferrin level). This results in a reduction of transferrin saturation to <15%.

PC 21

1. Megaloblastic anaemia
2. Red blood cells (RBCs) are macrocytic and oval (macro-ovalocytes). Neutrophils are larger than normal (macropolymorphonuclear) and some hypersegmented, having ≥5 lobes (normally 3–4 lobes) neutrophils.
3. The characteristic large cells are megaloblasts. These cells are large with a deeply basophilic cytoplasm, prominent nucleoli and a distinctive, fine nuclear chromatin pattern.

PC 22

1. Sickle cell anaemia.
2. Point mutation in the sixth codon of β-globin chain that leads to the replacement of a glutamine residue with a valine residue.
3. These crises are episodes of hypoxic injury and infarction which cause severe pain. The affected organs are bones, lungs, liver, brain, spleen and penis.
4. Mixing of blood sample with an oxygen-consuming reagent such as metabisulphite induces sickling of red cells. This is known as **sickling test**. It can be done with 2% metabisulfite or dithionite.

PC 23

1. Hereditary spherocytosis
2. There are intrinsic defects in the red cell due to diverse mutations which lead to an insufficiency of membrane skeletal components. The pathogenic mutations commonly seen in ankyrin, spectrin, band 3 and band 4.2.
3. Aplastic crises are usually triggered by acute parvovirus infection. This virus infects and kills red cell progenitors (normoblasts), causing red cell production to cease.
4. Osmotic fragility test which is increased in hereditary spherocytosis.

> **Note**
> Spherocytes on peripheral blood smear are not pathognomonic of hereditary spherocytosis (HS) as it may be found in autoimmune haemolytic anaemia, ABO haemolytic disease (but not with RH haemolytic disease) of newborn, G6PD deficiency and infections/burns.

PC 24

1. β-Thalassemia major
2. β-Thalassemia minor (trait)
3. Anisopoikilocytosis, target cell, microcytes, basophilic stippling, and fragmented red cells.
4. The marrow is hypercellular and active. The expanding marrow erodes existing cortical bone and induces new bone formation, giving rise to a "crew-cut" appearance.

PC 25

1. β-Thalassemia minor (thalassemia trait).
2. The person will be heterozygous β-thalassemia ($β^0/β$, or $β^+/β$). One β globin chain will be normal, other is defective.
3. Anaemia will be either absent or if present mild.

4. It will reveal increase in HbA_2 ($\alpha_2\delta_2$) to 5.4% of the total haemoglobin (normal 2.5 + 0.3%). Adult haemoglobin or HbA will be 84% of total haemoglobin (normal 96%).

PC 26

1. Lung (pulmonary) infection, bronchopneumonia type.
2. Focal opacities due to consolidation in right lung.
3. *Staphylococcus aureus*
4. There will be suppurative, neutrophil-rich exudate which fills the bronchi, bronchioles and adjacent alveolar spaces.

PC 27

1. Bilateral 'fluffy or wooly' opacities predominantly in the upper zones with fibrotic infiltration. Diagnosis is pulmonary tuberculosis (Koch).
2. Erosion of blood vessels by the active pulmonary lesion, particulary bronchial artery is the source of haemoptysis.
3. Ziehl-Neelsen or ZN stain (acid-fast stain) is used to detect the organism, i.e. tubercle bacilli. The acid fastness of tubercle bacilli is due to mycolic acids, cross-linked fatty acids and other lipids in the cell wall of the bacilli. The bacilli take up stain by heated carbolfuchsin and resist decolourisation by weak acids and alcohol unlike other organisms, which cannot resist decolourisation. So, tubercle bacilli are acid fast as well as alcohol (ethanol) fast.

Note

False positive AFB (acid-fast bacilli) staining in ZN stain may be seen due to Nocardia, Legionella, Cryptosporidium, Isospora, Rhodococcus and some protozoa.

PC 28

1. Emphysaema of lung, a type of COPD (chronic obstructive pulmonary disease)
2. These patients over ventilate and remain well oxygenated as well as tachypnoea.
3. Protease-antiprotease imbalance hypothesis. There is destructive effect of high protease coupled with low antiprotease lead to tissue damage.
4. Death is due to:
   i. Respiratory acidosis and coma
   ii. Right-sided heart failure, and
   iii. Massive collapse of the lungs secondary to pneumothorax.

PC 29

1. Bronchial asthma
2. Status asthmaticus
3. Major basic protein of eosinophils.
4. These are collections of crystalloids, made up an eosinophil lysophospholipase binding protein called galectin.

PC 30

1. Lung cancer (carcinoma).
2. Initially FNAC may be done to determine the malignant nature of the neoplasm. But final diagnosis should be made after lung biopsy and histopathologic examination.
3. There are five main histologic types:
   i. Adenocarcinoma
   ii. Squamous cell carcinoma or epidermoid carcinoma
   iii. Small cell carcinoma
   iv. Large cell carcinoma
   v. Combined carcinoma, e.g. adenosquamous carcinoma (combination of adenocarcinoma and squamous cell carcinoma).

PC 31

1. Congestive heart failure (CHF) due to right-sided heart failure.
2. Congestive heart failure (CHF) due to left sided-heart failure.

   In the lung, some RBCs extravasate into pulmonary oedema fluid within the

alveolar spaces, where they are phagocytosed and digested by macrophages, which store iron of haemoglobin in the form of haemosiderin. These haemosiderin laden macrophages are known as **heart failure cells**.
3. In the liver, congestion is most prominent around central veins within hepatic lobules, which show red-brown centrilobular discolouration. But the peripheral region becomes paler. This combination of dark and pale colour produces **nutmeg liver**.

PC 32

1. Myocardial infarction.
2. Cardiac-specific proteins, particularly troponin T and troponin I.
3. Gross features: Mottling with yellow-tan infarct centre.
   Microscopic features: Coagulation necrosis with loss of nuclei and muscle striations, dense neutrophilic infiltration into the infarcted area (interstitial).

PC 33

1. Infective endocarditis (subacute bacterial endocarditis).
2. *Streptococcus viridans* in case of previously damaged valves. *Staphylococcus aureus* in both normal and abnormal valves. But *S. viridans* is more common organism and less virulent.
3. There are vegetations which contain fibrin (thrombotic debris), inflammatory cells and bacteria or other organisms.
4. In RHD, vegetations are small, warty and present along the lines of closure of valve leaflets. In infective endocarditis they are large, irregular and present on the valve-cusps that can extend onto the chordae.

PC 34

1. Peptic ulcer disease.
2. *Helicobacter pylori* or *H. pylori* (spiral-shaped or curved bacilli)
3. - Duodenum (first part)
   - Stomach (lesser curvature near the junction of body and antrum).
   - Margins of jejunostomy
   - Gastro-oesophageal junction in GERD or Barrett's oesophagus.
   - In ileal Meckel's diverticulum containing ectopic gastric mucosa
   - Stomach, duodenum and/or jejunum (multiple ulcers) in Zollinger-Ellison syndrome.

PC 35

1. Ulcerative colitis, a type of inflammatory bowl disease (IBD).
2. There are diffuse inflammatory infiltrates which are limited to the mucosa and superficial submucosa. There are cryptitis, crypt abscess, architectural crypt distortion and epithelial metaplasia. But noncaseating granuloma is absent unlike Crohn's disease.
3. Migratory polyarthritis, sacroiliitis, ankylosing spondylitis, uveitis, skin lesions, pericholangitis and primary sclerosing cholangitis.

PC 36

1. Acute proliferative (poststreptocoal/postinfectious) glomerulonephritis or nephritic syndrome.
2. - Anti-streptolysin O (ASO)
   - Anti-deoxyribonuclease B (anti-DNAse B)
   - Anti-streptokinase (ASKase)
   - Anti-nicotinyl adenine dinucleotidase (anti-NADase)
3. The glomeruli are enlarged and hypercellular with diffuse involvement. The diffuse hypercellularity of glomerular tuft is due to proliferation of mesangial, endothelial and occasionally epithelial cells (acute proliferative lesions). Also, there are infiltration of leukocytes, mainly neutrophils and sometimes monocytes (acute exudative lesions).

There may be interstitial oedema and inflammation and the tubules often contain red cell casts.

PC 37

1. Nephrotic syndrome
2. In children, most common cause is minimal change glomerulonephritis. In adults, most common cause is membranous glomerulonephritis and focal segmental glomerulosclerosis.
3. A highly selective proteinuria consists mostly of low-molecular weight proteins (albumin 70kD; transferrin 76kD molecular weight). In non-selective or poorly selective proteinuria there are other proteins like high molecular weight globulins in addition to albumin.

PC 38

1. Pyogenic osteomyelitis (bacterial osteomyelitis).
2. *Staphylococcus aureus* is the commonest pathogen (80–90% of the cases).
3. In the neonate, the metaphyseal vessels penetrate the growth plate, resulting in frequent infection of the metaphysis, epiphysis, or both.
    But in children, pathogenic organism typically affects the metaphysis as metaphyseal vessels do not penetrate growth plate.
    Again, in adults, bacteria infect epiphyses and subchondral regions due to closure of growth plate and the metaphyseal vessels reunite with their epiphyseal counterparts.
4. In sickle cell disease, Salmonella bacteria are the causative organism.

PC 39

1. Ewing's sarcoma
2. The tumour arises from medullary cavity in diaphysis and usually affects long tubular bones, especially the femur and the flat bones of pelvis.
3. The tumour is composed of sheets of uniform small, round cells which are slightly larger than lymphocytes having scant cytoplasm, that may appear clear because it is rich in glycogen. There may be presence of **Homer-Wright rosettes** (where the tumour cells are arranged in a circle about a central fibrillary space) which are indicative of neural differentiation. The tumour contains fibrous septae and a little stroma. Necrosis may be present. Mitotic figures are a few in number.

PC 40

1. Prostatic adenocarcinoma
2. Gleason system is used for prostatic adenocarcinoma. According to this system, prostate cancers are divided into 5 grades on the basis of glandular patterns of differentiation.
3. In most laboratories, serum PSA level of 8 ng/ml is used as a cut-off.
    However, upper age specific reference range is better:
    - For men 40–49 years: 2.5 ng/ml
    - For men 50–59 years: 3.5 ng/ml
    - For men 60–69 years: 4.5 ng/ml
    - For men 70–79 years: 6.5 ng/ml
4. AMACR (alpha-methyl-coenzyme A-racemase), which is positive in 82–100% of prostatic adenocarcinoma.

PC 41

1. Hepatocellular carcinoma (HCC)
2. Serum α-fetoprotein (AFP).
3. Four major etiologic factors:
    i. Chronic viral infection (HBV, HCV)
    ii. Chronic alcoholism
    iii. Non-alcoholic steatohepatitis (NASH)
    iv. Food contaminants (primarily aflatoxins)
4. HCC appears grossly as (1) a unifocal large mass, (2) multifocal (widely distributed variable size nodules), (3) a diffusely infiltrative cancer.

Note

False positive AFP may be seen due to yolk sac tumours, embryonal carcinoma, and many non-neoplastic like cirrhosis, massive liver necrosis, chronic hepatitis (specially HCV infection), normal pregnancy, fetal distress or death and fetal neural tube defects such as anencephaly and spina bifida.

PC 42

1. human immunodeficiency virus (HIV) infection causing AIDS (acquired immunodeficiency syndrome).
2. HIV 1 group M subtype C is the commonest type.
3. p24 is the most readily detected viral antigen and is the target for the antibodies, used to diagnose HIV infection.
4. Candidiasis is the most common fungal infection in AIDS in India. *Pneumocystis jiroveci* (previously *carini*) is most common fungal infection in AIDS in world.

PC 43

1. Keloid scar.
2. There is excessive formation of the repair components (here collagen) leading to abnormality of the repair process and leads to complication of would healing.
3. Hypertrophic scar.
4. In hypertrophic scar, the scar tissue is restricted to the original wound and regress.

   In keloid, the scar tissue grows beyond the boundaries of the original wound and does not regress.

PC 44

1. Squamous cell carcinoma (keratinizing type)
2. Human papillomavirus, strain HPV 16 and HPV 18 (also HPV 31 and HPV 33).
3. • Squamous cell carcinoma (arise from ectocervix)
      – Keratinizing or nonkeratinizing type
      – Verrucous
      – Papillary transitional
      – Lymphoepthelioma-like
   • Adenocarcinoma (arise from endocervical glands)
      – Mucinous
      – Endometrioid
      – Clear cell
      – Serous
      – Mesonephric
      – Well differentiated villoglandular
      – Minimal deviation (adenoma malignum)
   • Other tumours/carcinomas
      – Adenosquamous
      – Glassy cell
      – Carcinoid tumour
      – Neuroendocrine
      – Small cell
      – Undifferentiated

PC 45

1. Haemophilia A (factor VIII deficiency)
2. X-linked recessive trait. So, it mainly affects males and homozygous females.
3. Mutations in factor VIII, which is an essential cofactor for factor IX in the coagulation cascade. The genetic lesions include deletions, nonsense mutations that create stop codons and mutations that cause errors in mRNA splicing.
4. Bleeding time (BT) and prothrombin time (PT) will be normal, whereas partial thromboplastin time (PTT) will be prolonged.

PC 46

1. Gaucher disease showing Gaucher cells in marrow.
2. It is autosomal recessive disorder resulting from mutations in the gene encoding glucocerebrosidase. So, glucocerebrosides accumulate in massive amounts within phagocytic cells.
3. Gaucher cells are found in spleen, liver, bone marrow, lymph nodes, tonsils, thymus are Peyer's patches.

4. There are 3 subtypes:
   Type I: Chronic non-neuropathic form
   Type II: Acute neuropathic form
   Type III: Intermediate between type I and type II.

PC 47
1. Urinary tract infection or UTI.
2. The specific gravity of urine will be increase (normal specific gravity of urine 1.016–1.025).
3. Urine culture test. More than 85% cases of UTI, causative organisms are gram-negative bacilli (*E. coli*, Proteus, Klebsiella)
4. Patient will develop chronic pyelonephritis. Grossly, the kidneys are usually irregularly scarred. If bilateral involvement, then they are asymmetric. The characteristic findings are coarse, discrete, corticomedullary scars overlying dilated, blunted or deformed calyces and flattening of the papillae.

PC 48
1. Iron deficiency anaemia
2. i. Increased blood loss: Menstruation in reproductive females
   ii. Increased requirements: Pregnancy, lactation and adolescence
3. i. Red cell indices: MCV↓, MCH↓, MCHC↓
   ii. Biochemical:
      - Total iron binding capacity (TIBC) is high (normal 250–450 µg/dl).

Note

Other parasites which cause anaemia are:
- *P. falciparum* (malaria): Normochromic anaemia
- *L. donovani* (kala-azar): Normochromic anaemia
- *Schistosoma haematobium*: Normochromic anemia
- *Trichuris trichiura*: Normochromic anaemia
- *T. gambiense* (sleeping sickness): Normochromic anaemia
- *Diphyllobthrium latum* (*D. latum*): Megaloblastic and pernicious anaemia.

- Serum ferritin is very low (normal 30–250 ng/ml)
- Serum iron level is low (normal 40–140 µg/dl)

4. Parasitic worms (helminths), specifically hookworms, which include:
   1. *Ancylostoma duodenale*
   2. *Necator americanus*
   3. *Ancylostoma ceylanicum*.

PC 49
1. Caseating granulomatous lymphadenitis, possibly due to tuberculosis.
2. Tuberculosis is caused by *Mycobacterium tuberculosis* bacilli. The diagnosis can be confirmed by:
   i. Culture of the aspirate: In LJ media and BACTEC media, gives positive culture.

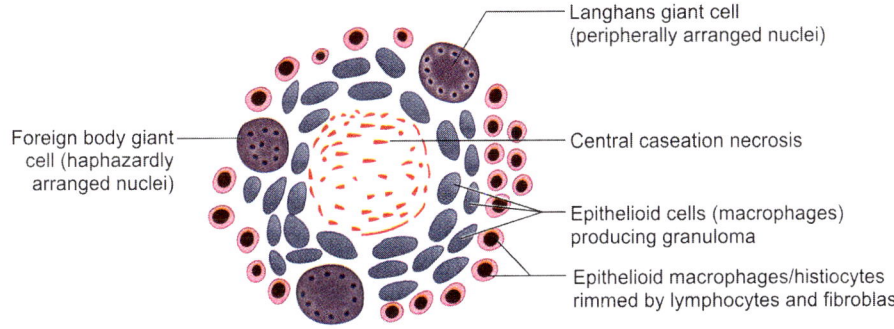

ii. ZN stain: Red-coloured tuberculous bacilli seen.
iii. Other: ESR will be high, Mantoux test may be positive. TB PCR may detect DNA of bacteria (insertion sequence IS 1081).

PC 50

1. Pyogenic (bacterial) meningitis. Because CSF pressure is highly increased (coming injet flow), CSF is hazy, glucose low (normal 40–80 mg%), protein content high (normal 15–45 mg/dl) and cell count is high (normal 1–4/mm^3).
2. Mostly neutrophils (>90%).
3. Severe headache, fever, vomiting, drowsiness, stupor, coma and occasionally convulsions. The most important clinical sign is stiffness of neck on forward bending (Kernig's sign) which is due to increased neck muscle tone and stiffness.
4. To find out the exact pathogen (bacteria), blood culture is needed followed by Gram stain (Gram +ve or Gram –ve bacteria).

Appendices

Appendix I: Common Instruments in Pathology

HAEMATOLOGY INSTRUMENTS/REAGENTS

Antisera (Antibody) for ABO and Rh Blood Grouping

- Blue-coloured vial: Antisera A
- Yellow-coloured vial: Antisera B
- Pink/red coloured vial: antisera AB
- Colourless vial: Anti-D (Rh) grouping

Uses

i. Antisera A, B, and AB for ABO blood grouping
ii. Anti-D for Rh grouping
iii. Both forward and reverse grouping can be done.

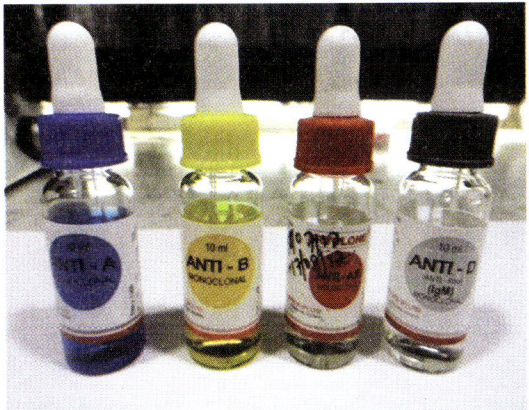

Fig. A1.1: Antisera for blood grouping

Bone Marrow Aspiration Needle

i. Klima's needle: In this needle, the adjustable guard is present along the length of the needle. This is more secure than the side guard present in Salah's BM aspiration needle. There is no side screw.

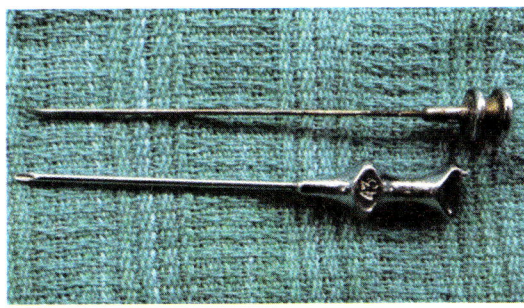

Fig. A1.2: Klima's needle

ii. Salah's needle: It has a guard which is fixed to the needle by a side screw.

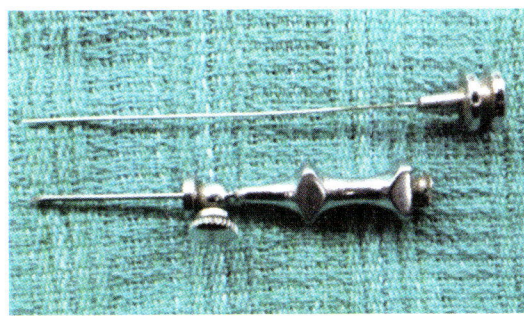

Fig. A1.3: Salah's needle

Parts of BM aspiration needle:
- Trocar
- Cannula/stylet
- Adjustable guard or side guard.

Ideal bone marrow needle:
- Should be stout
- 7–8 cm in length

- Well fitted stylet
- Edges well sharpened

DLC Counter (Manual) for Differential Leukocyte Count (DLC)

Use: To determine the relative number (percentage, %) of each type of white blood cell presents in the blood.

Instrument: Made of steel with pressing keys and a knob at both ends.

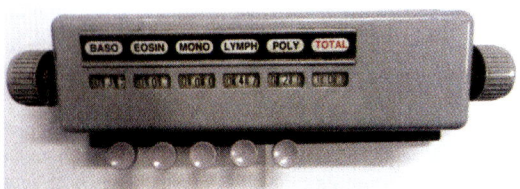

Fig. A1.4: DLC counter

Graduated Pipette (1 ml)

Instrument: Glass pipette with etched marking of 0.1 each.

Use: Dispensing required small volume of liquid.

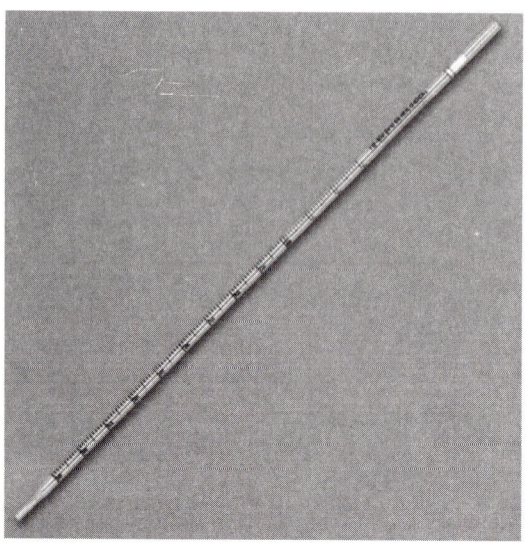

Fig. A1.5: Graduated pipette (1 ml)

Lancet (Blood Lancet)

Instrument: Similar to a small scalpel but with a double-edged blade or needle. It is made of metal having a sharp-pointed end with fixed depth. Blood lancet is generally disposable.

Uses
i. To make punctures, such as a finger prick to collect capillary blood.
ii. Also used to prick the skin in skin testing for allergies.

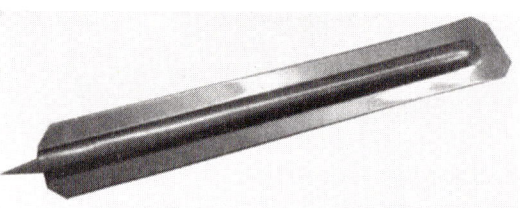

A

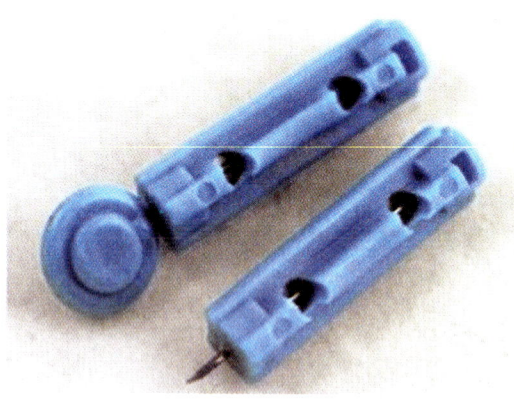

B

Fig. A1.6A and B: Blood lancet

Neubauer (Improved) Counting Chamber or Haemocytometer

Hemo means blood; Cyto means cell; Meter means measurement/counter. Thus, it is an instrument used to count the blood cells.

Instrument: It is a thick crystal slide (made up of crystal glass). Generally, it measures 30 × 70 mm with a thickness of 4 mm. Two type: (i) Simple counting chamber (rarely used) which has one counting area in the central part, (ii) double chambers (commonly used) which have two counting areas that can be loaded independently. The depth is 0.1 mm in the double chambers, there is an H-shaped grove and on both sides two counting areas present.

Neubauer chamber's counting grid is 3 × 3 mm in size. The grid has 9 square divisions of width 1 mm.

Uses

i. Usually used for counting blood cells (WBC, RBC or platelets)
ii. Sperm counts
iii. Cell count in body fluids

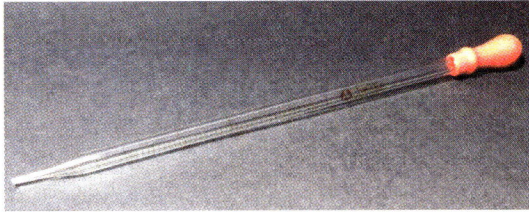

Fig. A1.8: Pasteur pipette

RBC Pipette

Refer to Chapter 4; Total count of WBC, RBC and Platelets (page 50).

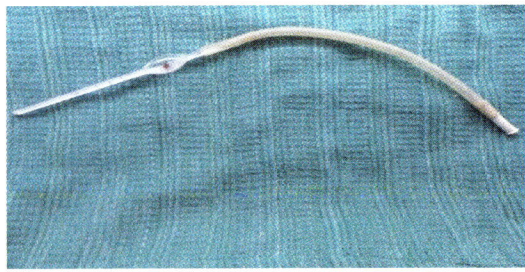

Fig. A1.9: RBC Pipette

Sahli's Pipette, Haemoglobinometer Tube and Comparator Box

Refer to Chapter 6; Haemoglobin Estimation (page 68).

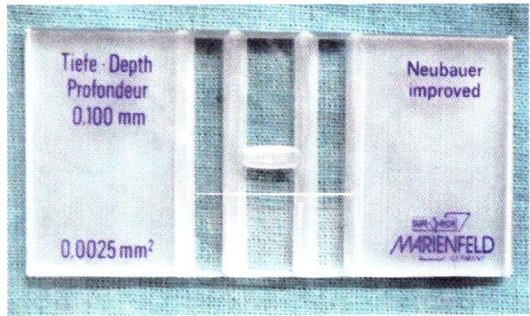

Fig. A1.7: Improved Neubauer chamber

Pasteur Pipette

Instrument: Also know as droppers or eye droppers. They are usually glass tubes tapered to a narrow point and fitted with a rubber bulb at the top. The combination of the Pasteur pipette and rubber bulb has also been referred to as a **teat pipette**. It has been named after French scientist Louis Pasteur. Pasteur pipette made of plastic is also available.

Uses

i. Used for filling Wintrobe's tube with blood.
ii. Used to transfer small quantities of liquids or chemical solutions without exposing it to the external environment.

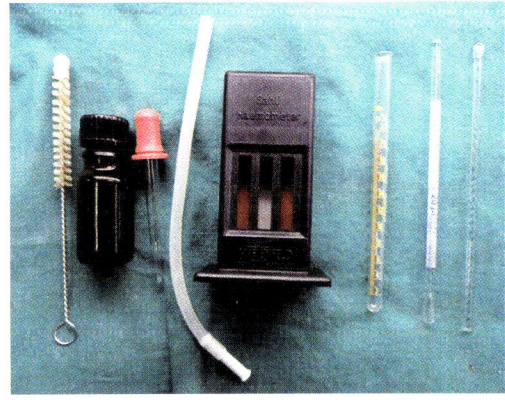

Fig. A1.10: Sahli's method instrument

Stopwatch

Instrument/device: It is a handled timepiece. Both manual and automatic versions are available. In manual timing, the clock is started and stopped by a person pressing a button. In automatic device, both starting and stopping are triggered automatically by sensors.

Uses

i. Used to determine the timing of the end point of in tests for coagulation studies and haemostasis.
ii. Also used to record timings in sports (stop clock)

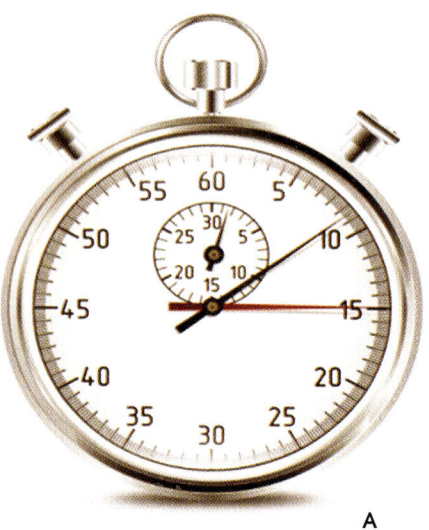 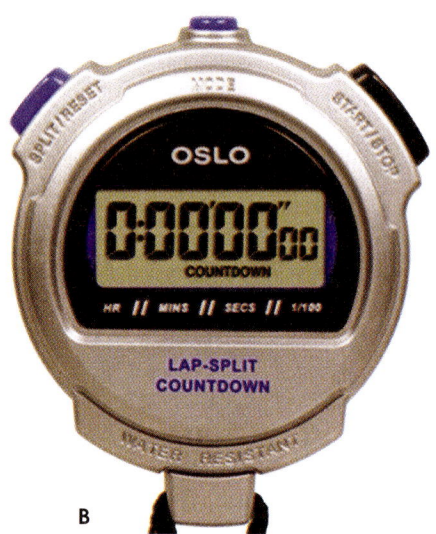

Fig. A1.11A and B: (A) Manual stopwatch; (B) Automatic stopwatch

Thermometer for Water Bath

Instrument: Usually glass thermometer with precision (markings).

Use: For placing in water bath to take temperature recording.

Trephine Biopsy (Jamshidi Type) Needle

Instrument: Made of stainless steel with tapering end to reduce crush artifact. It has needle stilette and a guard.

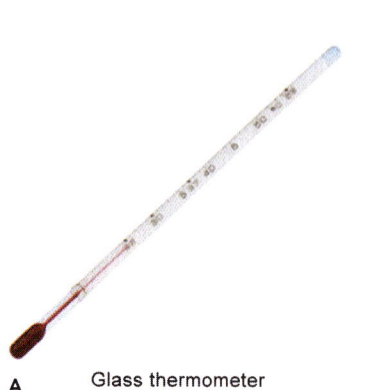 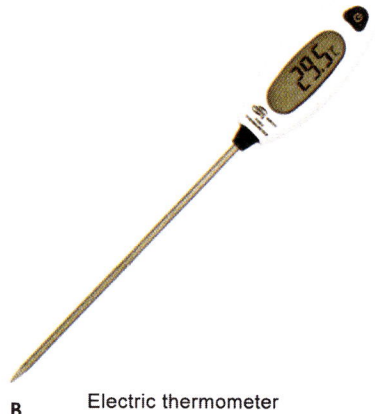

A   Glass thermometer   B   Electric thermometer

Fig. A1.12A and B: Thermometer

Uses

i. To obtain bone marrow tissue. It is cylindrically shaped solid piece of bone marrow, 2 mm wide and 2 cm long (80 μl).

ii. Bone marrow tissue obtained is processed by paraffin embedding technique for microscopic examination.

iii. Can also be used for immunohistochemistry (IHC), flow cytometry (immunophenotyping) and PCR (polymerase chain reaction).

Vacutainers with Vacupuncture Needle

Schematic diagram of using vacutainer tube and vacutainer needle.

Vacutainer needle + vacutainer holder + vacutainer tube.

Refer to Chapter 1; Blood Collection and Anticoagulants (page 13).

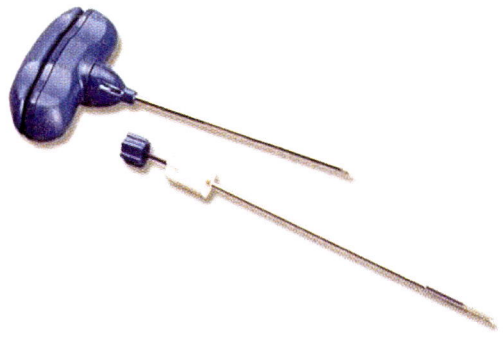

Fig. A1.13: Jamshidi needle

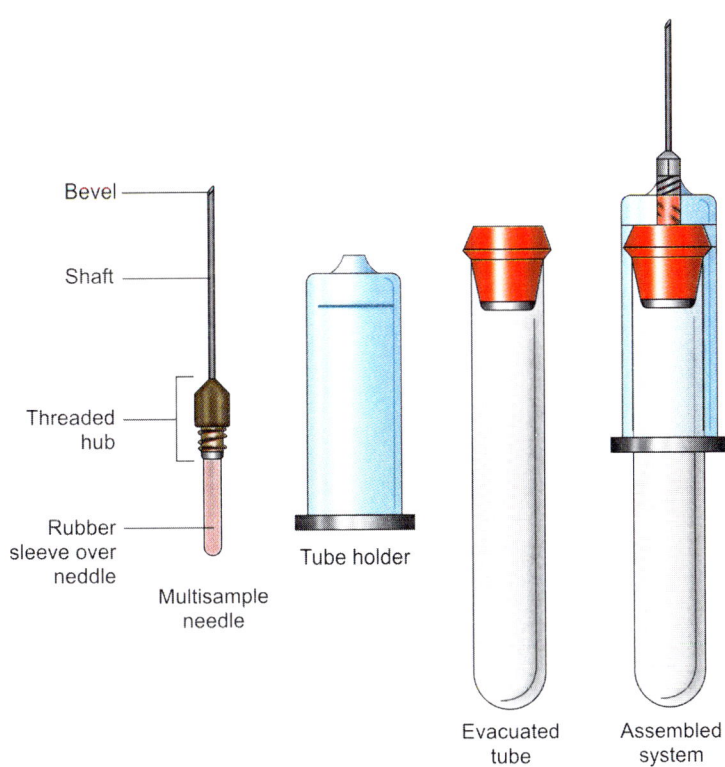

Fig. A1.14: Vacutainers with vacupuncture needle

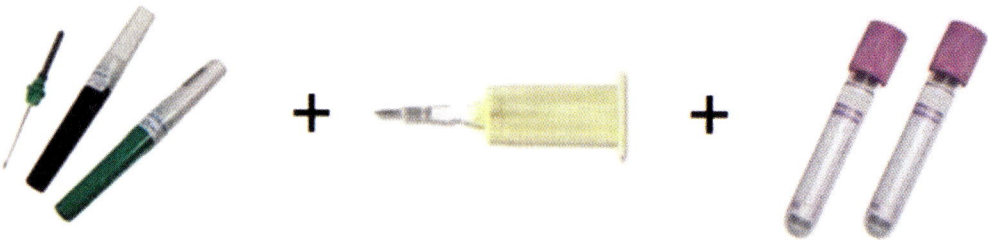

Fig. A1.15: Vacutainers system

Westergren's Pipette

Refer to Chapter 5; ESR and PCV (page 57).

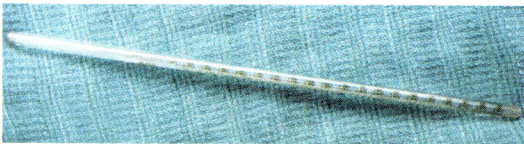

Fig. A1.16: Westergren's pipette

Westergren's Stand

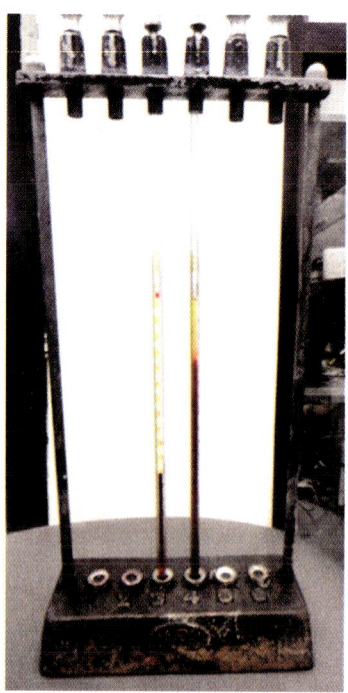

Fig. A1.17: Westergren's stand or ESR stand

Instrument: Made of stainless steel base with top support. Multiple ESR pipettes can be placed within it in a vertical position. Usually up to 6 ESR pipettes can be placed.

Use: To record ESR in Westegren method./

Wintrobe (Haematocrit) Tube

Refer to Chapter 5; ESR and PCV (page 60).

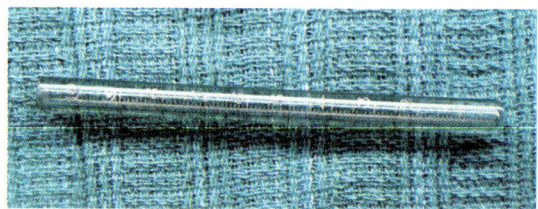

Fig. A1.18: Wintrobe's tube

Wintrobe's Stand

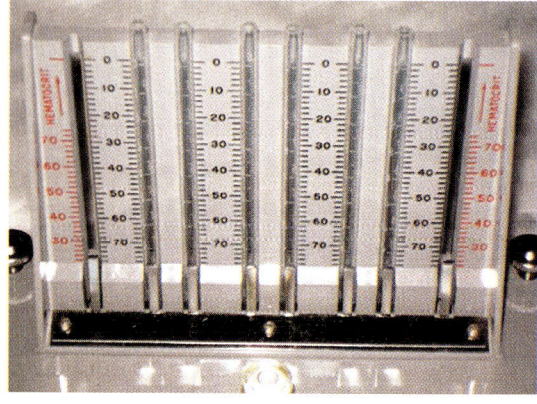

Fig. A1.19: Wintrobe's stand

Instrument: Made of good quality metal (stainless steel) and coated with enamel. Usually 2 to 8 Wintrobe's tubes can be placed.

Use: To record ESR in Wintrobe's method.

CLINICAL PATHOLOGY INSTRUMENTS/REAGENTS

Dipstick for Urine

Reagent strip: A standard urine test strip may comprise up to 10 different chemical reagents which react (change color) when immersed in, and then removed from, a urine sample. The test is read after 30 to 120 seconds.

Use: To determine pathological changes in patient's urine in standard urinalysis (proteins, glucose, ketone, haemoglobin, bilirubin, urobilinogen, acetone, leukocyte, pH and specific gravity).

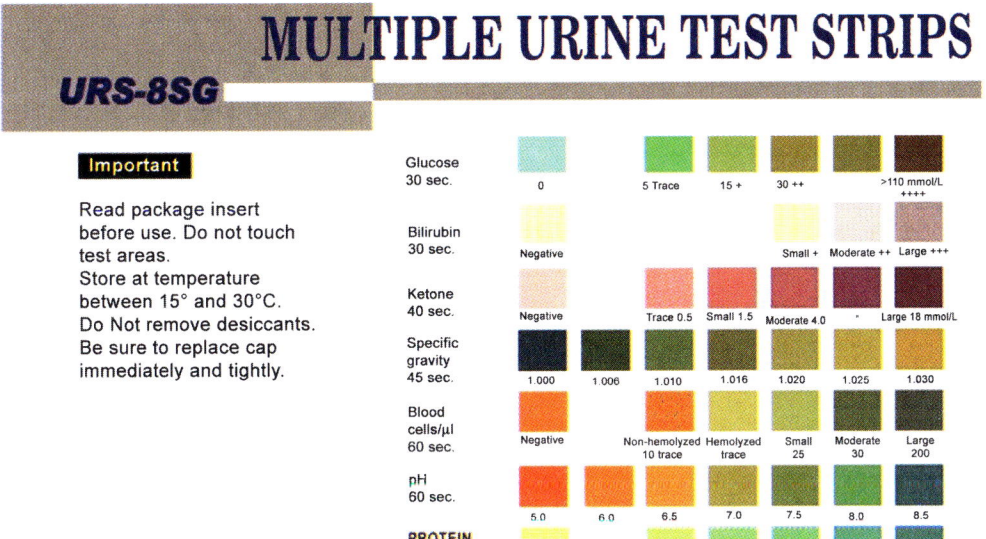

Fig. A1.20: Dipstick (multistick)

Esbach's Albuminometer

Refer to Chapter 9; Urine Examination (pages 110 and 114).

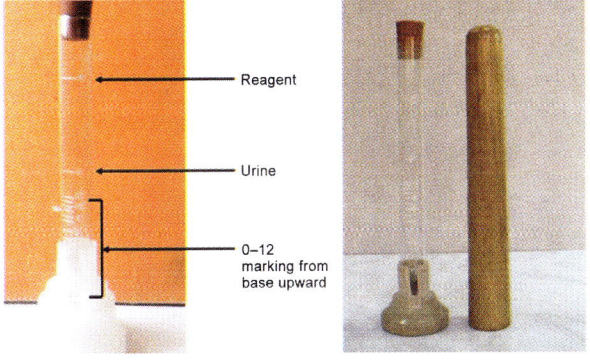

Fig. A1.21: Esbach's albuminometer

Lumbar Puncture Needle

It is a sterile long slender needle with a stilette. It is about 10 cm long and has a bore of 1–1.5 mm.

Refer to Chapter 10; LP Needle, CSF and Body Fluids (page 129).

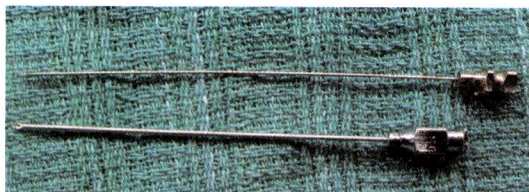

Fig. A1.22: LP (lumbar puncture) needle

Urinometer (Hydrometer)

Refer to Chapter 9; Urine Examination (page 107).

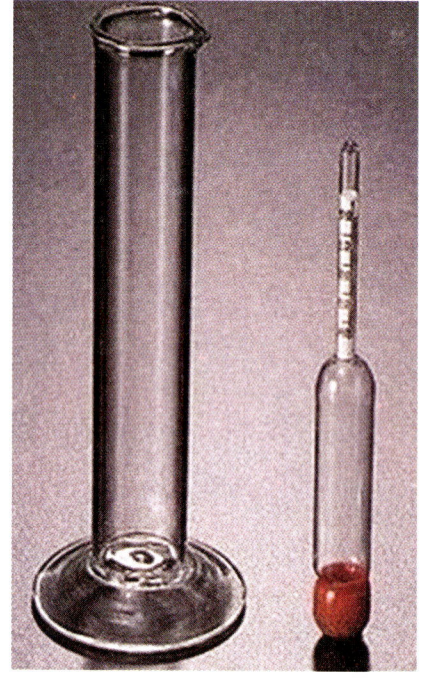

B

Fig. A1.23A and B: Urinometer (hydrometer)

HISTOPATHOLOGY

Block Moulds (Leuckhart's (L) Mould Method)

Description: L-shaped heavy brass. Two such pieces are used and placed as required to make paraffin block. It is named after Leuckhart invention in 1881.

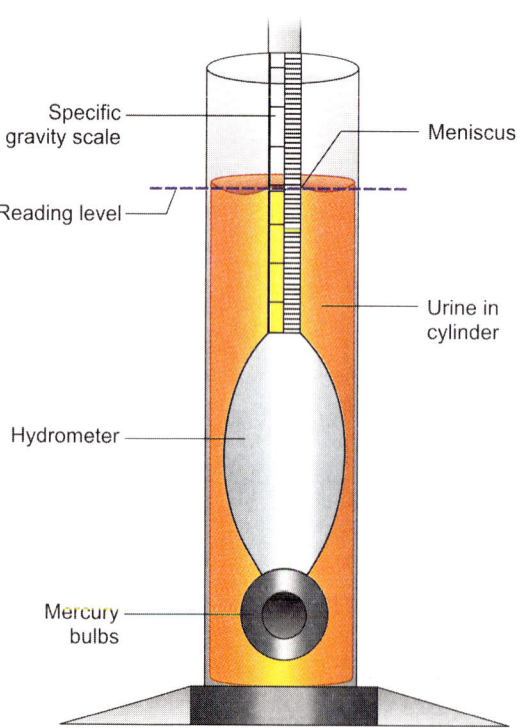

A

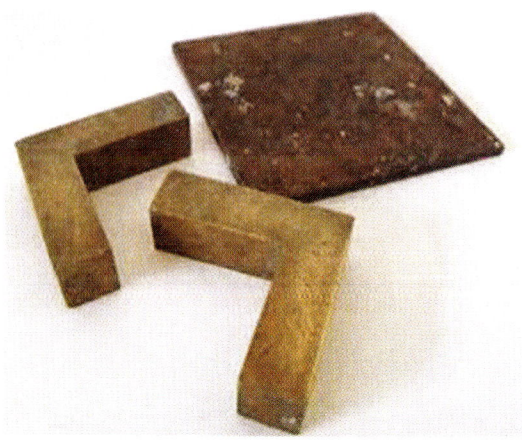

Fig. A1.24: Leuckhart's (L) mould

Use: Tissue embedding. After adding fixative, biopsies are embedded in paraffin/wax for subsequent tissue sectioning in microtome.

Block Moulds (Plastic) or Cassettes

Description: Made of plastics and light weight.

Use: Same as metal block moulds

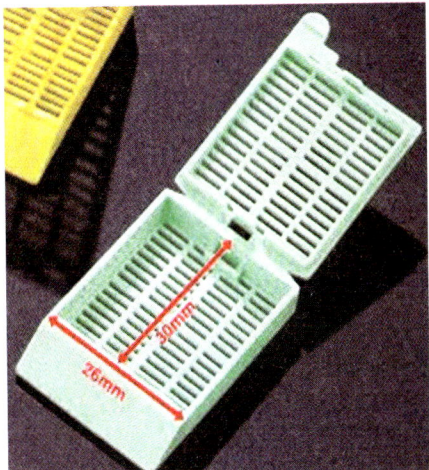

Fig. A1.25: Plastic mould

Microtomy Blade (High and Low Profile)

Description: High profile disposable blades (Leica 818) are ultra-fine yet durable, the 80 mm long × 14 mm high × 0.35 mm thick blades, can make very thin sections. Low profile (Leica 819) disposable blades are 80 mm long, 8 mm high and 0.25 mm thick.

Both high and low profile blades are made of stainless steel.

Use: Microtome and cryostat sectioning.

Microtome Knife (Plain Wedge Type)

Description: It is made up of stainless steel. It is wedge-shaped and uses in rotary microtome. High and low profile placed within knife for section cutting.

Use: Microtome and cryostat section cutting.

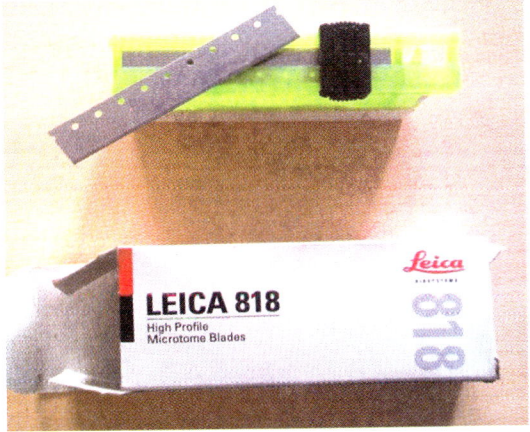

Fig. A1.26: Microtome blade (high profile)

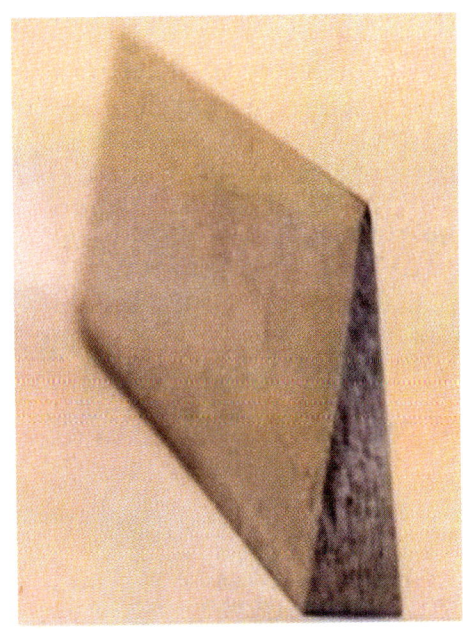

Fig. A1.27: Microtome knife

Tissue Capsule (Stainless Steel) Cassette

Description: This capsule is autoclavable, made of stainless steel, and resistant to most of the common laboratory acids and chemicals. There are many holes embedded on its lid and base to facilitate the fluid flow in it. It has secure positive snap cap.

Use: Paraffin wax embedding for tissue processing.

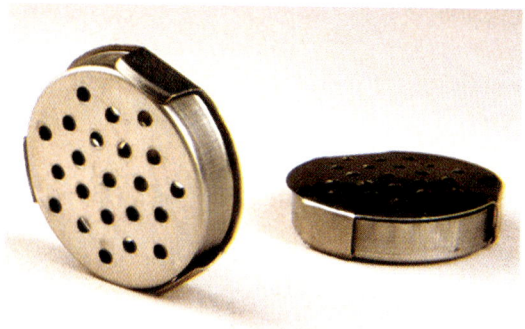

Fig. A1.28: Stainless steel cassette

CYTOPATHOLOGY

Ayre's Spatula

Description: It is a wooden spatula with U-shaped opening on one side and a flat surface on another. The broad end is for vaginal sample collection and the narrow end is for cervical sample collection.

Use: It is rotated 360° to collect cervical/vaginal cells for Pap (Papanicolaou) staining. It is being replaced by cytobrush and Ayre's bury device/spatula.

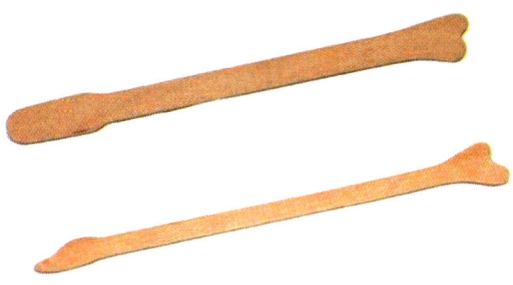

Fig. A1.29: Ayre's spatula

Coplin Jar

Description: It is a covered glass (or plastic) vessel that is rectangular in cross section and grooved inside for holding microscope slides vertical during processing or staining. It can hold up to 10 slides of the size 1 × 3 inches.

Use: For fixation of slides (alcohol), staining of smears or histologic sections.

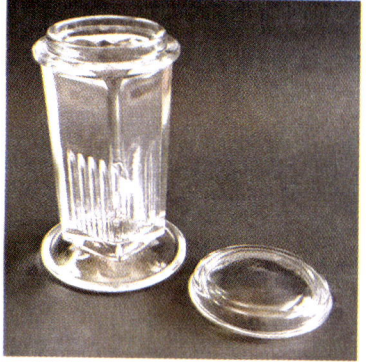

A

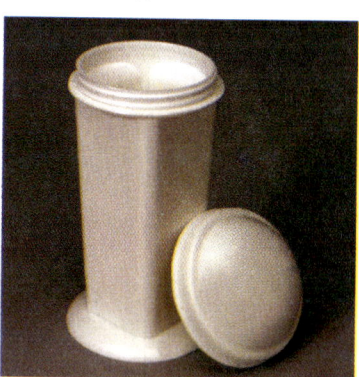

B

Fig. A1.30A and B: (A) Coplin jar (glass), (B) Coplin jar (plastic)

Franzen Handle (Syringe Holder)

Description: Made up of stainless steel and can hold 10/20 ml syringe. It can produce a good negative pressure. The holder leaves one hand free to immobilize and to feel the target lesion. Other hand is used for aspiration (negative pressure).

Use: To aspirate material during FNAC and making smears.

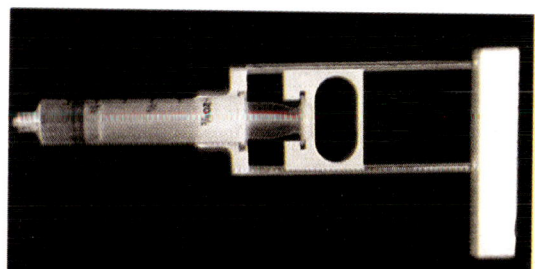

Fig. A1.31: Franzen handle (syringe holder)

Appendix II: Reference Values (Range)

NORMAL REFERENCE VALUES IN HAEMATOLOGY

Parameters	Males	Females
• Haemoglobin (Hb)	13–18 g/dl	11–16 g/dl
• Haematocrit (PCV)	41–53 %	36–46 %
• ESR i. Westergren method	0–10 mm/1st hour	0–20 mm/1st hour
ii. Wintrobe method	0–7 mm/1st hour	0–14 mm/1st hour
• Mean corpuscular volume (MCV)	78–98 fl	78–98 fl
• Mean corpuscular haemoglobin (MCH)	28–32 pg	26–34 pg
• Mean corpuscular haemoglobin concentration (MCHC)	31–36 g/dl	31–36 g/dl
• Serum iron	80–180 µg/dl	30–160 µg/dl
• Total iron binding capacity (TIBC)	250–450 µg/dl	228–428 µg/dl
• Transferrin saturation	30–35 %	30–35%
• Serum ferritin	36–300 ng/ml (mean 90)	10–200 ng/ml (mean 18)
• Prothrombin time (PT)	11–14 seconds	11–14 seconds
• Activated partial thromboplastin time (APTT or PTTK)	35–45 seconds	35–45 seconds
• Haemoglobin A_1C	4–6 %	4–6 %
• Serum fibrinogen	200–400 mg/dl	150–400 mg/dl
• RBC count	4.5–5.5 million/mm^3	3.8–5.2 million/mm^3
• WBC count or total leukocyte count (TLC)	4,000–11,000/mm^3 (4–11 × 10^9/L)	4,000–11,000/mm^3 (4–11 × 10^9/L)
• Platelet count	1,50,000–4,00,000/mm^3 (150–400 × 10^9/L)	1,50,000–4,00,000/mm^3 (150–400 × 10^9/L)
• Reticulocyte count (adult and children)	0.5–2.0 %	0.5–2.0 %
• Reticulocyte count (infants)	2–6 %	2–6 %
• Absolute eosinophil count	40–450 cells/mm^3	40–450 cells/mm^3

Differential leukocytes count (DLC)

- Neutrophils (polymorphs) — 40–70 % (2,00–7,500/mm^3 or µl)
- Lymphocytes — 20–40 % (1.500–4,00/mm^3 or µl)
- Monocytes — 2–10 % (200–800/mm^3 or µl)
- Eosinophils — 1–6 % (40–450/mm^3 or µl)
- Basophils — <1% (10–100/mm^3 or µl)

Critical values in haematology

Laboratory test values/findings	Risk/clinical significance
• Haemoglobin <7g/dl	• Myocardial ischaemia
• Haemoglobin >20 g/dl	• Hyperviscosity syndrome
• Total leukocyte count <2,000/mm^3	• Infections (especially when neutrophil) count falls below 500/mm^3)
• Total leukocyte count >50,000/mm^3	• Leukaemia, leukaemoid reaction
• Platelet count <40,000/mm^3	• Critical count, platelet/blood transfusion required
• Platelet count <20,000/mm^3	• Spontaneous bleeding
• Platelet count <10,000/mm^3	• Serious haemorrhage
• Platelet count <1,00,000/mm^3 (thrombocytopenia)	• Bleeding time increased
• Platelet count >10,00,000/mm^3 (thrombocytosis)	• Thrombosis
• Prothrombin time >30 seconds or >3 times control valve	• Bleeding
• Plasma fibrinogen <100 mg/dl	• Bleeding
• Activated partial thromboplastin time (APTT) ≥75 seconds	• Bleeding
• D-dimer: Positive	• Disseminated intravascular coagulation (DIC)

Lipid profile

Component	Reference value	
	Conventional	SI unit
• Total serum cholesterol		
i. Desirable for adults	<200 mg/dl	<5.17 mmol/L
ii. Borderline high	200–239/dl	5.17–6.18 mmol/L
iii. High and undesirable	>240 mg/dl	>6.21 mmol/L
• Triglycerides	<160 mg/dl	>1.55 mmol/L
• HDL cholesterol		
i. Low (undesirable)	<40 mg/dl	<1.03 mmol/L
ii. High, protective range	>60 mg/dl	1.55 mmol/L
• LDL cholesterol		
i. Desirable range	100–130 mg/dl	<3.34 mmol/L
ii. Borderline high	130–159 mg/dl	3.36–4.11 mmol/L
iii. High	160–189 mg/dl	4.11–4.20 mmol/L
iv. Very high	>190 mg/dl	>4.21 mmol/L

Clinical chemistry

Component	Specimen	Reference value	
		Conventional units	SI units
• Alpha fetoprotein (AFP)	Serum	0–8.5 ng/ml	0–8.5 µg/L
• Aminotransferases (transaminases)			
i. Aspartate (AST, SGOT)	Serum	12–38 U/L	0.20–0.65 µkat/L
ii. Alanine (ALT, SGPT)	Serum	7–41 U/L	0.12–0.70 µkat/L
• Amylase	Serum	20–96 U/L	0.34–1.6 µkat/L
• Bilirubin	Serum		
i. Total		0.3–1.3 mg/dl	5.1–22 µmol/L
ii. Direct (conjugated)		0.1–0.4 mg/dl	1.7–6.8 µmol/L
iii. Indirect (unconjugated)		0.2–0.9 mg/dl	3.4–15.2 µmol/L
• Calcium (total)	Serum	8.7–10.2 mg/dl	2.2–2.6 mmol/L
• C-reactive proteins (CRP)	Serum	0.2–3.0 mg/L	0.2–3.0 mg/L
• Glucose (fasting)	Plasma		
i. Normal range		70–100 mg/dl	<5.6 mmol/L
ii. Impaired fasting glucose (IFG)		101–125 mg/dl	5.6–6.9 mmol/L
iii. Diabetes mellitus		>126 mg/dl	>7.0 mmol/L
• Glucose (2 hours postprandial or PP)	Plasma		
i. Normal		<140 mg/dl	<7.8 mmol/L
ii. Impaired glucose tolerance (IGT)		140–200 mg/dl	7.8–11.1 mmol/L
iii. Diabetes mellitus		>200 mg/dl	11.1 mmol/L
• Phosphatases	Serum		
i. Acid phosphatase		0–5.5 U/L	0.90 µkat/L
ii. Alkaline phosphatase		33–96 U/L	0.56–1.63 µkat/L
• Prostatic specific antigen (PSA)	Serum	0–4.0 ng/ml	0–4.0 µg/L
• Proteins (total)	Serum	6.7–8.6 g/dl	67–86 g/L
i. Albumin		3.5–5.5 g/dl	35–55 g/L
ii. Globulins		2.0–3.5 g/dl	20–35 g/L
iii. Albumin/globulin ratio		1.5–3:1	
• Troponins, cardiac (c Tn)			
i. Troponin I (c Tn I)	Serum	0–0.08 ng/ml	0–0.8 µg/L
ii. Troponin T (c Tn T)	Serum	0–01 ng/ml	0–0.1 µg/L
• Rheumatoid factor (RF)	Serum	<15 IU/ml	<15 KIU/L
• Blood urea nitrogen (BUN)	Blood	7–20 mg/dl	2.5–7.1 mmol/L
• Uric acid	Serum		
i. Males		3.1–7.0 mg/dl	0.18–0.41 µmol/L
ii. Females		2.5–5.6 mg/dl	0.15–0.33 µmol/L

Urea and electrolytes

Analyte	Reference value	
	Conventional units	SI units
• Sodium	136–146 mEq/L	136–146 mmol/L
• Potassium	3.5–5.0 mEq/L	3.5–5.0 mmol/L
• Chloride	95–107 mEq/L	95–107 mmol/l
• Urea	20–40 mg/dl	3.3–6.6 mmol/L
• Creatinine	0.6–1.2 mg/dl	53–106 µmol/L

Index

A

10% formalin (4% formaldehyde) 146
24 hours specimen 104
3-aminopropyltriethoxysilane (APES) 153
A1 and A2 87
ABH substances 87
ABO and Rh systems 85
ABO system 86
Absence of H genes 86
Absolute eosinophil count (AEC) 54
Absolute indications for bone marrow
    aspiration 45
Acanthocytes 23
Acetic acid 146
Acetone 148
Acid haematin or Sahli method 68
Acidic urine 108
Acquired immunodeficiency syndrome
    (AIDS) 254
Activated partial thromboplastin time
    (APTT) 81, 82
Acute appendicitis 170
Acute lymphoblastic leukaemia (ALL) 255
Acute myeloid leukaemia (AML) 255
Acute proliferative (poststreptococal/
    postinfectious 258
ADA (adenosine deaminase) 141
Adenocarcinoma 139, 191
Adenocarcinoma of stomach 169
Adult and childhood polycystic kidney 222
Advantages of
    cyanomethaemoglobin method 70
    frozen sections 157
    gel card method 96
Agar 150
Agranulocytes 24
Agranulocytosis 27
Albuminometer 114
Alcohol fixative 147
Alcohol 146
Alimentary glycosuria 127

Alkaline haematin method 71
Alkaline urine 108
All bone marrow 18
Alum haematoxylin 158
Amyloidosis 254
Anisochromia 23
Anisocytosis 23
Anticoagulants 7
Antisera (antibody) 263
Apoptotic body 253
Arneth
    count 25
    index 25
Arterial puncture 4
Atheroma of aorta 206
Automated methods of ESR 59, 63
Automated tissue processing 151
Ayre's spatula 187, 272

B

Barr body 25
Barr body sex chromosome 182, 184
Basal cell carcinoma 179
Basal–parabasal cells 186
Base sledge microtome
Basophilia 30
Basophilic stippling 23
Basophils 30
Bence Jones proteinuria 116
Benedict's qualitative test 108
Benedict's quantitative test 109
Benign hyperplasia of prostate (BHP) 176, 232
Benzidine test 119
β-Thalassemia major 256
β-Thalassemia minor (thalassemia trait) 256
Bleeding time 76, 82
Block moulds (plastic) 270, 271
Blood 3
Blood collection tubes 10
Blood group 85
Blood transfusion 94

Blood–brain barrier 129
Blueing 158
Body cavity fluid 133
Bombay blood group 87, 98
Bombay blood group (Oh) type 86
Bone marrow aspiration 35
Bone marrow aspiration needle 263
Bone marrow examination 35
Bone marrow films 18
Bone marrow trephine biopsy 37
Bouin's fluid 147
Bradshaw test 116
Bread and butter 207
Brodie's abscess 225
Bronchiectasis 209
Bronchogenic carcinoma 213
Brushing 181
Buccal smear method 183
Buffy coat 11
Burr cells 23

C

Cabot rings 24
Calcium chloride ($CaCl_2$) 79, 81
Capillary haemangioma 180
Capillary tube method for PCV 61
Capillary tube methods of Wrights 79
Carbowax 150
Carboxyhaemoglobin (HbCO) 66
Carcinoma *in situ* 189
Carcinoma of
  breast 229
  cervix 228
  penis 230
Caries spine 225
Carnoy's fixative 146
Cassette 271
Casts 121
Cause of
  prolonged prothrombin time (PT) 80
  haematuria 119
  haemoglobinuria 119
  ketonuria 117
  lymphocytosis 28
  neutropenia 27
  pleural, peritoneal and pericardial effusion 136
  prolonged APTT 82
  prolonged bleeding time 77
Cavernous haemangioma 180
Celloidion 150
Cerebrospinal fluid (CSF) 129
Cervical smear 185

Charging (filling) 51
Chemical (iron content) method 71
Chemical theory of Romanowsky staining 21
Chemstrip 118
Chimerism 99
Chloroform 149
Choice of fixative 148
Chronic
  cholecystitis 174
  glomerulonephritis 220
  lymphocytic leukaemia 255
  myeloid leukaemia 255
  pyelonephritis 220
Chyluria 123
Classic seminoma 231
Classification of
  decalcifying agents 155
  fixatives 146
Clear cell carcinoma of kidney 170
Clearing 148, 149
Clearing agent in tissue processing 156
Cleft-like retraction artefact 179
Clinical chemistry 275
Cloaca 224
Clot retraction study 84
Clotting time or coagulation time 77, 82
Cobweb 132
Cold
  abscess 225
  agglutinins 92
Collagen fibres 166
Collection of
  cervical Pap smear 188
  exfoliated cells 181
Colloid goitre (nodular goitre) 177
Colorectal cancer 218
Colour 106
Column agglutination method 96
Comparator box 68
Complications of gall stone 236
Composition of
  RBC fluid 52
  WBC diluting fluid 50
Contraindications of
  bone marrow 37
  bone marrow aspiration 45
  doing FNAC 201
  doing LP 132
Coplin jar 272
Copper sulphate method 73
Coulter analyzers 53
Counting chamber 47

Counting of
  leukocytes 51
  RBCs 52
Cover glass method 14, 16
Critical values in haematology 274
Crush preparations 18
Crystals found in
  acid urine 123
  alkaline urine 123
CSF findings in some common disorders 134
CSF pressure 132
Cyanomethaemoglobin method 69, 73
Cytobrush 187
Cytology 181
Cytology of body fluids (effusions) 191
Cytopathology 181
Cytoplasmic vacuoles 26
Cyto-spatula 187

D

Decalcification 155,156
Decreased ESR 59
Dehydration 148
Dermoid (teratoma) tumour of ovary 228
Different stages of lobar pneumonia 209
Differential leukocyte count (DLC) 24, 273
Dioxane (diethyl dioxide) 149
Dipstick for urine 269
DLC counter 264
Döhle bodies 26
Dolichos biflorus 87
Double oxalate 12
Double oxalate (Wintrobe's mixture) 8, 12
DPX or distrene dibutylpthalate xylol 155
Dry tap 45
Duct carcinoma of breast 175, 198
Duke method for BT 77
During blood grouping 99
Dysmorphic erythrocytes 121

E

Ear lobe puncture 6
EDTA 7
Effect of storage of blood 10
Elastic fibres 166
Electronic method for
  blood cell count 53
  counting WBC 54
Embedding 148, 149
Emphysema 210
Emphysema of lung 168

Eosinophilia 29
Eosinophilic leukaemoid reactions 31
Eosinophils 29
Epithelial and stromal components 169
Erythrocyte sedimentation rate 56
Erythrocytes 22
Esbach's albuminometer 269
Esbach's method 114
ESR 56
Ethyl alcohol (ethanol) 148
Ewing's sarcoma 259
Examination of stained blood films 22
Excess EDTA 13
Exfoliative cytology 181, 201
Extrinsic pathway of coagulation 83
Exudate 135

F

False positive results (ABO grouping) 92
Fatty
  casts 122
  liver 174, 233
Faulty staining 21
Fehling's test 109
Fibrinous pericarditis 207
Fibroadenoma of breast 175, 198
Fibrocaseous tuberculosis of lung 211
Fibroid uterus (leiomyoma) 227
Field's stain 20
Fine needle aspiration cytology (FNAC) 194
Finger prick (stick) 6
Fish-mouth appearance 205
Fixation of blood films 17
Fixative for Pap smears 200
Fixatives used in cytology 184
Flea-beaten kidney 222
FNAC technique 194
Formal saline (10%) 146
Formalin fixatives 146
Forward grouping 88
Franzen handle (syringe holder) 272
Frozen section 157
Functional proteinuria 128

G

Gall stones 235
Ganglion (ganglion cyst) 199
Gastric carcinoma 214
Gaucher
  cells 260
  disease 260

Gel card method 96
Gelatin 150
Gerhardt's ferric chloride test 118
Giant cell tumour (of bone) 171
Giant cell tumour of bone (osteoclastoma) 226
Giemsa stain 20
Globulin test in CSF 141
Gomori's silver impregnation stain 164
Graduated pipette 264
Granular casts 122
Granular contracted kidney 219
Granulocytes 24
Granulomatous lymphadenitis 196

H

H and E stain 166
H antigen 87
H gene 86
H substance 86
H substance (H antigen) 98
Haematoxylin 158
Haematuria 118, 125
Haemoglobin (Hb) pipette 74
Haemoglobin A 67
Haemoglobin A2 67
Haemoglobin Bart 67
Haemoglobin colour scale (HCS) method 73
Haemoglobin estimation 65
Haemoglobin F 67
Haemoglobin H 67
Haemoglobin M (HbM) 66
Haemoglobin S 67
Haemoglobinometer
   pipette 68
   tube 68
Haemoglobinuria 119, 125
Haemophilia A 260
Harris alum haematoxylin 159
Heart failure cells 258
Heat and acetic acid test 112
Heavy proteinuria 115
Heel puncture 5
Heinz bodies 66
Heller's nitric acid test 113
HemoCue 73
HemoCue method 72
Heparin 7
Hepatocellular carcinoma (HCC) 259
Hereditary spherocytosis 256
High grade SIL 189
Histoclear 149

Histological techniques 145
Hodgkin lymphoma 255
Homer-Wright rosettes 259
Howell-Jolly bodies 24
Human haemoglobin 66
Hyaline casts 122
Hydronephrosis 221
Hyperchromia 22
Hypersegmented neutrophils 25
Hypochromia 22
Hyposthenuric 106

I

Ideal gauge needle 12
Ideal peripheral blood smear 32
Immature teratoma 229
Impregnation 148, 149
Imprint cytology 182
Improved Neubauer chamber 46
In Pap smears 202
In peripheral blood smear (PBS) 34
Indications for collection of CSF 132
Indications of
   bone marrow aspiration 37
   bone marrow biopsy 37
   FNAC 194
   trephine or bone marrow biopsy 45
Infective
   endocarditis 258
   organisms 202
Intermediate squamous cell 186
International normalized ratio (INR) 80
Interventional cytology 201
Intrinsic 83
Investigations of synovial fluid 135
Involucrum 224, 225
Iron deficiency anaemia 256, 261
Iron
   haematoxylin 158, 159
   status 40
ISI (international sensitivity index) value 80
Islam's bone marrow aspiration needle 37
Islam's needle 41
Isopropyl alcohol 149
Isosthenuric 106
ITP 255
Ivy's method for BT 76

J

Jamshidi needle 41
Jaundice 254

K

Kaolin 81
Keloid scar 260
Ketonuria 117
Klima bone marrow aspiration needle 36
Knife materials 153

L

Landsteiner 85, 93
Large white kidney (RPGN) 220
LBC 187
Lee and White method 78
Left-sided colorectal carcinoma 219
Left ventricular hypertrophy (LVH) 206
Leiomyoma 173
Lepidic pattern of growth 214
Leuckhart's embedding iron 154
Leuckhart's (L) mould 270
Leukoerythroblastic reaction 26
Light's criteria for pleural fluid 140
Lines of Zahn 253
Lipid profile 274
Lipoma 179
Liquid-based cytology 187
Lobar pneumonia 209
Low and fixed specific gravity of urine 127
Low grade SIL 189
Lumbar puncture method 129
Lumbar puncture needle 129, 270
Lymphocytes 27
Lymphocytic leukaemoid reactions 31
Lymphocytopenia 28
Lymphocytosis 28

M

MacNeal stain 19
Macrocytes 23
Macronodular 233
Macrovesicular steatosis 234
Major basic protein 29
Major crossmatch 100
Malignant melanoma 178
Manual processing 150
Marrow aspiration 35
Masson's trichrome staining 167
Mature cystic teratoma 229
May-Grünwald-Giemsa stain 20
May-Hegglin anomaly 26
MCH 64
MCHC 64
MCV 64
Megaloblastic anaemia 256
Mesothelial cells 139, 192
Mesothelioma 139, 192
Metachromasia 30
Metastatic adenocarcinoma 192
Metastatic deposit in lymph node 177
Methaemoglobin (Hi) 65
Methanol 149
Method of
   ABO blood grouping 88
   PCV determination (Wintrobe tube) 61
Methods of
   ESR estimation 56
   haemoglobin estimation 67
MGG stain 194
Microalbuminuria 128
Microcytes 23
Micronodular 232
Micronodular cirrhosis 232
Microplate method 92
Microscopic examination of urine 120
Microtome 156
Microtome knife 153, 271
Microtomes 152
Microtomy 152
Microtomy blade 271
Microtyping system 96
Microvesicular steatosis 233, 234
Mild dysplasia 189
Miliary tuberculosis of lung 212
Minimal proteinuria 116
Minor crossmatch 100
Mitral stenosis 205
Mixed or micro-macronodular cirrhosis 233
Moderate dysplasia 189
Moderate proteinuria 116
Modified Drabkin's solution 70
Modified Westergren method 57
Monocytes 28
Monocytosis 28
Mordant 158, 167
Mounting media 154
Mucin clot test (Ropes test) 133, 137
Multiple myeloma 255
Multistix 118
Myeloid–erythroid ratio (M:E ratio) 40
Myocardial infarction 258

N

N/10 HCl 74
NAP score 255
Necrosis 253

Nephrotic syndrome 259
Neubauer chamber 46
Neubauer (improved) counting chamber or haemocytometer 264
Neurofibroma 199
Neutral buffered formalin (10%) 146
Neutropenia 26
Neutrophil (leukocyte) method 184
Neutrophilia 26
Neutrophilic leukaemoid reactions 31
Normal range of
   ESR 58
   PCV 62
Normal reference values in haematology 273
Normal synovial fluid 135
Normal values of CSF 131
Normochromia 22
Normocytes 23
Nutmeg liver 258

O

Oil red O stain 163
Oliguria anuria 106
One unit of blood 99
Organised elements in urine 120
Original Drabkin's solution 70
Orthotoluidine test 119
Osgood and Haskin's test 117
Osteogenic sarcoma 171, 226
Osteomyelitis 225
Osteomyelitis and sequestrum 224
Other names of FNAC 200
Oxalate 8
Oxyhaemoglobin method 71

P

Packed cell volume 60
Papanicolaou stain 185
Papillary carcinoma of thyroid 197
Pappenheimer bodies 23
Paraffin
   section cutting 153
   wax 149
Paraplast 150
parasites 34
Parts of bone marrow needle 44
PAS (periodic acid–Schiff) reagents 161
PAS positive substances 162
Pasteur pipette 265
Patterns of different proteinuria 115
Pelger-Huët anomaly 26
Peptic ulcer 214

Peptic ulcer disease 258
Periodic acid–schiff (PAS) stain 161
Peripheral palisading 179
pH (reaction) of urine 107
Philadelphia chromosome (Ph) 255
Phospholipid 81
Plasma 3, 12
Platelet adequacy and platelet count 33
Platelet count (manual method) 52
Platelet dust 34
Platelet-poor plasma (PPP) 79
Platelet satellitism 33
Platelets (thrombocytes) 31
Pleomorphic salivary adenoma 169
Pleomorphic salivary adenoma of salivary gland 200
Poikilocytosis 23
Polychromasia 22
Polycystic kidney 222
Polyuria 106
Portal cirrhosis 173
Post-chromatin 146
Posterior superior iliac spine 44
Post-fixation 146
Postural proteinuria 128
Potassium and sodium oxalate 8
Pott's disease 225
Preparation of marrow films 39
Preparation of thick film 17
Preparing red cell suspension 88
Preservation of urine 105
Primary fixatives 145
Primary intestinal tuberculosis 217
Principle of
   PAS staining 166
   reticulin staining 166
Progressive staining 158
Proliferative endometrium 171
Prolonged coagulation time 79
Prostatic adenocarcinoma 259
Proteinuria 112
Prothrombin
   index 80
   time 79, 82
Prussian blue stain 40
PSA level 259
Puncture of
   ilium 37
   the sternum 38
Pyogenic (bacterial) meningitis 262
Pyogenic osteomyelitis 259
Pyuria 121

R

RBC (red blood cell or erythrocyte) casts 122
RBC pipette 48, 265
Reactions 94
Reactive mesothelial cells 192
Reagent strip method 110, 114, 118
Reagent strips/dipsticks 107
Rectangular (boxcar) nuclei 207
Red blood cell count (manual method) 51
Red cell indices 64
Red infarcts 253
Reference values of CSF 130
Refractometer 107
Regressive staining 158
Renal cell carcinoma 223
    glycosuria 127
    tuberculosis 223
Reporting of bone marrow films (myelogram) 40
Resins 150
Reticulin fibres 166
Reticulocyte 65
Reverse grouping 88, 99
Rh D antigen 93, 94
Rh factor 93
Rh grouping method 94
Rh positive (Rh+) 94
Rh system 93
Rheumatic heart disease (RHD) 208
Right-sided colorectal carcinoma 219
Romanowsky stains 19
Rotary
    microtome 152, 156
    rocking microtome 152
Rothera's test 117
Rouleaux formation 24, 92

S

Sahli method 73
Salah bone marrow aspiration needle 36
Salicylaldehyde method 118
Schilling count 26
Schistocytes (cell fragment) 23
Scrape method 181
Scrape or brush cytology 182
Secondary
    fixatives 146
    tuberculosis 217
Secretors and nonsecretors 87
Secretory endometrium 172
Sections 152
Seminoma of testis 176, 231
sequestrum 224, 225
serofibrinous pericarditis 208
Serum 3, 12
Serum grouping (reverse grouping) 92
Sickle cell anaemia 256
Sickling test 256
Skin puncture 5
Slide method (ABO grouping) 90
soap-bubble appearance 227
Sodium fluoride 9
Solid phase adherence technology 97
Some common FNAC findings (microscopic) 196
Special stains for bone marrow smear
        examination 45
Specific gravity 106
Specific gravity method 71
Specific gravity of normal urine 107
Spectroscopic method 71
Sperm count 55
Spherocytes 23
Spider web coagulum 132
Spinner or spin method 14, 16
SpinThin method 189
Spurious/pseudo anaemia 75
Stages of sedimentation (ESR) 58
Staining method using alum haematoxylin and
        eosin 159
Staining of blood smear 19
Standardized template method for BT 76
Steps in tissue processing 148
Stirrer 69
Stopwatch 265
Subgroups of A 87
Subtypes of blood group A 98
Sudan black B stain 163
Sugar in urine 111
Sulfhaemoglobin (SHb) 66
Sulphosalicylic acid test 112
Superficial squamous cells 185
SurePath 188
SurePath method 188
Synovial fluid 135, 138

T

Tallqvist method 73
Target cells (leptocytes) 23
TB (tuberculosis) spine 225
Test 108
Test for blood 119
Test for reducing substance 108
Tests for Bence Jones protein 116

Thalassaemia major 67
Thermometer for water bath 266
Thick coverslip 49
Thick smear 16
ThinPrep 188
ThinPrep method 188
Thrombocytopenia 32
Thrombocytosis (thrombophilia) 32
Thromboplastins 79
Tissue capsule 271
Tissue processing 147
Toluene (toluol) 149
Toluenesulphonic acid (TSA) test 117
Total leukocyte count (TLC) 24
Toxic granules 26
Transudate 135
Trephine biopsy 35
Trephine biopsy (Jamshidi type) needle 266
Trisodium citrate 7
Tube method (ABO grouping) 91
Tubercular ulcer 216, 217
Tuberculosis of
  lung 168
  lymph node 177
Tubidimetric method 115
Türk cells 27
Types of fixatives 145
Typhoid ulcer 215, 217

U

Universal
  donor 95
  recipient 95
Urea and electrolytes 276
Urinalysis 103, 125
Urinary tract infection or UTI 261
Urine 103
Urine and pregnancy test 123
Urine
  collection 103, 105
  report 105
  volume 106

Urinometer (hydrometer) 107, 270
Use of ESR 58

V

Vacupuncture needle 267
Vacutainer 13, 267
van Slyke's oxygen capacity method or gasometric method 71
Venipuncture 3
Verhoeff's van Gieson stain 163
Verrucous carcinoma 231
Vibratome 153
Virchow's triad 253

W

Warm antibodies 93
Watered silk appearances 227
Waxy casts 122
WBC (leukocyte) casts 122
WBC pipette 48
Wedge method 14
Weigert's iron haematoxylin 160
Westergren method 57
Westergren's pipette 268
Westergren's stand 268
White blood cell count (manual method) 49
White blood cells (WBCs) 24
White infarct 253
WHO haemoglobin colour scale method 71
Wintrobe (haematocrit) tube 60, 268
Wintrobe's method 58
Wintrobe's stand 268
Wright's stain 20

X

Xanthochromia 132
Xylene (xylol) 149
Zenker's fluid 147
Zeta crit 60
Zeta potential 56
Zeta sedimentation rate (ZSR) 59
Ziehl-Neelsen or ZN stain 257